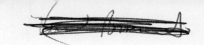

Manual of Pediatric Nursing Procedures

MANUAL OF
Pediatric Nursing Procedures

Nedra Skale, MS, RN, CNA

Nurse Clinician, Division of Pediatric Surgery
Department of Surgery, Humana Hospital—Michael Reese
Chicago, Illinois

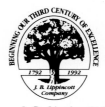

J. B. Lippincott Company

Philadelphia
New York
London
Hagerstown

Sponsoring Editor: Barbara Nelson Cullen
Developmental Editor: Marian A. Bellus
Project Editor: Elizabeth A. Durand
Indexer: Helene Taylor
Designer: Anne O'Donnell

Design Coordinator: Doug Smock
Production Manager: Caren Erlichman
Production Coordinator: Kevin P. Johnson
Compositor: Bi-Comp, Incorporated
Printer/Binder: Courier/Kendallville

6 5 4 3 2 1

Library of Congress Cataloging-in-Publication Data

Skale, Nedra.
    Manual of pediatric nursing procedures / Nedra Skale.
        p.   cm.
    Includes bibliographical references and index.
    ISBN 0-397-54782-X
    1. Pediatric nursing—Handbooks, manuals, etc.   I. Title.
    [DNLM: 1. Pediatric Nursing—methods—handbooks.   WY 39 S626m]
RJ245.S56   1992
610.73′62—dc20
DNLM/DLC
for Library of Congress   91-18393
                                                                        CIP

Any procedure or practice described in this book should be applied by the health-care practitioner under appropriate supervision in accordance with professional standards of care used with regard to the unique circumstances that apply in each practice situation. Care has been taken to confirm the accuracy of information presented and to describe generally accepted practices. However, the authors, editors, and publisher cannot accept any responsibility for errors or omissions or for any consequences from application of the information in this book and make no warranty, express or implied, with respect to the contents of the book.

Every effort has been made to ensure that drug selections and dosages are in accordance with current recommendations and practice. Because of ongoing research, changes in government regulations and the constant flow of information on drug therapy, reactions, and interactions, the reader is cautioned to check the package insert for each drug for indications, dosages, warnings and precautions, particularly if the drug is new or infrequently used.

To my mom

and to all those children and their families
who have been and will be touched
by a patient, kind, understanding and caring nurse.

Contributors

Eva Alcantara, BSN, RN
Clinical Nurse II
Pediatric ICU
Humana Hospital—Michael Reese
Chicago, Illinois

Anita Barlan, BSN, RN
Clinical Nurse II
Pediatric ICU
Humana Hospital—Michael Reese
Chicago, Illinois

Dionisia Bizarra, BSN, RN
Clinical Nurse II
Neonatal Stepdown Unit
Humana Hospital—Michael Reese
Chicago, Illinois

Norma J. Coe, BSN, RN
Clinical Nurse II
Pediatric ICU
Humana Hospital—Michael Reese
Chicago, Illinois

Joan Fogata, BSN, RN
Clinical Nurse II
Pediatric ICU
Humana Hospital—Michael Reese
Chicago, Illinois

Audrey Klopp, PhD, RN, ET
Clinical Nurse Specialist/ET
Humana Hospital—Michael Reese
Chicago, Illinois

Pamala LaScala, BSN, RN
Clinical Nurse II
Infant/Toddler Unit
Humana Hospital—Michael Reese
Chicago, Illinois

Susan P. Maloney, BSN, RN
Nurse Clinician
Pediatric Cardiology
Humana Hospital—Michael Reese
Chicago, Illinois

Johnnie M. Morgan, BS, RN
Assistant Nurse Manager
Adult Medical Unit
Humana Hospital—Michael Reese
Chicago, Illinois

Mary V. Muse, MSN, RN
Nurse Manager
School Age/Adolescent Unit
Humana Hospital—Michael Reese
Chicago, Illinois

Michele Knoll Puzas, MHPE, RN, C
Nurse Clinician
Pediatric Nursing
Humana Hospital—Michael Reese
Chicago, Illinois

Ruth Novitt Schumacher, MSN, RN
Lecturer
University of Illinois at Chicago
School of Nursing
Chicago, Illinois

Nedra Skale, MS, RN, CNA
Nurse Clinician
Pediatric Surgery
Humana Hospital—Michael Reese
Chicago, Illinois

Jackie Starck, BSN, RN
Clinical Nurse III
Infant/Toddler Unit
Humana Hospital—Michael Reese
Chicago, Illinois

Jeffrey Zurlinden, MS, RN
Project Coordinator
Chicago Community Programs for
Clinical Research on AIDS
Chicago, Illinois

List of Reviewers

Ruth Bindler, *RN, RS*
Associate Professor
Intercollegiate Center for Nursing
Education
Spokane, Washington

Viginia P. Bowler, *MSN, RN*
Instructor, Nursing Program
Pima Community College
Tucson, Arizona

Marlene L. McClure, *MSN, RN*
Associate Professor
Department of Nursing
Pittsburg State University
Pittsburg, Kansas

Eileen Liscik O'Brien, *PhD, RN*
Associate Professor
School of Nursing
University of Maryland
Baltimore, Maryland

Beth Richardson, *MSN, RN, CPNP, DNS (CANDIDATE)*
Associate Professor
Indiana University School of Nursing
Indianapolis, Indiana

Preface

As a nurse clinician, educator and administrator, I share the concerns of others that standard procedures are used without thought to the impact of the process on the child and family. Most procedure manuals are step-by-step recipe books with no tie to the nursing process or how the procedure in question fits into the comprehensive care of the child.

Staff must become sensitive to the meaning of hospitalization and treatment to children. They must develop skills and techniques for working constructively with children and their families and use their understanding of growth and development to identify problems that were present before hospitalization as well as those induced by illness. They need to know how to help children master the stresses of hospitalization and how to recognize obstacles to optimal health. Until this occurs, we will see a continuation of arbitrary and disease-oriented management of children.

We do not intend to give all concepts or theories related to each procedure. We expect students and practicing health team members to use the material and references as a basis for application to individual situations and as a stimulus for ideas related to new ways of delivering health care. We invite the users of this manual to use the procedures and teaching guides as written or to adapt them to their institution policies. We are seeking improved methods of providing health care to large groups while keeping the care personal, individual, and cost effective.

Pediatric nurses attain necessary skills from a variety of sources. This book is a collection of the most common pediatric procedures and teaching guides. It organizes each procedure so that the practitioner has a clear definition/purpose of the procedure, understands what assessments need to be made before the procedure takes place, and knows the universal standards to be taken into consideration along with applicable nursing diagnoses and the equipment needed. The steps in the procedure are then listed, accompanied by rationale and expected outcomes. Lastly, home care considerations and family education, along with up-to-date references, are included. The thread that ties all these procedures together is the family unit and how nursing can be practiced within this unit.

Nedra Skale, RN

Acknowledgments

This text is the creation of talented individuals whom I wish to acknowledge for their assistance in the completion of this project.

From J. B. Lippincott Company:

Barbara Cullen
Editor

Marian Bellus
Developmental Editor

Elizabeth Durand
Project Editor

Susan Hermansen
Art Director

Heidi Beck Crooks, former Vice President for Nursing at Michael Reese Hospital and Medical Center; currently Associate Director of Nurses, University of California, Los Angeles.

Peggy Levine, photographer

Dimitri Karetnikov, illustrator

Roseann O'Malley, typist

Without their many hours of dedicated time and effort, this book would not have been published.

Thank you one and all.

Contents

Introduction

It is the intent of this book to present the most common pediatric nursing procedures in a concise and straightforward format that will facilitate competent performance of nursing skills. The nurse is reminded to involve the child and family in all aspects of care. Key features include:

- The steps of the nursing process as an organizational framework
- An abundance of photographs and drawings to fully illustrate the nursing actions involved with the various steps of each procedure
- Procedures written to encompass the skills necessary to care for both well and ill children
- Reproducible parent teaching guides that can be photocopied and distributed to parents
- Procedures that are user-friendly for students and experienced nurses alike.

A procedure may be defined as a series of steps by which a desired result is accomplished. The procedures developed in this book not only detail the steps in the procedure but also take the practitioner through an expanded look at the nursing process as it relates to each procedure. Steps in the nursing process are used to describe the nurse's responsibility in carrying out the procedure. Each procedure follows a consistent format, as outlined below:

Definition/Purpose: It is the responsibility of the nurse to understand the reasons for performing a procedure and the ways in which his or her actions affect the overall health of the child. This section defines the procedure and gives the reason for its performance.

Assessments: The nurse is responsible for gathering in an organized and systematic way information about the child's current and past health status. This includes physical findings, psychosocial factors, developmental factors, the child's and the family's understanding of the current condition and treatment, and the ability and readiness of the child and the family to participate in the care. Understanding past experiences, cultural differences, and developmental levels will help predict the child's responses to nursing procedures and how the desired goals can best be achieved.

Standard of Care: It is the responsibility of the nurse to recognize certain elements of the procedure that are accepted practice. Accepted practice is defined as this: Nursing care administered according to the standard must result in a positive outcome for the patient and family. These elements are highlighted in this section and are not repeated in the text of the procedure.

Nursing Diagnoses: In order to deliver care effectively, the nurse must identify nursing diagnoses that direct the care in terms of goals and interventions. The nursing diagnoses identified must be phrased in the correct NANDA terms and consist of actual or high risk problems that nurses are licensed to treat and for which they are legally and professionally accountable.

Planning: It is the responsibility of the nurse to gather the appropriate equipment needed to perform the procedure in a timely manner.

Interventions: Here the nurse is responsible for putting the plan of care into action by taking actual bedside actions and documenting the results of the action. Rationales are given where appropriate. Expected outcomes reflect observable behaviors so that the nurse, child, and family can measure progress.

Family Education and Home Care Considerations: Lastly, the nurse is responsible for evaluating the effectiveness of the procedure and for determining what follow-up care and teaching is needed.

The procedures in this book all follow the above format. The first two units deal with general procedures: the remaining units are organized by body systems. Procedures are organized into the appropriate unit followed by teaching guides.

It must be emphasized here that for infection control purposes the procedure on Universal Precautions needs to be applied to every situation where applicable.

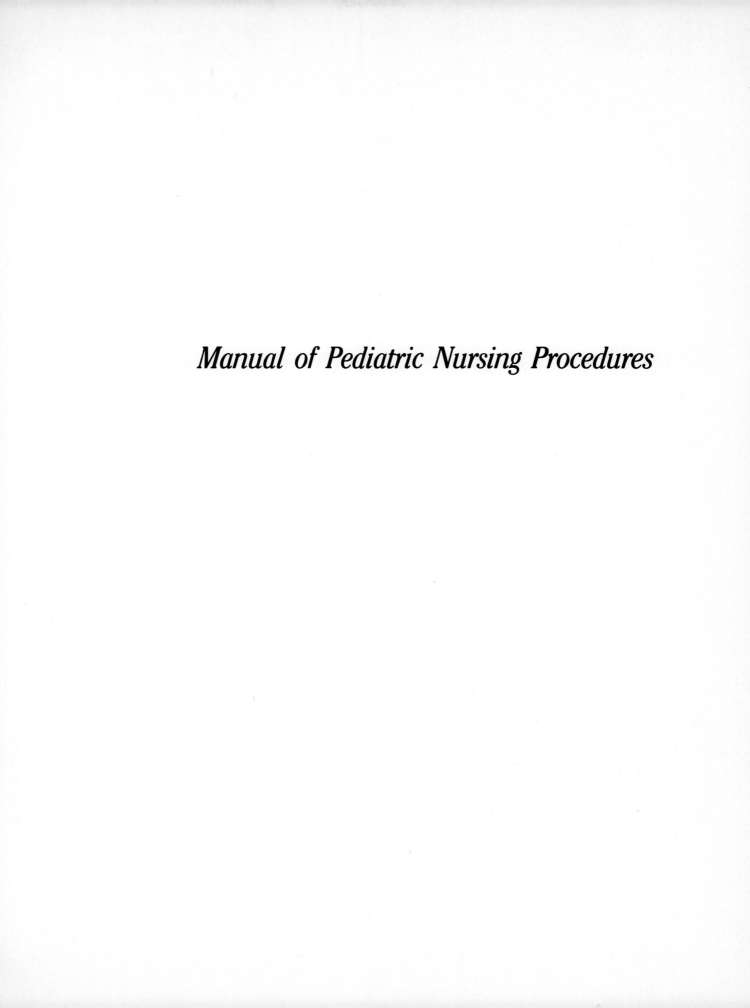

Manual of Pediatric Nursing Procedures

Administration Procedures

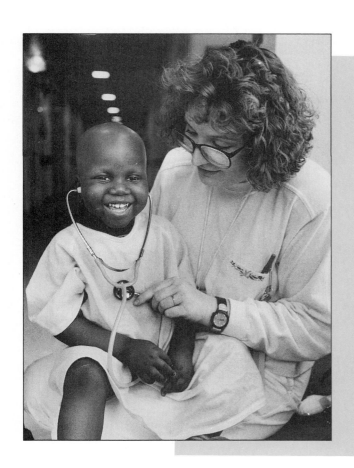

Unit I

Patient Admission

1

Definition/Purpose

Admission of a child to a health care facility differs from that of an adult due to the state of rapidly changing physical, cognitive, and emotional factors which are evident.

The ability to provide comprehensive care will be determined in large part by the extensive data base gathered on admission. The data base consists of information about the child and family useful for health maintenance, or for evaluation and treatment of a sick child. These data should be separated according to content—history, physical examination, and tests. It is important to record the data on a systemic, comprehensive form that ensures the information is easily retrievable for patient care, teaching, and research (Fig. 1-1). Incomplete or inaccurate records can lead to inadequate identification of problems, poor formulation of management, and lack of follow-up.

NURSING ADMISSION ASSESSMENT

Adm. Date _3-1-91_

Adm. Time _5 PM_

Adm. From _ER_

Accompanied by _Mother_

T _39.5_ Ax

_____ Oral

P _182_

R _46_

BP _102/64_ Extremity _RA_

Ht _82 cm_

Wt _11 kg_

Allergies: None _____ Yes _✓_
Dilantin
Ampicillin

Oriented to:
unit	✓	visiting	✓
playroom	✓	safety	✓
smoking	✓	isolation	NA
ID band	✓	I & O records	✓

(continued)

History

Current problem: _Fever x 2 days;_
vomiting x 2 days;
diarrhea x 3 days

Previous admission: _10-4-'90 Trache_
inserted for subglottic stenosis;
11-10-90 Gastrostomy inserted for
nutrition due to ↓ po intake; 1-2-91
10-day admission for pneumonia (RSV+)

Physical Impairments:
Mental retardation; cerebral
palsy; seizure disorder

Family Background

	Name	phone no.
Mo	_June_	_797-1111_
Fa	_Samuel_	_794-0101_
Guardian	_NA_	

Siblings

Name	Age
John	_5 years_
Emily	_1 mo_

Language spoken: _English_

Special Considerations: _John's being_
tx for TB x 4 months

Diet

Appetite: Good _____ Fair _____ Poor _____

Formula: Type _Pediasure_

or   Amount _1 can_

Tube   Frequency _QID_

Feeding

Diet: Regular for age _____

Other: _Follow each tube feed with 75cc H₂O_

Medications

		Frequency/Times
Name	Dose	Administered
Phenobarbital	_30 mgm_	$9^A + 9^P$
Depakene	_100 mgm_	$9^A + 5^P + 9^P$
	(all via G-tube)	

Swallows tablets   Y _____   N ✓

Crushed _____ mixed with _____

Liquid _____ using syringe _____

spoon _____

Communicable Diseases

	Had	Exposed	Date
Rubella	__	____	____
Chicken Pox	✓	____	_1-91_
Measles	__	____	____
Mumps	__	____	____
MRSA	__	____	____

Elimination

Pattern: Regular ✓ _1 x day_

Irregular _____

Cloth diapers _____ Enuresis _____

Dispos. diapers ✓ Constipation ✓

Potty trained _____ Diarrhea _____

Ostomy _____ Other _____

(continued)

Immunizations UTD _____✓_____

Status unknown _____

Comments: _____

_____

_____

_____

Menses Y (N) LMP _____

Birth Control Y (N) Type _____

Special word for _____

Developmental

School Y (N) Grade: _____

Special learning needs: _____

_____

_____

Hearing impaired Y (N)

Speech impaired (Y) N

Method of expressing pain: _Cry_

Comfort measures: _Likes to be held;_
likes to listen to music

Fears/Dislikes: _Needles_

Hobbies/Activities: _Likes to play with blocks_

Aware of reason for current

hospitalization (Y) N NA

(family aware)

Self Care Y (N)

Uses:

WC (Y) N

Braces Y (N)

Splints (Y) N
(when sleeping)

Discharge Plans

Date	Plan	Date Accomplished
3-1-91	Rehydrate child as ordered by physician	3-3-91
3-1-91	Reestablish intact skin around trache	3-4-91
3-2-91	Reinstruct family on skin care around trache	3-5-91

Needs Assistance in:

Feeding	Y	N
Bathing	(Y)	N
Dressing	(Y)	N
Elimination	(Y)	N
Ambulation	(Y)	N
	(O)	

Summary

2-yr-old alert, black female admitted for dehydration. Mucous membranes dry, skin turgor poor with tenting of skin on abdomen. No tears. Mother reports decreased urination during last 2 days. IV in (L) arm infusing at 50 cc/hr. IV with good blood return — no redness or swelling

(continued)

Crutches   Y   (N)

Eyeglasses   Y   (N)

Contacts   Y   (N)

Hearing Aid   Y   (N)

Dental Aid   Y   (N)

Smokes: Y   (N)

Has: Gastrostomy tube Size ___14F___

Tracheostomy tube Size ___1.0___

Pharyngostomy tube Size _____

Implantable venous port
                             Y   (N)

Pacemaker   Y   (N)

noted. G-tube in place with intact skin around stoma. No drainage or redness around stoma. Trache in place with skin excoriation around stoma. Lungs clear bilaterally. Secretions from trache are thick green/foul smelling. Culture of secretions sent to lab. On admission to unit, had 100 cc liquid green stool — hematest —. Bowel sounds hyperactive.

MIC G-tube in place with 5cc H_2O in balloon. Last changed by mother on 2-20-91. Shiley trache without inner cannula in place. Last changed by mother on 2-28-91.

Admission Assessment by: ___Sarah Leepe___, RN

(Depending on the hospital, this information may be entered into a computerized system or recorded on a hard copy which is placed in the charts.)

Standard of Care

1. The data should be collected during the earliest contacts with the child and family, since they provide baseline information against which to measure and assess the significance of change.
2. An adequate data base cannot be gathered simply by using a questionnaire or by asking direct questions. Skillful, nonstructured observation and interviewing should be used to gather data.
3. The Registered Nurse is accountable for the nursing assessment. However, some portions of the assessment may be delegated to other health care members, and then verified or validated by the professional nurse (assessment requires a signature by a Registered Nurse).
4. All the data gathered will become a permanent part of the child's medical record.

Assessment

The following assessment outline needs to be completed on all children upon their admission to the hospital:

1. Identifying data—includes a restricted range of information to provide an orienting context for interpreting a medical record:
   a. Age
   b. Sex
   c. Race
   d. Religion
   e. Marital status and number of children, if appropriate
   f. Serious and chronic illnesses
   g. Primary language
   h. Country of origin
2. Chief Complaint—includes a brief description of the parents' or child's perception of the primary reason for the admission
   a. Reason for admission
   b. Duration of symptoms, location, quality, quantity, and course of the illness
3. Historians—includes those people accompanying the child to the hospital and any other sources (medical records, consultants, letters from schools) of medical information
4. Sources of Health Care—includes the prior sources of health care and the reasons why there is a change to a new health care facility
5. Past Health History—includes a well-organized, concise presentation of the health history
   a. Birth history
   b. Maternal obstetric history
   c. Maternal pregnancy/labor–delivery
   d. Child's condition at birth (birth weight, number of days in hospital at birth)
   e. Common childhood illnesses
   f. Serious illnesses
   g. Surgical procedures
   h. Accidents and injuries
   i. Allergies
   j. Immunizations
6. Patient Profile—includes a well-organized picture of the child's current life situation
   a. Social history—household members, physical characteristics of the home, primary caregivers, day care, school, economic situation, and agencies involved with the family

    b. Developmental history—general description of the child's personality, fears, habits, play, relationships, language and communication, motor skills, and adaptive or problem-solving ability

7. Family Medical History—includes significant features of the medical history of all immediate family members (parents, siblings, grandparents)

8. Review of System—includes a thorough checklist of questions about recent symptoms that are applicable to children
    a. General appearance—overall state of health, frequent infections, exercise tolerance, weight gain or loss, fatigue, fevers, night sweats
    b. Vital signs
    c. Integument—acne, rashes, tendency to bruise, dryness, pigment changes, deformities of nails, hair growth or loss
    d. Musculoskeletal—weakness, lack of coordination, muscle pains, fractures, sprains, abnormal gait, stiffness, cramps
    e. Lymph nodes—enlarged nodes or masses, discharge
    f. Head—headache, dizziness
    g. Skull—injury
    h. Eyes—visual problems, strabismus, eye infections, edema of lids, excessive or lack of tearing, use of glasses
    i. Ears—pain, discharge, hearing loss
    j. Nose—nosebleeds, congestion, obstruction
    k. Mouth—problems with teeth, bleeding gums
    l. Throat—sore throats, choking, hoarseness
    m. Neck—pain, limited movement, thyroid enlargement, masses, torticollis
    n. Breasts—enlargement, discharge, masses
    o. Respiratory—cough, colds, wheezing, shortness of breath, sputum production
    p. Cardiovascular system—cyanosis, fatigue, murmur, anemia
    q. Gastrointestinal—nausea, vomiting, diarrhea, constipation, blood in stool
    r. Genitalia—menarche, date of last menstrual period, vaginal discharge, pruritus, sexual activity, pain on urination, hematuria, nocturia, change in size of scrotum
    s. Rectum/anus—prolapse, bleeding
    t. Extremities—injury
    u. Nervous system—seizures, tremors, speech problems, loss of memory, fears

Nursing Diagnoses

The following is a list of possible diagnoses and could apply, depending on the child's age, clinical situation, and physical condition:

Anxiety

Fear

Impaired adjustment

Ineffective family coping

Parental role conflict

Planning

In planning to admit a child to your unit, obtain an admission sheet and all other instruments that you will need to examine the child (thermometer, pajamas, etc.) and make the child and parents comfortable.

Interventions

PROCEDURE	**RATIONALE/EXPECTED OUTCOME (EO)**

Infants. (0–8 months)

1. Do as much of the physical exam and assessment as possible with the infant held in the parent's lap.

The infant's major concern is whether or not to trust people. Infants have definite preferences and exhibit no hesitation in letting anyone know about those preferences. They rely on continuity and their primary nurturers. This will also allow the interviewer to assess the parent–child bond (eye contact, physical touch).

EO: The child and parent will experience decreased fear and anxiety if the admission assessment is accomplished in a well-organized fashion that takes into account the child's age and developmental level.

2. Avoid abrupt and jerky movements. Use a quiet tone.

3. Let the older infant touch the instruments before examiner uses them (Fig. 1-2).

This will gain the infant's cooperation

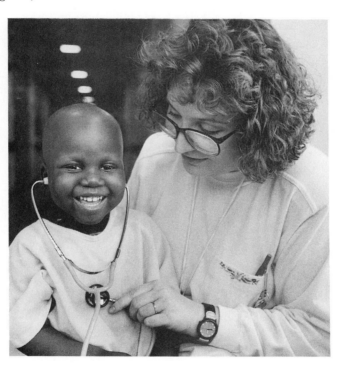

Figure 1-2.

4. Perform the least distressing task first (for example, listen to the heart before taking a rectal temperature or looking into an infant's ears). Maintain eye contact.

Evaluation that needs to be accomplished when the child is quiet should be done first.

Infants. (9–12 months)

5. Gather as much information as possible about the infant by just observing—no touching.

6. Keep the parent within the child's range of vision.

At this age, anything or anybody not within view is assumed to be gone.

EO: The child or parent will plan for the adaptation required by the change in the child's health status.

PROCEDURE	**RATIONALE/EXPECTED OUTCOME (EO)**

Toddler. (1–3 years)

7. Expose only part of the child's body at any one time.

At this age, the child does not like to be nude. He or she may object to being without clothing.

EO: The family will discuss their current concerns and questions with the health care team members.

8. Carry out the easiest procedures first, and quickly finish with the more distasteful ones.

9. Never give a choice when there is none. State commands in a positive manner. Do not beg or plead.

The toddler strives for autonomy and wants to make choices. "No" is a favorite word.

10. Allow the toddler to hold familiar objects.

The toddler can deal with symbols (familiar objects from home such as a favorite toy or blanket).

EO: The child will have familiar objects from home to hold and play with while in the hospital.

Preschoolers. (3–5 years)

11. The examiner can ask children of this age questions and sometimes get a reliable response.

Although this age group has acquired language, the examiner must not be misled into thinking that adult thought processes are occurring.

12. The preschooler needs feedback and explanations of what needs to be accomplished.

The preschooler is egocentric and experiences a large variety of terrors and fantasies. Preschoolers feel that skin holds them together and any threat to its integrity will make them fall apart. Also, illness may mean retribution for being "bad."

EO: The child will be given feedback and explanations of what is expected.

School Age

13. The physical examination can progress along an adult pattern from head to toe, after giving a brief explanation of each procedure.

Children at this age can accept information but may not yet be able to integrate it into their surroundings. Until the age of 9, children have little knowledge of their bodies or how they function; however, never underestimate their responses.

14. A concern for privacy is important. Provide privacy by closing bedside drapes or the door to the room and provide an examination gown.

Adolescent

15. Ask the parent to leave the room during an examination.

Adolescents want identity and independence.

EO: The parent will understand the need for the adolescent to take control of some aspects of care in such ways as requiring privacy during examinations or choosing treatment times if possible.

16. Give adolescents feedback about what is normal about their bodies.

This is an age of idealism. Even if the adolescent is ill, find some aspect of the exam that is normal and expand upon it.

17. Encourage good health habits at this time.

This age group is receptive to wellness teaching.

Patient/Family Education: Home Care Considerations

1. Explore alternative support systems for the child's current health problem.
2. Encourage the family to bring toys or special items from home to provide for continuity.
3. Encourage the family to participate in play activities with the child to strengthen family relationships (for example, by accompanying the child to the playroom).
4. Discuss health topics with the family that are relevant to the age and development of the child (safety, diet, skin care).

References

Ferhold, J.D. (1980). *Clinical assessment of children.* Philadelphia: J.B. Lippincott Company.

Gavey, J. (1988). Baby admissions. *Nursing Times, 84*(49) 43–45.

Johnson, S.H. (1986). *Nursing assessment strategies for the family at risk.* (2nd ed.). Philadelphia: J.B. Lippincott Company.

McFarlane, J. (1974). Pediatric assessment and intervention. *Nursing '74,* December, 66–68.

Moore, A. (1989). Crisis intervention: A care plan for families of hospitalized children. *Pediatric Nursing, 15*(3), 234–236.

Schoonover, L.A., Gooden, M.D., & Moore, P. (1982). Assessment: A nursing model. *Nursing Management, 13*(4), 18–22.

Yoos, L. (1981). A developmental approach to physical assessment. *Maternal–Child Nursing, 6*(3), 168–170.

Patient Transfers

2

Definition/Purpose

The transfer of a child from one nursing unit to another or from one institution to another disrupts the child's and family's normal routine in relation to the hospital setting. The goal is to afford the family a smooth transition while communicating all necessary information to a new set of caregivers.

Standard of Care

1. The child will be transported in the manner most appropriate to his or her physical condition, safety, and comfort. Appropriate warmth and temperature stabilization are essential to pediatric patients, particularly young infants.

Assessment

1. Assess the pertinent history and physical findings to determine the appropriate mode of transport for the child, the number and type of supportive relationships that will help the child cope with change, and the child's ability to verbalize concerns.
2. Assess psychosocial and developmental factors relative to the degree of perceived disruption, feelings, and attitudes, as well as patterns of coping, dependency, and socialization.
3. Assess the family's knowledge of the need for the transfer and their ability to help the child adjust.

Nursing Diagnoses

The following is a list of possible diagnoses and could apply, depending on the child's age, clinical situation, and physical condition:

Impaired adjustment

Anxiety

Fear

High risk for injury

Planning

In planning to transfer a child, the following equipment must be gathered:

Transfer form or checklist

Appropriate mode of transportation

Interventions

PROCEDURE	RATIONALE/EXPECTED OUTCOME (EO)

1. Check with the admitting office of the receiving unit or hospital for accommodations.

EO: The child's transfer will be accomplished in an organized manner.

2. Notify the unit charge nurse on the receiving unit of the transfer and arrange a time of transfer.

A meeting should occur between the sending and receiving nurses before the transfer of children who have complex nursing requirements. A telephone conversation may be adequate for less complex cases.

3. Notify the unit charge nurse of any special equipment that will be needed for the child, such as a suction machine or special bed.

4. Explain to the child and family the reason for the transfer and the area of relocation.

Explanations may clarify information and help lessen fears.

EO: The child or family will have decreased anxiety relative to the transfer.

5. Assemble all the child's equipment and belongings.

6. Ensure that adequate blankets, head coverings, and other devices are used to maintain the child's temperature.

Infants have difficulty maintaining their temperature.

7. Provide the following on the transfer form (Fig. 2-1):
   a. A nursing summary of child's past and current problems and status
   b. Current vital signs
   c. Active nursing diagnoses with care plan
   d. Child's and family's understanding of the illness and treatment.
   e. Current treatments: medications, dressing changes, feedings, etc. (See example.)

This ensures that the nurses assuming the child's care will have all relevant information necessary to plan and deliver care.

EO: The child's care will continue to be delivered in a safe manner.
EO: The child will have continuity of care.

MICHAEL REESE HOSPITAL AND MEDICAL CENTER
DEPARTMENT OF PEDIATRIC NURSING
PICU TRANSFER SUMMARY

DATE/TIME: _3-1-91 (2 PM)_   TRANSFER TO: _7E_

_2-25-91_   _15 mo_   _F_   VITAL SIGNS: _36⁶ (R)_   _124_   _36_
    ADMISSION DATE   AGE   SEX   T   P   R

DIET: _Clear liquids_   ALLERGIES: _None_

PO: _✓_ NG: ___ NJ: ___ G Tube: ___

MEDICAL DIAGNOSES: _GSW to chest with pneumothorax (40%)_

NURSING DIAGNOSES: # _Altered gas exchange_
Altered skin integrity   # _Altered level of comfort_
    (see attached care plan)

(continued)

BRIEF HISTORY OF PRESENT ILLNESS/CONDITION: *15-mo-old who was shot in the chest while being held by mother. Entrance wound under Ⓡ armpit, exit wound through Ⓛ shoulder*

SURGERY/SPECIAL PROCEDURES/COMPLICATIONS: (Dates)

Ⓡ chest tube placed 2-25-91; removed 2-28-91 with full lung expansion

SPECIAL PRECAUTIONS: (Needles, Bld, Isolation) *None*

MEDICATION	TIME	DOSE	ROUTE	SPECIAL EQUIPMENT NEEDED
Tylenol elixir	*PRN (pain)*	*160 mg*	*PO*	*IV pump* *Oxygen*

ASSESSMENT

CARDIAC
Rate *124* B/P *96/52*
Temp. *36.6 Ⓡ* Other _____

RESPIRATORY
Rate *36* Range *24-40*
Breath Sounds *Decreased breath sounds in RUL. Upper airway congestion*
O₂ mode *1 L per nasal cannula*

RENAL
Fluid Restriction *None*
Previous 24° I/O = *1475/1210*
Today from 6ª I/O = *425/125*

In = *325* IV, *100* PO

Out = *125* Urine, *0* Stool

= *0* NG, *0* Other

FRO *Neg.* Sugar *Neg.* BLD *Neg.*

GI
Stool X *1*
Type: *brown/soft*

Heme *No* CS *No*
Other _____

(continued)

IV FLUIDS

\# __4__ , __200__ cc Bag __20__ cc Burette

rate __10 cc__, site __Ⓛ hand__

tubing changed __3-1-91__
Date

\# _____ , _____ cc Bag _____ cc Burette

rate _____ , site _____

tubing changed _____
Date

NEURO/PSYCHE

Alert active child. Not afraid of strangers

LAB DATA (2-28-91)

Na 140; K 4.2; Cl 104; Hb 10.6; Hct 38
CXR: Minimal infiltrate RUL, rest of lung fields clear

NOTIFIED OF TRANSFER

S/O __Mother__
Relationship

__3-1-91__   __10 AM__
Date   Time

Family Knowledge of Illness/Prognosis: *Father of child in jail for shooting; mother supportive of child; maternal GM also involved. Social worker and protective services involved.*

PROCEDURE	RATIONALE/EXPECTED OUTCOME (EO)
8. Ensure that all scheduled medications and treatments are completed up to the time of transfer. Clarify orders for those medications or treatments scheduled during the time of the transfer to ascertain who is responsible for them.	The time taken by the transfer may interfere with scheduled treatments or medications.
9. Obtain the appropriate mode of transportation.	
10. Escort the child with his or her belongings to the new unit.	
11. Introduce the child and family to the receiving nurse and give a report on the child's status.	*EO: The child will be allowed time to adjust to the new environment and people.*

Patient/Family Education: Home Care Considerations

1. Give careful, age-appropriate explanations; encourage questions and verbalization of any concerns.
2. Provide positive reinforcement to child and parents; involve the family in the transfer process.

References

Kanter, R.K. (1989). Adverse events during inter-hospital transport: Physiologic deterioration associated with pretransport severity of illness. *Pediatrics, 84*(1), 43–48.

Tompkins, J.M. (1990). Interhospital transport of seriously ill or injured children. *Pediatric Nursing, 16*(1), 51–53.

Patient Discharge

Definition/Purpose

The discharge of a child from the hospital can be both a happy and an anxiety-producing experience. As health care providers, we must ensure the child a safe discharge and provide the child and family with the knowledge and skills necessary to continue care at home.

Standard of Care

1. Discharge planning will begin on the day of admission with a nursing care plan that includes a discharge section.
2. Minors will be discharged only to their legal guardians, unless other arrangements have been made ahead of time and are documented in the medical record.
3. Prior to discharge, the child and family will have learned the skills necessary for follow-up care at home.

Assessment

1. Assess the pertinent history and physical findings for information that the family will need upon discharge.
2. Assess psychosocial and developmental factors related to anxiety regarding treatment, body image disturbances, hopelessness, fear of dying, and habits or rituals that would affect a discharge plan.
3. Assess the child's and family's knowledge of the reason for hospitalization and the follow-up care needed.

Nursing Diagnoses

The following is a list of possible diagnoses and could apply, depending on the child's age, clinical situation, and physical condition:

Anxiety

Fear

Self-care deficit

Planning

In planning to discharge a child, gather the following equipment:

Medical record

Discharge form and instructions

Appropriate method of transport

Interventions

PROCEDURE	**RATIONALE/EXPECTED OUTCOME (EO)**

1. With confirmation of the diagnosis, incorporate discharge planning into the initial nursing care plan.

Establishment of short- and long-term goals determines the discharge plan.

EO: The child's discharge planning will begin on admission and be incorporated into the nursing care plan.

2. Using available resources, plan and implement a teaching program for the child and parents in the assessment and care of the child, the use of equipment, the administration of medications, and other related activities.

Discharge planning focuses on those procedures that parents or children are expected to continue at home.

EO: The child and family will have a decreased level of anxiety regarding discharge as a result of predischarge teaching.

3. Plan opportunities for parents to demonstrate their understanding and skills in providing the care and observation needed when the child returns home. Document instructions and parents' understanding of skills.

4. Contact the discharge planner so that the family obtains the necessary equipment and supplies for home care.

EO: The child will have the supplies needed for care at home.

5. Review any care given immediately prior to discharge.

6. Write a discharge note in the medical record including the following:
   a. Instructions given on diet
   b. Instructions given on activity
   c. Instructions given on medications, including dosage, schedule (time of last dose given and when next dose to be given), and side effects
   d. Instructions given on treatments, observations needed for the child's specific problem, and when to notify the physician
   e. Instructions regarding resumption of school or day care
   f. Instructions given family on when and where to return to see the doctor
   g. How the child left the hospital (walking, wheelchair, etc.) and condition at discharge (suture line healed, cast intact, etc.)

The medical record should reflect the instructions given to the family.

EO: The child's medical record will reflect the instructions given to the family, along with the condition of the child at the time of discharge.

7. Have parent or guardian sign appropriate discharge papers; give family written instructions (Fig. 3-1).

Michael Reese Hospital and Medical Center

Department of Nursing

DISCHARGE INSTRUCTIONS/SUMMARY FORM

1. Activity Level and Special Instructions for Self Care: *No tub bath; sponge bath only until return to see doctor. Leave dressing in place—do not remove No bike riding. May return to school but no physical education.*

(continued)

2. Diet/Instructions: *Regular food for age*

3.

MEDICINE & DOSAGE	ROUTE & SPECIAL INSTRUCTIONS	TIME	REASON	NOTIFY DOCTOR IF
Ampicillin	*by mouth*	6^A–12^P	*for infection*	
	every 6 hours	6^P–12^A		
	* *Finish entire bottle of medicine**			
	Notify doctor for fever, vomiting, or drainage from wound			

4. I may contact *Dr. Hamilton* Phone *222-0001* if I have any questions/problems.

5. Return Appointment with *Dr. Hamilton* Date *5-9-91* Phone *222-0001*

6. I have received a copy of and understand the above instructions:

George Apple — father   *Jane Tepper, RN*   *5-1-91*

Patient or Authorized Party   Physician/Nurse   Date

7.   PATIENT

13-yr-old discharged with father. Child afebrile, well hydrated, pain free. Dressing to lower right quadrant of abdomen dry, intact, without redness or drainage. Both parent and child instructed on the importance of finishing antibiotic for total of 10 days.

(Continue Summary Note on back of form)

8. Mode of Discharge: W/C ☐   Ambulatory ☐   Carried ☐   Ambulance ☐

PROCEDURE

8. Assist the family in gathering the child's belongings, and escort them to the door if necessary.

RATIONALE/EXPECTED OUTCOME (EO)

Patient/Family Education: Home Care Considerations

1. Establish appropriate referrals, which may include formal referrals to a nursing agency, physical therapist, or tutor, or informal referrals such as introducing the family to others who have had similar experiences.

2. Instruct the family on whom to contact if questions arise; supply them with key telephone numbers.

References

Scharen, K., Beich, M., Envoy, K., et al. (1990). Evaluating written discharge instructions in a pediatric setting. *Journal of Nursing Quality Assurance, 4*(4), 63–71.

Smith, B. (1990). Effective discharge planning and home health care: How-to's for the staff nurse. *Advanced Clinical Care, 5*(1), 6–8.

Taylor, C., Lillis, C., & LeMone, P. (1989). *Fundamentals of nursing: The art and science of nursing care.* Philadelphia: J.B. Lippincott Company.

Informed Consent

4

Definition/Purpose

Every child is guaranteed freedom from bodily contact by another person unless consent is granted by his or her legal guardian. In health care settings, informed consent is needed for admission and routine treatment, for specialized diagnostic procedures (many involving sedation or the injection of dyes), for surgical treatment, and for experimentation or photography involving the child.

Obtaining informed consent is the responsibility of the person who will execute the procedure or conduct the research study. The nurse's responsibility is to check that a signed and witnessed consent is in the child's record and to respond to questions the guardian has about the consent. The use of a printed consent form should not take the place of the actual explanation given to the guardian about the procedure, its risks and benefits, and alternative treatments. The nurse signs the consent form as a witness to the guardian's signature of the form, not as the person obtaining consent.

Standard of Care

1. An informed consent is required for all routine health care services and for nonroutine diagnostic treatment, research procedures, photography, or release of medical records.
2. A signed consent is not needed in an emergency if there is an immediate threat to health or life and the guardian authorized to consent cannot be reached.
3. A signed consent is not needed for action taken in response to an unanticipated complication during surgery if the guardian cannot be reached or the delay that would be caused by attempting to contact the guardian threatens the child's health or life.
4. Minors cannot sign an informed consent for themselves unless they are married, pregnant, or self-supporting. Always consult the legal affairs department to clarify a minor's status.
5. A guardian's refusal to sign a consent should be documented. If the physician feels that the refusal will threaten the health or life of the minor, the legal affairs department and child protective agency should be notified so that a court order can be obtained for the procedure.
6. A consent must be written, signed by the child's guardian, and be specifically for the procedure performed. If signed, in person, by the guardian, one witness is needed. If a telephone consent is obtained, two witnesses are needed.
7. Once signed, nothing can be added to the consent without the guardian's knowledge and approval.

Assessment

1. Assess whether the four elements of an informed consent have been ensured:
   - Disclosure
   - Comprehension

- Competence
- Voluntariness.

2. Assess whether the minor's legal guardian is consenting to the procedure. If there is reasonable doubt as to the validity of a guardianship, request legal documents to verify guardianship (for example, birth certificate, legal documents with guardian's name).

Nursing Diagnoses

The following is a list of possible diagnoses and could apply, depending on the child's age, clinical situation, and physical condition:

Anxiety

Fear

Decisional conflict

Altered family processes

Planning

When planning to obtain a signature on an informed consent, the following tools are needed:

Consent form (completely filled in)

Ballpoint pen

Legal documents with proof of guardianship (if doubt arises).

Interventions

PROCEDURE

Ensure an Informed Consent by:

1. Disclosure (by the physician)
   a. The guardian is informed of the child's current medical status and anticipated course of treatment.
   b. The guardian is informed of the risks and benefits of the treatment alternatives.
   c. The guardian is told that no outcomes can be guaranteed.
   d. The guardian is given a professional opinion as to the best alternative.

2. Comprehension
   a. Impediments to comprehension such as anxiety, fear, cultural barriers, terminology, and time spent on the explanation are assessed.
   b. The nurse must convey information to aid understanding.

3. Competence
   a. The nurse assesses the competence of the parent/guardian in making a decision.

   b. The nurse assesses the possible deleterious effects of the decision on the child.

RATIONALE/EXPECTED OUTCOME (EO)

The parent/guardian must be given complete, up-to-date information on the child's condition and intended treatment to decrease anxiety/fear of the unknown and to make the best decision for the child's well-being.

EO: The parent/guardian will be able to make an informed decision on the care of the child.

Nurses may know an explanation was given but find the parent/guardian still has a misunderstanding related to the treatment.

EO: The parent/guardian will have their questions answered in language that they can understand.

The parent/guardian's ability to make a decision may be clouded by anxiety, fear, medication, depression, disorientation or confusion.

The parent/guardian is able to communicate and understand the information presented. The parent/guardian

PROCEDURE

    c. The nurse will obtain an interpreter or person to use sign language if necessary.

4. Voluntariness
   a. The nurse determines that the consent for the procedure was freely given.
   b. The nurse does not coerce or manipulate the guardian to sign the consent.

5. If the nurse has reservations about any of the above four elements of a consent, the physician must be notified before the procedure is performed.

6. If the guardian refuses to sign the consent, the physician should be notified so that the consequences of refusal can be discussed. The guardian should sign a release form indicating refusal to consent and releasing the hospital from responsibility for the outcome of this act. This becomes a permanent part of the medical record. If refusal is life-threatening, the physician will notify the child protection agencies for court approval to perform the procedure.

RATIONALE/EXPECTED OUTCOME (EO)

has the ability to reason and deliberate.

EO: The nurse will assess the competence of the person making the decision and will notify the physician or legal department if questions arise.

Threatening a parent/guardian in a manner that creates fear of battery is an assault.

EO: The decision to sign the consent by the parent/guardian is a freely given, well-informed decision.

Consequences of not obtaining an informed consent can include battery charges against the hospital staff.

Religious or cultural reasons are sometimes given for refusal of a procedure (for example, blood transfusion). The parent/guardian, however, may not object to a court approving the procedure.

EO: The child will receive the treatment necessary to maintain health.

Patient/Family Education: Home Care Considerations

1. The family will be informed of an impending procedure, its risks and benefits, and alternative treatments.

References

Curtin, L.L. (1982). Informed consent: Rights, responsibilities, and roles. *Nursing Management, 13*(10), 7–8.

Cushing, M. (1984). Informed consent: An MD responsibility. *American Journal of Nursing, 84*(4), 437–440.

Ferrari, M.R. (1986). Avoiding legal risks in pediatrics. *Nursing Life, 6*(2), 24–25.

Northrop, C. (1986). Avoid the perils of misinformed consent. *Nursing '86, 16*(10), 43.

Rhodes, A.M. (1987). Consent for medical treatment. *Maternal-Child Nursing, 12*(2), 133.

Springer, E.W. (1970). *Nursing and the law.* Pittsburgh, PA: Aspen.

Taylor, C., & Hobaugh, R. (1986). The role of the critical care nurse in developing informed consent. *Dimensions in Critical Care Nursing, 5*(2), 98–105.

Taylor, C., Lillis, C., & LeMone, P. (1989). *Fundamentals of nursing: The art and science of nursing care.* Philadelphia: J.B. Lippincott Co.

General Assessment Procedures

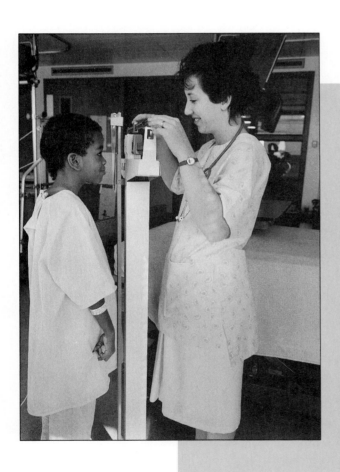

Unit II

Apgar Scoring

5

Definition/Purpose

The Apgar score is the most useful guide for evaluating the newborn infant's need for resuscitation. The Apgar system is used to evaluate the infant at 1 and 5 minutes of age. The 1-minute score correlates with acidosis and survival; the 5-minute score correlates with neurologic outcome. The Apgar scoring system evaluates color, tone, grimace, respiration, and pulse. These are listed in order of importance, from least to the most important. Each system receives 0, 1, or 2 points, and the points are then totaled for the final score.

Asphyxia is defined as a failure to provide the cell with oxygen and remove carbon dioxide. Both circulation and ventilation are essential to avoid asphyxia. There are multiple stimuli at birth to alter the circulation and initiate respirations. The actual stimuli for initiating respiration are thought to include a rise in pco_2, interruption of umbilical circulation, and tactile and temperature stimulation. Neonatal asphyxia can result from multiple factors (for example, prolapsed cord, sepsis, meconium aspiration, or abnormal presentation). It is important to realize when evaluating a neonate in distress or full arrest that the asphyxial event may have begun in utero. It is difficult to document the beginning of the hypoxic period.

Standard of Care

1. Every infant will be assessed at the 1- and 5-minute intervals after birth and have an Apgar score recorded in the medical record.

Assessment

1. Assess the pertinent history and physical findings for maternal medications or anesthesia, length of labor, and fetal tolerance of labor. Assess length of time between rupture of membranes and delivery and the weight, length, heart rate, respirations, temperature, blood count, general appearance, condition of the cord, response to stimuli, activity pattern, and the presence of meconium on the infant.

2. Assess the parental preparation for the infant and parents' available support systems.

3. Assess the family's knowledge of the needs of the infant and the lifestyle changes anticipated.

Nursing Diagnoses

The following is a list of possible diagnoses and could apply, depending on the child's age, clinical situation, and physical condition:

Ineffective airway clearance

High risk for altered body temperature

Decreased cardiac output

Planning

When assisting in the delivery of a baby, the following equipment needs to be gathered in order to assign Apgar scores:

Stethoscope

| **PROCEDURE** | **RATIONALE/EXPECTED OUTCOME (EO)** |

1. Become familiar with the Apgar scoring system (Table 5-1).

Table 5-1. Apgar Scoring

	0	1	2
Appearance	Blue, pale	Pink body, blue hands/feet	Pink
Pulse	Absent	<100/minute	>100/minute
Grimace (irritability)	None	Some grimace	Cough/cry
Activity (muscle tone)	Limp	Slight flexion	Active, good flexion
Respirations	Absent	Slow, irregular	Crying, rhythmic

2. Become familiar with the implications of Apgar scores (Table 5-2).

Table 5-2. Implications of Apgar Scoring

Score	Implication	Action
0–3	Severe depression	Full resuscitation
4–6	Intermediate depression	Partial resuscitation
7–10	Responding well to transition	Support newborn's own effort

PROCEDURE

3. After delivery of the infant:
   a. Suction nose and mouth.
   b. Dry infant.
   c. Place under radiant warmer.

4. Assess 1-minute Apgar score.

5. If the 1-minute Apgar is 7–10, keep the infant warm and dry and continue to assess until the 5-minute Apgar is complete.

6. If the Apgar is 4–6 at 1 minute, the infant will be cyanotic, weak, limp, and hypoxic. Dry the infant, keep the infant warm, clear airway, and give oxygen.

7. If the initial Apgar is 0–3, rapidly dry and warm the infant and begin resuscitation. Administer appropriate drugs and fluids.

RATIONALE/EXPECTED OUTCOME (EO)

All infants are a bluish color at birth. By 2 minutes, most are pink.

EO: The child's airway will be cleared. The child will be dry and have a stable normal body temperature.

If it is evident prior to 1 minute that resuscitation is necessary, start resuscitation immediately. Pulse, respiratory rate, and muscle tone are better predictors of the need for resuscitation than the Apgar score.

If the score is normal at 1 minute and worse at 5 minutes, consider maternal drugs or congenital lesions.

EO: The child's Apgar score will be determined at 1 and 5 minutes of age.

If the heart rate is maintained over 100 beats per minute and if the respiratory rate is normal (30–60 breaths/minute), complete the initial assessment and transfer the infant to the nursery. If the heart rate falls below 100 beats/minute, begin to ventilate the baby.

EO: The infant will have the prescribed medications administered and the physiologic response noted.

PROCEDURE	**RATIONALE/EXPECTED OUTCOME (EO)**
8. Assess the Apgar at 5 minutes. If the Apgar is still below 7, continue CPR, intubate, ventilate, and monitor blood gases.	*EO: The child's heart rate will be maintained above 100; respiratory rate will be assisted and blood gases will be within the normal range.*
9. Document the scores and the interventions taken in the medical record.	*EO: The child's medical record will indicate the assessments made and the actions taken on behalf of the newborn.*

Patient/Family Education: Home Care Considerations

1. Describe the characteristics of the infant. Keep the parents informed of the infant's activity and progress.
2. Inform the parents of the Apgar scores and their implications for care.

References

Clark, D.A., & Hakanson, D.O. (1988). The inaccuracy of Apgar scoring. *Journal of Perinatology, 3*(8), 203–205.

Coen, R.W., Avroy, A., Fanaroff, M.D., et al (1988). A fast, efficient newborn exam. *Patient Care, 22*(11), 192–197, 200–204, 207.

Reeder, S., & Martin, L. (1992). *Maternity nursing: Family, newborn and women's health care.* (17th ed.). Philadelphia: J.B. Lippincott Company.

Temperature

6

Definition/Purpose

The body temperature normally remains within a fairly constant range, with a balance between heat production and heat loss regulated by the hypothalamus. Heat is produced by exercise and the body's ability to metabolize food. Heat is lost through the skin, the lungs, and the body's waste products. When more heat is produced than is lost, the body's temperature will be elevated. When more heat is lost than produced, the body's temperature will be subnormal. An instrument used to measure heat is a thermometer. Temperature measurement is possible by means of esophageal, intravascular, and tympanic sites as well as the traditional oral, axillary, and rectal routes. In all cases, the goal remains to obtain an accurate temperature as safely and conveniently as possible.

Standard of Care

1. Take axillary, rectal, or tympanic temperature in children under 4–6 years of age or in a child of any age who is uncooperative or unconscious.

2. Take axillary, rectal, or tympanic temperatures on all children who are receiving oxygen therapy or who are tachypneic. Results obtained from two research studies indicate that there is a significant difference between temperatures taken orally and those taken by the axillary or rectal method. This difference is related to ventilatory cooling of the mouth due to oxygen therapy or tachypnea.

3. Oral or tympanic temperatures may be taken on children over the age of 6 years, if patients are cooperative.

4. "Normal" body temperature is 37°C (98.6°F) orally, up to 38°C (101°F) rectally, and 36°C (96.8°F) axillary. A child with a rectal temperature exceeding 38°C (100.4°F) or an oral temperature of 37.9°C (100.2°F) is considered febrile (Table 6-1).

Table 6-1. Average body temperature in well children under basal conditions

Age	Temperature	
	°F	°C
3 months–6 months	99.4	37.5
1 year	99.7	37.7
3 years	99.0	37.2
5 years	98.6	37.0
7 years	98.3	36.8
9 years–11 years	98.1	36.7
13 years+	97.8	36.6

Assessment

1. Assess the child's usual pattern of behavior for developmental level and previous experience with health care settings and temperature determination in particular.

2. Assess level of consciousness, pertinent history, and physical findings that would help determine the correct means of taking a temperature (for example, no rectal

temperatures on children with colon or rectal surgery or diarrhea, or on oncology patients.)

3. Assess the family's ability to measure the child's temperature, recognize hypo/hyperthermia as a symptom of an illness, and respond appropriately.

Nursing Diagnoses

The following is a list of possible diagnoses and could apply, depending on the child's age, clinical situation, and physical condition:

Pain

High risk for altered body temperature

Fear

High risk for injury

Planning

When planning to take a child's temperature, assemble the following equipment:

Water soluble lubricant

Thermometer

• Rectal or stubby bulb (Fig. 6-1)

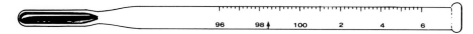

Figure 6-1. Stubby/rectal bulb.

• Oral bulb (Fig. 6-2)

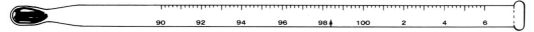

Figure 6-2. Oral bulb.

• Electronic (interchangeable oral and rectal probes) (Fig. 6-3)

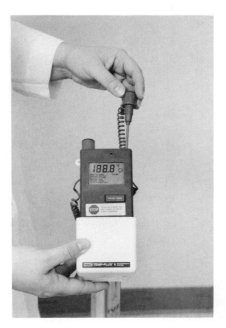

Figure 6-3.

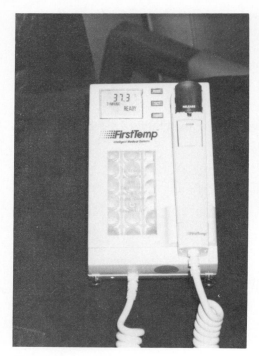

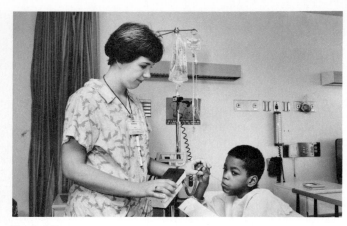

Figure 6-5.

Figure 6-4.

- Tympanic probe (Fig. 6-4)
- Gloves (Some institutions advocate wearing gloves when taking a temperature because of the contact with stool, urine, and saliva.)

PROCEDURE	**RATIONALE/EXPECTED OUTCOME (EO)**

1. Prepare the child in a developmentally appropriate manner.

   EO: The child will cooperate with the temperature determination as developmentally able.

2. Oral determination
   a. Wash hands.
   b. Select an instrument (oral/stubby or electric).
   c. If the thermometer has been stored in chemical solution, rinse it with water and wipe it dry with a soft tissue.

   A chemical solution may irritate the mucous membranes and have an objectionable taste.

   d. Shake a glass thermometer until the mercury is below the 95°F mark or the 35.5°C mark. Firmly hold the non-bulb end of the thermometer and briskly snap the hand at the wrist. If using an electronic thermometer, remove from charger and slide cover over probe.

   This action moves the mercury bulb end.

   e. If the child is over the age of 6 years, place the bulb under the right side of the child's tongue. Have child close mouth around the thermometer.

   The right side of the tongue is specified so that the bulb is placed close to the sublingual artery, thus gaining a more accurate temperature.

   f. Leave the thermometer under the tongue for 3–5 minutes. Stay with the child while thermometer is in place (Fig. 6-5).

   EO: The child will remain free from injury.

   g. If an electric thermometer is used, use the oral probe with a disposable plastic probe cover. The thermometer will signal when the peak temperature has been reached.

PROCEDURE

    h. Remove the thermometer from the mouth and read the temperature.

    i. After use, wipe thermometer with soft tissue, rinse in cold water, and store according to policy.

3. Rectal determination
    a. Wash hands.
    b. Select an instrument (rectal/stubby or electric) and provide privacy for the child.

    c. Rinse, wipe, and shake the rectal thermometer as suggested in the procedure for obtaining an oral temperature. If an electronic thermometer is used, remove from charger and slide cover over probe.

    d. Lubricate the bulb with a water soluble gel.

    e. Infant—Place infant prone; spread the buttocks with one hand and insert the thermometer slowly and gently with the other hand. The bulb should be inserted into the rectum about $\frac{1}{4}$–$\frac{1}{2}$ inch. If resistance is felt, remove thermometer and choose another route (Figs. 6-6 and 6-7).
    Older child—Position child on side; separate buttocks to expose the anal opening; gently insert the thermometer into the rectum about 1–$1\frac{1}{2}$ inches.

RATIONALE/EXPECTED OUTCOME (EO)

EO: The child will have an accurately measured temperature.

Wiping off contaminated particles helps to reduce the spread of organisms.

Insertion of a rectal thermometer represents an invasion of the child's body and may cause an increase in the normal fear of body mutilation; therefore, take a rectal temperature only when deemed necessary.

This reduces friction and helps to insert the thermometer and minimize irritation of the mucous membranes in the anal canal.

EO: The child will experience minimal discomfort.

EO: The parent or child will express fear or concerns to the staff.

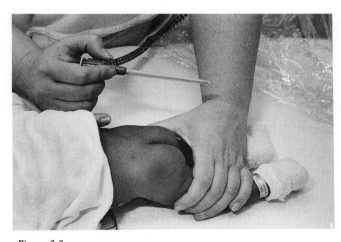

Figure 6-6.

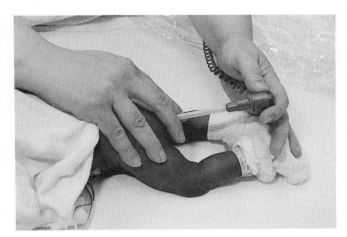

Figure 6-7.

    f. Hold thermometer in place for 3–4 minutes or until electronic thermometer signal is heard. Never leave child alone with a rectal thermometer in place.

Allowing sufficient time for the thermometer to register results in a more accurate measurement of body temperature.

PROCEDURE

    g. Remove the thermometer gently in a straight line. Wipe it off with a soft tissue. If using an electronic thermometer, insert probe into base and store in charger. Read the temperature.

    h. Reposition child in a comfortable position and clean thermometer according to policy.

4. Axillary determination
    a. Wash hands.
    b. Select instrument—follow institution policy concerning whether to use a rectal or oral thermometer.
    c. Rinse, wipe, and shake the thermometer as suggested in the procedure for obtaining an oral temperature. If an electronic thermometer is used, remove from charger and place cover on probe.

    d. Place the bulb under the arm, well up into the armpit. Bring the child's arm down close to the body and hold in place.

    e. Leave in place 10 minutes or until electronic thermometer signal is heard.

5. Tympanic determination
    a. Wash hands.
    b. Select the contact infrared tympanic thermometer.
    c. Place the probe tip covered by a polyethylene speculum into the outer third of the external auditory canal.
    d. The scan button on the handle is pressed and the machine accumulates emitted infrared energy for 1 second.
    e. The base displays the temperature.
    f. Record temperatures; replace handle in base after removing speculum.

RATIONALE/EXPECTED OUTCOME (EO)

Fecal matter on the thermometer makes it difficult to read.

When the bulb rests against superficial blood vessels in the axilla and skin surfaces are brought together to reduce air surrounding the bulb, a more accurate measurement is obtainable.
EO: The child will have an accurately measured temperature.

Special circumstances, such as children with otitis media or sinusitis, or the premature infant with small external ear canals, need further study to determine accuracy in these situations. The temperature of the tympanic membrane reflects core body temperature, since the tympanic membrane shares the blood supply with the hypothalamus, the center of core body temperature regulations.

EO: Children of all ages will have temperatures measured safely and conveniently.

Patient/Family Education: Home Care Considerations

1. Teach the child or family how to take an accurate temperature
    a. Which method to use (oral, rectal, axillary) according to age, developmental level, and level of cooperation
    b. Correct technique as stated above
    c. How to read the thermometer:
       • Hold the thermometer in the right hand, at the end away from the bulb, between the thumb and index finger (Fig. 6-8).

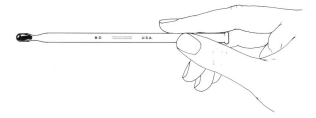

Figure 6-8.

- Turn the thermometer between thumb and index finger until you see the numbers on the bottom and the scale markings on the top (Fig. 6-9).

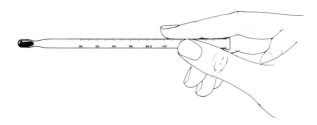

Figure 6-9.

- Hold the thermometer below eye level and turn it slowly until you see a wide mercury band between the scale and the numbers (Fig. 6-10).

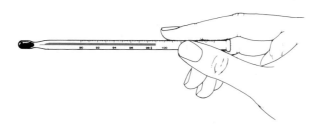

Figure 6-10.

- Read the temperature at the end of the mercury band. Fahrenheit scales are usually marked in intervals of $\frac{2}{10}$ of a degree. The scale reads 100.2°F. Centigrade scales are usually marked in $\frac{1}{10}$ of a degree. The scale reads 37.5°C.

2. Educate parents about normal diurnal variation of body temperature and which temperatures are considered a fever.
   a. A rectal temperature above 38°C (101°F) is considered febrile.
   b. An oral temperature above 37.9°C (100.2°F) is considered febrile.

3. Educate the parents on the common signs of fever. (The child's clinical presentation is a more accurate index of disease severity than the degree of fever.)
   a. Pinkish, red, flushed skin that is warm to touch
   b. Restlessness or excessive sleepiness
   c. Irritability
   d. Thirst
   e. Poor appetite
   f. Headache
   g. Excessive perspiration
   h. Glassy eyes and a sensitivity to light
   i. Increased pulse and respiratory rate
   j. Disorientation and confusion
   k. Convulsions

4. Explain the importance of administering an antipyretic at the correct dose and appropriate time interval. Teach the parents about the use of aspirin and its relationship to Reye's syndrome; tell them not to use aspirin with children under age 16 for varicella, flu, or viral illness.

5. Educate the parents that bathing and sponging with cold water or alcohol to reduce a fever makes the child uncomfortable; alcohol subjects the child to irritation of the respiratory tract due to the smell, and bathing with either alcohol or cold water can cause shivering, thus increasing body temperature. Give only a tepid sponge bath for a temperature above 40°C (104°F).

6. Educate the parents on the common signs of hypothermia:

   a. Pale, cold skin that is clammy to touch
   b. Listlessness
   c. Slow pulse and respiratory rate
   d. Confusion ranging to disorientation.

7. Explain the importance of seeking medical attention for hypothermia or hyperthermia.

References

Abrams, L., Buchholz, C., McKenzie, N., & Merenstein, G. (1989). Effects of peripheral IV infusion on neonatal axillary temperature measurement. *Pediatric Nursing, 15,* 630–632.

Barber, N., & Kilmon, C.A. (1989). Reactions to tympanic temperature measurement in an ambulatory setting. *Pediatric Nursing, 15,* 477–481.

Bliss-Holtz, J. (1989). Comparison of rectal, axillary and inguinal temperatures in full-term newborn infants. *Nursing Research, 38,* 85–87.

Donahue, A. (1983). Tepid Sponging. *Journal of Emergency Nursing, 9,* 78–82.

Durham, M., Swanson, B., & Paulford, N. (1986). Effect of tachypnea on oral temperature estimation: A replication. *Nursing Research, 35*(4), 211–214.

Erickson, R. (1976). Thermometer placement for oral temperature measurements. *International Journal of Nursing Study, 13,* 199–208.

Erickson, R. (1980). Oral temperature differences in relation to thermometer and technique. *Nursing Research, 29,* 157–164.

Lewis, L. (1984). *Fundamental skills in patient care.* Philadelphia: J.B. Lippincott Company.

Robichaud-Ekstrand, S., et al (1989). Comparison of electronic and glass thermometers: Length of time of insertion and type of breathing. *Canadian Journal of Nursing Research, 21,* 61–73.

Younger, J.B., & Brown, B.S. (1985). Fever management: Rationale or ritual. *Pediatric Nursing, 11,* 26–29.

Pulse

7

Definition/Purpose

The measurement of vital signs must be looked at in relation to each child's chief complaint and past medical and social history. Every clinical situation is unique. It is often forgotten how much clinical information can be obtained by documenting the presence or absence of pulses at a specific location as well as their rate, pattern, and cadence.

Bradycardia is defined as a persistent heart rate (pulse) of less than 100–120 beats per minute (bpm) in the neonate and infant and less than 80 bpm in the child. Transient bradycardia can be normal in the neonate during feeding or sleeping; therefore, the term "bradycardia" is only applied to persistent decrease in heart rate.

Tachycardia is defined as a pulse over 200 bpm in the neonate and infant and above 140–160 bpm in the child. Transient tachycardia may occur with crying or other activity that increases the demand for oxygen. For instance, the child's heart rate will increase 10 bpm for each degree Celsius elevation in temperature. Heart rate elevation will also be seen if ventricular stroke volume decreases, as in congestive heart failure, tamponade, or low cardiac output (Table 7-1).

Table 7-1. Normal Pulse Ranges in Children

Age	Normal Range	Average
0–24 hours	70–170 bpm	120 bpm
1–7 days	100–180 bpm	140 bpm
1 month	110–188 bpm	160 bpm
1 month–1 year	80–180 bpm	120–130 bpm
2 years	80–140 bpm	110 bpm
4 years	80–120 bpm	100 bpm
6 years	70–115 bpm	100 bpm
10 years	70–110 bpm	90 bpm
12–14 years	60–110 bpm	85–90 bpm
14–18 years	50–95 bpm	70–75 bpm

Standard of Care

1. The pulse rate is taken as part of the measurement of routine vital signs.

2. The pulse rate is counted for a full minute in a neonate, infant, or young child. It is counted for 30 seconds in the older child, and then is multiplied by 2.

3. A satisfactory pulse can be taken radially in children over 2 years of age. In infants and young children the apical pulse is more reliable.

4. Apical pulse rates should be obtained from all cardiac patients (those with congestive heart failure, congenital anomalies, or arrhythmias) or children on digitalis preparations.

Assessment

1. Assess the pertinent history for the reason the child is hospitalized, medications

taken, previous surgical procedures, allergies, fluid shifts or imbalances, respiratory illnesses, or anemic episodes.

2. Assess the physical findings for tachycardia, bradycardia, abnormal quality of the pulse, pulse deficit from arms to legs (usually brachial or radial compared with femoral), and unequal or nonpalpable pulses, including carotid, brachial, radial, femoral, popliteal, posterior tibial, and dorsalis pedis.

3. Assess the child's and family's knowledge of the admitting diagnosis, medication regimen (if any), and future plans for care.

Nursing Diagnoses

The following is a list of possible diagnoses and could apply, depending on the child's age, clinical situation, and physical condition:

Anxiety

Fear

Decreased cardiac output

Planning

In planning to take a pulse rate, the following equipment is needed:

Stethoscope

Pen and paper.

PROCEDURE

RATIONALE/EXPECTED OUTCOME (EO)

Infant and Young Child and All Cardiac Patients—Apical Rate

1. The apical rate should be taken before any other vital sign measurement is attempted. Approach the child in a quiet gentle manner.

Taking the temperature or blood pressure may agitate the child and make him or her cry, thus making it more difficult to hear.

EO: The infant will be approached in a quiet, gentle manner and have his or her pulse counted.

2. Place the stethoscope between the left nipple and sternum (Fig. 7-1).

The point of maximum intensity is located lateral to the nipple at the third or fourth interspace.

3. Count the beats for 1 minute.

Since arrhythmia is normal at this age, counting for less than 1 minute may lead to an inaccurate rate.

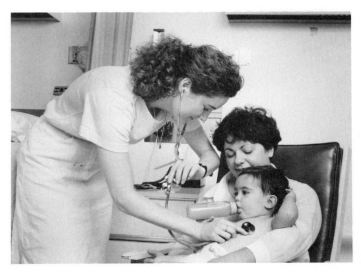

Figure 7-1.

Figure 7-2.

PROCEDURE	**RATIONALE/EXPECTED OUTCOME (EO)**

Older Child—Radial Rate

4. Place the first, second, or third finger along the child's radial artery and press gently against the radius. Rest the thumb in opposition to the fingers on the back of the child's wrist (Fig. 7-2).

The fingertips will feel pulsations. If the thumb is used for palpation, the caregiver's own pulse may be felt.

EO: The child's radial pulse will be counted accurately.

5. Apply only enough pressure so that the child's pulsating artery can be felt.

Too much pressure obliterates the pulse. Too little pressure will make the pulse imperceptible.

6. Count the arterial pulsations for 30 seconds and multiply by 2 to calculate the rate for one minute. If the pulse rate is abnormal, palpate the pulse for 1 full minute.

When the pulse is abnormal, longer counting and palpation are necessary to identify unusual characteristics of the pulse.

7. Assess rhythm, (regularity versus irregularity), amplitude (strength of pulsation), and elasticity of the vessel (distention of vessel) while counting the rate.

Irregularity in heart rate may disrupt the cardiac output. Amplitude indicates the quality of the heart's contraction. Elasticity of the blood vessel does not affect the pulse but does reflect the status of the vascular system.

8. Accurately record the following in the medical record:
   a. Rate
   b. Quality of the pulse
   c. Location felt
   d. Regularity or irregularity of rate
   e. Activity of child at time pulse is taken.

This provides accurate documentation.

EO: The child's medical record will reflect the pulse rate, how and where it was taken, and any irregularities.

9. Report any changes in pulse characteristics to the physician immediately.

Changes in pulse rate may indicate changes in the physical examination.

EO: The child will have his or her cardiac output monitored through changes in rate and quality and location of pulsations.

Patient/Family Education: Home Care Considerations

1. Inform the parents of the need to monitor their child's pulse.

2. Teach the parents how to count their child's pulse if they will need to record this measurement at home (for example, child on digoxin). Instruct them on what is an acceptable range and when to notify their physician.

References

Bates, B. (1991). *A guide to physical examination and history taking.* (5th Ed.). Philadelphia: J.B. Lippincott Company.

Birdsall, C. (1985). How do you interpret pulses? *American Journal of Nursing, 85*(7), 785–786.

Ferholt, J.D. (1980). *Clinical assessment of children.* Philadelphia: J.B. Lippincott Company.

Gift, A.G., & Soeken, K. L. (1988). Assessment of physiologic measurements. *Heart and Lung, 17*(2), 128–133.

Hollerbach, A.D., & Snead, N.V. (1990). Accuracy of radial pulse assessment by length of counting interval. *Heart and Lung, 19*(3), 258–264.

Stone, S. (1986). A new concept in routine vital sign measurement. *Nursing Management, 17*(2), 28–29.

Suddarth, D. (1991). *The Lippincott manual of nursing practice.* (5th ed). Philadelphia: J.B. Lippincott Company.

Taylor, C., Lillis, C., & LeMone, P. (1989). *Fundamentals of nursing: The art and science of nursing care.* Philadelphia: J.B. Lippincott Company.

Respirations

8

Definition/Purpose

Respiration is the act of breathing. Inhalation is the act of breathing in, and exhalation is the act of breathing out. The respiratory centers in the medulla oblongata and in the pons are sensitive to the amount of carbon dioxide in the blood and thus control respirations. The process of exchanging oxygen and carbon dioxide between the body cells and the blood is called internal or tissue respiration, while the process of exchanging oxygen and carbon dioxide between the lungs and blood is called external respiration.

Standard of Care

1. The respiratory rate is counted for 1 full minute during infancy and early childhood because of the irregularity of the respirations.
2. The respiratory rate is counted for 30 seconds in the older child.
3. Compare the respiratory rate to the normal range for age.
4. Respiratory rate counting is often accompanied by auscultation of the lungs.

Assessment

1. Assess level of consciousness and pertinent history and physical findings that would explain variations in the respiratory effort of the child.
   a. Assess type of respiration (Table 8-1).

Table 8-1. Types of Respiration

	Description	Possible Etiology
Eupnea	Normal, quiet effortless respirations	
Tachypnea	Rapid rate	Fever, infection, anxiety, shock, heart failure, alkalosis, certain poisonings
Bradypnea	Slow rate	Tumors of the brain, poisoning by opiates
Apnea	Cessation of respirations	May be normal in neonates if less than 15 seconds. If periods of apnea continue, the cause must be investigated.
Asphyxia	Prolonged interference with aeration of blood	Obstruction of airway, depression of respiratory center, lack of oxygen, lack of hemoglobin
Hyperpnea	Increased rate or depth of respirations, gasping in nature	In metabolic acidosis, hyperpnea is called Kussmaul respirations, as seen in diabetic patients.
Cheyne-Stokes respirations	Respirations increase in force and frequency to a certain point, then decrease until they cease altogether. After a brief period of apnea, the cycle is repeated.	

(continued)

Table 8-1. (*continued*)

	Description	Possible Etiology
Blot respirations	Irregular periods of apnea, alternating with periods in which four or five breaths of identical depth are taken.	Increased intracranial pressure

    b. Assess quality of respirations:

        Labored respirations: Note the time of onset, duration, predisposing factors, any retractions or nasal flaring.

        Noisy breathing: Describe sound heard to differentiate a snore of nasal obstruction from a stridor of laryngeal or tracheal origin.

        Wheezing: Prolonged and high-pitched sound. Timing suggests diagnosis.

            Inspiratory—upper airway obstruction (croup, epiglottitis)

            Expiratory—early phase of bronchospasm, intrathoracic obstruction (asthma)

            Inspiratory and expiratory—progressive bronchospasm or midtracheal lesion

        Paroxysmal: suggests impairment of diaphragm function.

  2. Assess the family's ability to count the respiratory rate and recognize deviations from the norm.

Nursing Diagnoses

The following is a list of possible diagnoses and could apply, depending on the child's age, clinical situation, and physical condition:

Fear

Potential for injury

Anxiety

Ineffective breathing pattern

Planning

When planning to take a child's respiratory rate, the following equipment is needed:

Watch with a sweep second hand or a digital watch with a "second" display

Stethoscope.

PROCEDURE	**RATIONALE/EXPECTED OUTCOME (EO)**
1. Approach the child in a quiet, non-threatening manner.	The child, if aware of the counting of respiratory rate, may alter the breathing rate. A true respiratory rate can be attained by unobtrusively observing the child while he or she is being held by a parent. *EO: The child and family will cooperate passively with this procedure.*
2. In the infant, note the rise and fall of the abdomen with each inspiration and expiration.	During infancy, the respiratory rate can be counted more easily by observing the abdomen because the respirations are abdominal in nature. *EO: The child's respiratory rate will be measured accurately.*
3. In the older child, note the rise and fall of the chest with each inspiration and expiration.	After infancy, the respiratory excursion is from the chest instead of the abdomen.

PROCEDURE	**RATIONALE/EXPECTED OUTCOME (EO)**
4. Using a watch with a sweep hand, count the number of respirations for 30–60 seconds, depending on the age of the child. Compare to the average rates at rest (Table 8-2).	A complete respiration consists of one inspiration and one expiration. Sufficient time is needed to observe the rate, depth, and quality of the respiratory effort.

Table 8-2. Average Respiratory Rates at Rest

Age	Rate (breaths/min)
Newborn	35
1–11 mo	30
2 yrs	25
4 yrs	23
6–8 yrs	20
10–12 yrs	19
14–18 yrs	16–18

5. Record the findings according to policy.	Notify the physician of any deviations.

Patient/Family Education: Home Care Considerations

1. Teach the family how to take an accurate respiratory rate:
   a. What constitutes a respiratory effort
   b. How long to count
   c. Normal versus abnormal rates.

2. Teach the family when to seek health care assistance:
   a. If the child is cyanotic
   b. If the respiratory rate is increased even when the temperature is within a normal range
   c. If the child has a persistent cough
   d. If the child is croupy or wheezing
   e. If the child grunts with each respiratory effort, suggesting respiratory distress syndrome (RDS), chest pain, pneumonia, or congestive heart failure
   f. If the child coughs out an increased amount of sputum or if sputum changes color from white to yellow or green, indicating an infection.

References

Lewis, L. (1984). *Fundamental skills in patient care.* Philadelphia: J.B. Lippincott Company.

Sconyers, S.M. (1987). The effect of body position on the respiratory rate of infants with tachypnea. *Journal of Perinatology,* Spring, 118–121.

Reeder, S., Martin, L. (1992). *Maternity nursing: Family, newborn and women's health care.* (17th ed.). Philadelphia: J.B. Lippincott Company.

Rosdahl, C. (1991). *Textbook of basic nursing.* (5th ed.). Philadelphia: J.B. Lippincott Company.

Blood Pressure

9

Definition/Purpose

The blood pressure is measured as part of the routine physical examination beginning at the age of 3 years and as part of the admission screening for all children admitted to the hospital. It is difficult to obtain an accurate blood pressure reading on an infant or small child, but the nurse is assisted by the correct equipment. The head of the stethoscope must not be too large for the size of the arm, and the cuff must be the appropriate width. A cuff that is too narrow will produce a falsely higher pressure, and a cuff that is too wide will produce a falsely lower pressure.

Systolic pressure is that point of the reading at which the sound is first heard. Diastolic pressure is that point of the reading at which the sound becomes muffled. The best approach calls for recording three numbers: the pressure at the appearance of the first consecutive sounds (systolic pressure), the pressure at the muffling of sounds, and the pressure at the cessation of sounds. The reading may be recorded as 112/76/62.

Methods for measuring the blood pressure include auscultation, palpation, Doppler, and flush. When deciding which method should be used either to measure or to estimate blood pressure, the decision must be based on the seriousness of the child's condition and how critical accuracy is in the blood pressure determination. For noncritically ill children, the auscultatory method is preferred over the other noninvasive methods. In critically ill children, the true blood pressure needs to be measured using intra-arterial devices.

Standard of Care

1. The cuff should be about the same width in proportion to the arm circumference as that used for the adult, or it should cover two thirds of the upper arm or thigh.

   Neonates—2.5 cm

   2 weeks to 1 year—5.0 cm

   1 to 13 years—6–10 cm

   Adult—10–13 cm.

2. Use the same size cuff for each reading.

3. The child should be at rest when the blood pressure is read. Excitement, discomfort, or distrust of the person taking the reading affects the blood pressure.

4. The blood pressure is measured before any anxiety-producing procedure is done.

Assessment

1. Assess the pertinent history and physical findings for the course of the illness, recent hospitalizations, plan of medical care, pain or discomfort, handicapping conditions, and physical or behavioral symptoms.

2. Assess developmental factors, including cognitive, social, and emotional level of functioning, coping mechanisms, daily routines, and the impact of the treatment on the child and family.

3. Assess the family's knowledge of the disease process, the need for compliance with a therapeutic regimen, and their ability to perform treatments and manage the child's health at home.

Nursing Diagnoses

The following is a list of possible diagnoses and could apply, depending on the child's age, clinical situation, and physical condition:

Anxiety

Pain

Altered tissue perfusion

Planning

When planning to measure a child's blood pressure, the following equipment must be gathered:

Stethoscope

Appropriate size cuff

Sphygmomanometer

Doppler blood pressure device

Elastic bandage.

PROCEDURE	**RATIONALE/EXPECTED OUTCOME (EO)**

Auscultation: Brachial Artery

1. Place the infant or child in a sitting or recumbent position. The forearm is supinated and slightly flexed.

Infants and small children may be quiet if the reading is taken while sitting in their parent's lap.

EO: The child's blood pressure will be measured using the most appropriate method taking into consideration the child's condition.

2. Remove all clothing from the upper extremity.

3. Demonstrate the equipment and procedure to the child using appropriate terminology. Check equipment for proper connection and function.

Excitement, discomfort, or distrust can affect the reading; thus, an explanation or demonstration of the equipment may allay fears.

EO: The child or family will express their concerns to the health care members and will in turn receive explanations to help decrease anxiety.

4. Place the correct size cuff around the upper arm, with the inflatable portion centered over the blood vessel. The lower edge should be 3 cm above the antecubital fossa (Fig. 9-1).

A cuff that is too narrow will cause a false elevated reading; a cuff that is too wide will result in a lower reading.

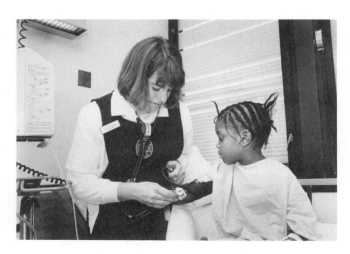

Figure 9-1.

PROCEDURE

5. Locate the artery by palpation at the antecubital fossa.

6. Close the air valve and rapidly inflate the cuff to 30 mm Hg above the expected systolic pressure or until the radial pulse disappears.

7. Place the stethoscope gently over the artery.

8. Slowly release the air valve, permitting the column of mercury to fall at a rate of 2–3 mm per heartbeat.

9. After readings have been made, the cuff is deflated and removed from the arm.

Auscultation: Popliteal Artery

10. Place the child in a prone position.

11. Place the correct size cuff around the thigh, with the lower edge about 2 cm above the popliteal space (Fig. 9-2).

RATIONALE/EXPECTED OUTCOME (EO)

If the head of the stethoscope presses too firmly, it will occlude the blood vessel.

With the gradual release of pressure on the blood vessel, the occluded lumen becomes patent. When the vessel opens, the pulse wave is transmitted to the periphery. At this point the vascular sounds become audible.

EO: The child's comfort will be restored with deflation and removal of the cuff from the limb.

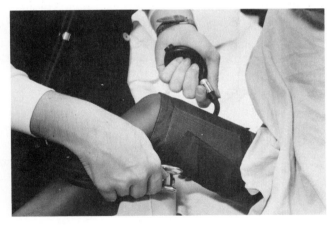

Figure 9-2.

12. The leg is slightly flexed, with the stethoscope over the popliteal artery. The subsequent procedure is identical to that for the brachial artery.

The systolic reading in infants is equal in the upper and lower extremities. After 1 year of age, the systolic reading will be higher in the arm than in the leg.

Palpation

13. The sphygmomanometer cuff is inflated until the radial pulse cannot be palpated.

14. With the palpating digit kept over the artery, pressure is released slowly until the pulse is felt. This endpoint is recorded as the systolic pressure.

The pressure of the cuff compresses the radial artery.

This point is 5–10 mm Hg lower than the systolic pressure measured by auscultation.

Doppler

15. Obtain the monitor, dual air hose, and the correct size cuff (Fig. 9-3).

16. Place the monitor on a firm, immobile surface.

This method is increasingly used for estimating blood pressure in children.

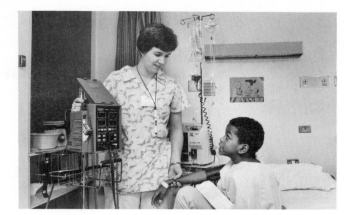

Figure 9-3.

PROCEDURE

17. Plug in the monitor and connect the dual air hose to the back of the monitor.

18. Screw the pressure cuff's tubing into the other ends of the air hose.

19. Wrap the correct size cuff around the child's limb.

20. Turn the power switch to the ON position. (Consult the manufacturer's instructions on your specific monitor regarding alarm limits and frequency of readings, etc.) Record the reading.

Flush. (*should be used in newborns or small infants whose pressure is difficult or impossible to obtain by other techniques*)

21. Place the child in a recumbent position.

22. Apply the cuff snugly to the distal forearm with the outer edge at the wrist. If lower extremity pressure is to be determined, the cuff is applied to the distal leg with the outer edge at the ankle.

23. Wrap the extremity distal to the cuff with an elastic bandage.

24. Inflate the cuff to 150–200 mm Hg and remove the elastic bandage.

25. Lower the cuff pressure by 5 mm Hg and leave at that level for 3–4 seconds. Repeat the procedure until flushing is observed in the blanched limb.

26. Repeat the procedure at least twice to confirm the reading.

RATIONALE/EXPECTED OUTCOME (EO)

About 20 seconds after the power is turned on, the cuff will inflate. For the first inflation the cuff is inflated to 160 mm Hg. It deflates in increments of 5–6 mm Hg. The cuff will completely deflate, and the systolic, mean arterial pressure, and heart rate will read out on the display.

Each subsequent inflation will be 35 mm Hg above the previous systolic reading.

Wrapping begins at the fingers or toes and progresses to the edge of the cuff. This forces the blood out of the extremity.

The hand or foot should appear pale in color and exsanguinated.

Flushing is a sudden pink color below the cuff edge, spreading distally. The monometer reading at this point is taken as the mean arterial blood pressure.

EO: The child's tissue perfusion will return to normal after the reading.

PROCEDURE

27. Upon concluding the blood pressure determination, record the following:
    a. Reading obtained
    b. Extremity used
    c. Type of method used
    d. Size of cuff used
    e. Person notified if reading is of concern.

RATIONALE/EXPECTED OUTCOME (EO)

For consistency of readings, all persons measuring a child's blood pressure need to be aware of the recorded information. Comparisons must be based on values obtained in similar ways (same extremity, same size cuff, etc.) (Tables 9-1, 9-2).

Table 9-1. Normal Blood Pressure Ranges

Age	Systolic (mm Hg)	Diastolic (mm Hg)
Newborn—12 hr (less than 1000 gm)	39–59	16–36
Newborn—12 hr (3000 gm)	50–70	24–45
Newborn—96 hr (3000 gm)	60–90	20–60
Infant	74–100	50–70
Toddler	80–112	50–80
Preschooler	82–110	50–78
School–age	84–120	54–80
Adolescent	94–140	62–88

Table 9-2. Mean Blood Pressure at Wrist and Ankle Using Flush Technique

Age	Wrist Range	Ankle Range
1–30 days	22–66	20–58
1–3 months	48–90	38–96
4–6 months	42–100	40–104
7–9 months	52–96	50–96
10–12 months	62–94	102

Patient/Family Education: Home Care Considerations

1. Assist parents with efforts toward planning for adaptation required by a child's changing health status.

2. Encourage the family to write down questions and concerns to discuss with health team members.

3. Teach parents to monitor their child's blood pressure at home, if necessary.

References

——— (1988). Taking accurate blood pressure readings. *Nursing, 18,* 32J, 32N.

Lynch, T.M. (1987). Invasive and non-invasive pressure monitoring in neonates. *Journal of Perinatal Neonatal Nursing, 1,* 58–71.

Rebenson-Piano, M., & Holm, K. (1988). Education of automatic blood pressure devices for clinical practice. *Dimensions of Critical Care Nursing, 7,* 228–235.

Weismann, D. (1988). Systolic or diastolic blood pressure significance. *Pediatrics, 82*(1), 112–114.

Height and Weight

10

Definition/Purpose

Physical growth measurements of children are performed regularly and provide valuable information in the total evaluation of children. Height (length) and weight are standard measurements that are frequently taken in health care agencies.

The median length of newborns in the United States is 49.9 cm (19¾ inches) for girls and 50.5 cm (20 inches) for boys. The first growth spurt takes place between birth and 1 year of age. During the first 6 months, length increases average 2.5 cm (1 inch), and by one year the increase in length is 50% of the birth length. Between the first and second year, the average increase in height is 10–12 cm (4–5 inches). After 2 years of age, the rate of growth slows until the second growth spurt, which occurs during adolescence.

The median birth weight is 3.23 kg (7 lbs) for Caucasian girls and 3.27 kg (7¼ lbs) for Caucasian boys. The weights of newborn Black, Asian, and Native American babies are lower. During the first few days of life, newborns usually lose about 10% of their birth weight due to fluid loss, but then steadily gain weight. By 6 months of age the birth weight has doubled; by 12 months it has tripled, and by 2 years it has quadrupled.

Many factors influence physical growth:

- Age
- Gestation (premature versus full-term birth)
- Sex
- Race
- Heredity
- Nutrition
- Illness
- Medical care
- Physical and emotional environments.

Growth charts give values for five centiles for stature and weight for each sex at two age intervals. The centile rank for a given child indicates the relative position that a child holds in a series of 100 children of the same age. Special consideration needs to be taken when plotting the growth of certain children, such as a preterm baby, a child with Down's syndrome, or a child with severe heart disease. For example, a girl with heart disease is expected to be about 1 cm smaller and 1 kg lighter, and a boy with heart disease 2 cm smaller and 1–2 kg lighter, than a child without heart disease. A child with Down's syndrome is expected to be smaller in linear growth but over the 95th percentile in weight.

Standard of Care

1. Infants must be weighed completely nude. The reference weight charts for infants from birth to 36 months old are compiled from nude weights.

2. The weight charts for the group from 3 to 18 years old include standardized examination clothing weighing 0.05 kg at 3 years to 0.3 kg from 6–18 years. Shoes should never be worn.

3. Weigh the child at the same time each day, usually before breakfast or feeding.

4. Use the same measuring device, if possible, for daily measures. Scales may need frequent calibration for accuracy.

5. Measurements must be compared to norms obtained in an identical manner (recumbent length is always greater than standing height). Plot values on growth chart.

Assessment

1. Assess prenatal history, birth, and neonatal course (weight at birth and discharge), past medical problems, height and weight of other family members, illnesses, nutritional intake, and developmental milestones.

2. Assess physical findings, including cardiac, respiratory, gastrointestinal, neurologic, and genitourinary status.

3. Assess developmental factors, including age when major milestones were achieved and the child's development compared to other siblings.

Nursing Diagnoses

The following is a list of possible diagnoses and could apply, depending on the child's age, clinical situation, and physical condition:

Fear

High risk for injury

Hypothermia

Planning

To weigh a child and measure his or her length, the following equipment must be available:

Scale

    Standing (platform)

    Infant

    Bed

Protector for the scale

Measuring boards—One for standing height and one for recumbent length

Growth charts.

PROCEDURE	**RATIONALE/EXPECTED OUTCOME (EO)**
1. Weigh the child.	
Infant Scale	
a. Balance scale with clean sheet of paper on bed of scale.	The protector sheet prevents the transfer of microorganisms from the scale.
b. Undress infant.	*EO: The child will be weighed accurately.*
c. Place infant on scale. Protect the infant from cold stress by increasing the temperature of the room before weighing. Place a hand over the body while balancing the weight on the scale.	*EO: The child will be protected from cold stress during the weighing procedure.* *EO: The child will be weighed without sustaining an injury.*

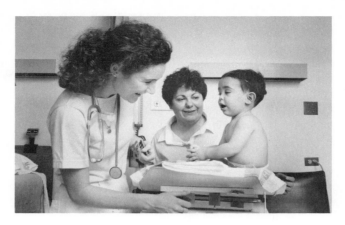

Figure 10-1.

PROCEDURE

The older infant may be weighed in a sitting position (Fig. 10-1).

d. Read weight, remove child from scale, and re-dress infant. Document weight.

Platform Scale

a. Place the scale next to the child's bed
b. Balance scale with protector sheet on footstand.
c. Assist the child onto the scale.
d. Make sure the child is not leaning on the bed or holding onto a piece of furniture. Many scales have a special handle that the child can hold onto.
e. Have child stand on the center of the platform (Fig. 10-2).
f. Read weight, assist child off scale, and document weight.

RATIONALE/EXPECTED OUTCOME (EO)

Standing in the center is necessary for accurate measurement and for safety.

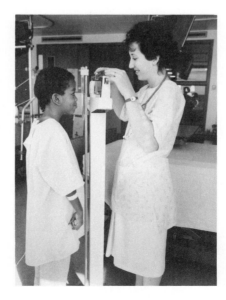

Figure 10-2.

PROCEDURE   **RATIONALE/EXPECTED OUTCOME (EO)**

Bed Scale

    a. Adjust the scale stretcher to a horizontal position and lock it in place.

    b. Balance scale with a protective cover over the stretcher.

    c. Turn the child to a lateral position, with the back toward the scale.

    d. Roll the base of the scale under the bed.

    e. Lock wheels.

    f. Lower the stretcher onto the bed.

    g. Roll child onto the stretcher.

    h. Move the weighing arms over the child and attach to stretcher.

    i. Pump the handle to raise the child 2 inches above the bed (Fig. 10-3).

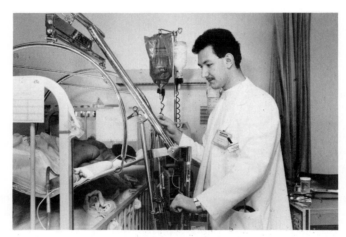

Figure 10-3.

    j. Ensure that the stretcher is not touching any part of the bed.

    k. Press the button to display the weight.

    l. Lower the child to the bed by using the pump handle.

    m. Detach the stretcher from the arms.

    n. Roll the child off the stretcher and document weight.

2. Measure the child's height.

Touching any equipment will affect the reading of the weight.

Standing

    a. Have the child take off his or her shoes.

    b. Have the child stand against a wall on which there is a ruler.

    c. The child's occiput, upper back, buttocks, and heels should touch the wall.

    d. A flat object is placed atop the head and against the ruler to obtain an accurate measurement. (The older child may stand on a scale.)

Height is measured from a standing position in children 3 years of age and older.

EO: The child's height will be measured accurately.

The child should look straight ahead, with the line of vision parallel to the floor.

PROCEDURE	RATIONALE/EXPECTED OUTCOME (EO)

Recumbent

a. Place the infant on a firm table.

b. Place the feet flat against a fixed upright surface at the zero mark of the ruler and measure from that point to the vertex against which a flat movable surface is placed.

c. Extend the infant's body fully by flattening the knees and maintaining the head in a midline position (Fig. 10-4).

Length is measured until the child can stand steadily.

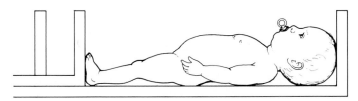

Figure 10-4.

d. A crown–rump position is measured the same as the recumbent length, except that the extremities are lifted up into the air and the footboard is pressed firmly against the buttocks while the sacrum is kept against the baseboard (Fig. 10-5).

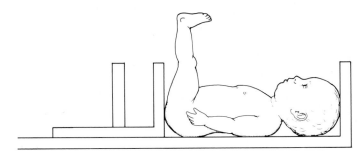

Figure 10-5.

Record measurements. Plot on growth charts.

Patient/Family Education: Home Care Considerations

1. Inform the parents of the child's measurements and where the child falls on the growth curve compared with other children of the same age.

2. Explain to the family the need to obtain weight measurements at the same time each day.

References

Arton, J. (1988). See how they grow . . . rate of growth of school children. *Nursing Times, 84*(14), 6–12, 36–38.

Burke, S.O., Roberts, C.A., & Maloney, R. (1988). Infant and child weights: Reliability and validity of scales. *Comprehensive Pediatric Nursing, 11*(4), 241–249.

Cronk, C., Crocker, A.C., & Pueschel, S. (1988). Growth charts for children with Downs syndrome: 1 month to 18 years of age. *Pediatric, 81*(1), 102–109.

Kavanaugh, K., Meier, P.P., & Engstrom, J.L. (1989). Reliability of weighing procedures for preterm infants. *Nursing Research, 85*(1), 178–179.

Head Circumference: Occipital-Frontal Circumference (OFC)

11

Definition/Purpose

The circumference of the head is a valuable tool in assessing the child's physical development as well as certain neurologic disorders. Subdural effusions and obstructive hydrocephalus can develop after meningitis, head trauma, or repair of meningomyelocele, and may be first detected by a rapidly increasing head circumference. On the other hand, a low OFC may indicate microcephaly.

Standard of Care

1. Measure the head circumference with a paper or flexible metal tape. Cloth tapes tend to stretch over time.
2. All infants should have their head circumference measured on admission to the hospital and on each well-child visit to the pediatrician. Head circumference should be plotted on a chart, along with the child's height and weight. OFC is usually measured up to 1–2 years of age.
3. Postoperative care of the infant neurosurgical patient should include a head circumference measurement on return from surgery and once during each shift thereafter. This may not be possible if a large head dressing is in place.
4. An infant being treated for meningitis should have a measurement of head circumference upon admission and one measurement every 8 hours thereafter.

Assessment

1. Assess the pertinent history and physical findings for symptoms leading to a neurologic disorder (indicated by recent signs of increased intracranial pressure or infection), general appearance, bulging fontanelle, poor feeding, and vomiting.
2. Assess the child's developmental factors, coping mechanisms, and previous hospital experience, and the family's knowledge of the illness and their willingness to learn.

Nursing Diagnoses

The following is a list of possible diagnoses and could apply, depending on the child's age, clinical situation, and physical condition:

Altered growth and development

High risk for injury

Planning

In planning to measure head circumference of an infant, the following equipment is needed:

Paper or flexible tape measure

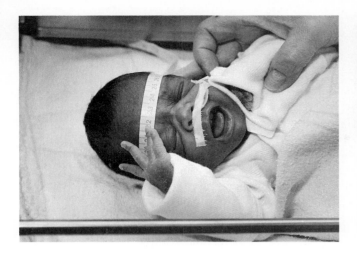

Figure 11-1.

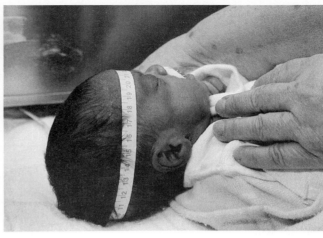

Figure 11-2.

Interventions

PROCEDURE	**RATIONALE/EXPECTED OUTCOME (EO)**
1. Gather the necessary equipment.	
2. Explain to the family the importance of the head circumference measurement.	*EO: The family will understand the importance of the head circumference measurement.*
3. The infant's head must be held completely still during the measurement.	A slight movement may displace the tape.
4. The tape is placed over the most prominent part of the occiput and around the forehead just above the supraorbital ridges.	*EO: The child's head circumference will be accurately measured.*
5. The tape is tightened snugly and the measurement taken over the forehead (Figs. 11-1 and 11-2).	Head circumference reflects intracranial volume; thus, it can be used to identify abnormal brain development.
6. Determine the infant's current developmental level based on norms (Tables 11-1 and 11-2).	*EO: The infant's development will be assessed using head circumference as one measurement.*

Table 11-1. Head Circumference Norms for Girls (in cm)

	Percentiles					
Age	3	25	50	75	90	97
Birth	32.5	33.9	34.7	35.4	36	36.6
3 months	37.9	39.2	40	40.8	41.7	42.3
6 months	40.9	42	42.8	43	44.5	45.4
9 months	42.6	43.8	44.6	45.4	46.3	47.2
12 months	43.6	45	45.8	46.7	47.7	48.4
15 months	44.3	45.6	46.5	47.4	48.4	49.1
18 months	44.9	46.2	47.1	48	49	49.8
2 years	45.8	47.2	48.1	49.1	50.1	50.9
3 years	46.8	48.4	49.3	50.3	51.1	52

Table 11-2. Head Circumference Norms for Boys (in cm)

	Percentiles					
Age	3	25	50	75	90	97
Birth	33	34.4	35.3	36.2	37	37.5
3 months	38.7	40	40.9	41.5	42.1	43.2
6 months	42.1	43.3	43.9	44.8	45.4	45.9

(continued)

Table 11-2. (*continued*)

Age	Percentiles					
	3	25	50	75	90	97
9 months	43.8	45.1	46	46.5	47.1	47.8
12 months	44.9	46.5	47.3	47.8	48.4	48.9
15 months	45.6	47.1	48	48.5	49.2	49.8
18 months	46.2	47.7	48.7	49.2	49.9	50.6
2 years	47	48.2	49.7	50.2	51	51.7
3 years	47.9	49.6	50.4	51.3	51.9	52.7

PROCEDURE	**RATIONALE/EXPECTED OUTCOME (EO)**
7. Plot head circumference on graphic sheet to determine what percentile the head size is in relation to age, height, and weight.	This will determine if the head circumference is above, below, or at the percentile norm.

Patient/Family Education: Home Care Considerations

1. Assist parents to individualize growth and development expectations for the child.
2. If pertinent, teach the parents the signs of increased intracranial pressure and when to seek medical attention.
3. Clarify and reinforce the information given to the parents by other health team members.

References

Ifft, D.L., Engstrom, J.L., Meier, P.P., et al (1989). Reliability of head circumference measurements for pre-term infants. *Neonatal Network, 8*(3), 41–46.

Reeder, S., Martin, L. (1992). *Materntiy nursing: Family, newborn and women's health care.* (17th ed.). Philadelphia: J.B. Lippincott Company.

Preoperative and Postoperative Care

12

Definition/Purpose

Preparation of the child and family for surgery must be designed after consideration of the child's cognitive and social levels of development and the family's perception of the child's health. During the preoperative period, the nurse, parent, and child have an opportunity to become acquainted and to establish a trusting relationship. When the nurse has assessed the level of knowledge and anxiety of the child and parents and their coping mechanisms, preoperative teaching can be tailored to their specific needs and preoperative care can be provided.

The postoperative responsibilities of the nurse include meeting the physical and psychologic needs of the child. The goal postoperatively is safe emergence of the child from anesthesia and an uneventful postoperative course. Children may need help in coping with a change in body image and must be encouraged to participate in their own care. Discharge planning after surgery should include both the child and the parents. Any limitations in activity are discussed, and appointments for follow-up care are given, and their importance is emphasized.

Standard of Care

1. A preoperative checklist should be placed on the front of the child's chart. As the required nursing responsibilities are carried out, each item on the list is checked off and dated.

Assessment

1. Assess the pertinent history and physical findings in relation to the reason for surgery, the child's response to the hospitalization, recent exposure to illness (especially upper respiratory infection and communicable diseases), any previous surgical procedures, vital signs, level of consciousness, level of hydration, weight, respiratory status, blood counts, etc.
2. Assess the child's developmental level and coping mechanisms, and the family's routine and habits.
3. Assess the child's and family's knowledge of the planned surgical procedure, the potential complications, and the convalescent period.

Nursing Diagnoses

The following is a list of possible diagnoses and could apply, depending on the child's age, clinical situation, and physical condition:

Anxiety

Fear

Pain

Ineffective breathing pattern

High risk for infection

Altered nutrition, less than body requirements

Fluid volume deficit

Fluid volume excess

Impaired skin integrity

Perceived constipation

Impaired verbal communication

Planning

When beginning to assess a child pre- or postoperatively, the following equipment is needed:

Flashlight

Stethoscope

Thermometer

Chem sticks for blood and urine testing

Watch with second hand

Intake/Output sheet

Preoperative teaching checklist

Depending on the complexity of the case, more or different equipment may be needed.

Interventions

PROCEDURE	**RATIONALE/EXPECTED OUTCOME (EO)**
Preoperative	
1. Orient the child and family to the nursing unit (Fig. 12-1).	
2. Discuss the surgical procedure with the child and parents, evaluating their understanding.	The child and family may not have an adequate understanding of hospital procedures or the preparation needed before a surgical intervention.
	EO: The family/child will demonstrate an understanding of the disease process, purpose of hospitalization, goals and complications of surgery, and the planned postoperative management.

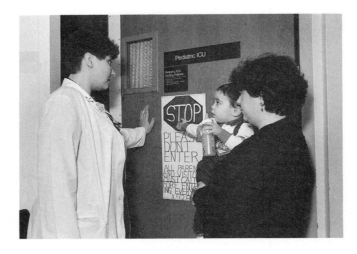

Figure 12-1.

PROCEDURE

3. Plan a preoperative teaching approach based on the child's prior preparation, level of comprehension, and previous experiences.

   a. Children under the age of 2 years usually do not have the ability to grasp the details of surgery but need reassurance that their parents will be waiting for them after the surgery and that they will return to home and friends soon. Allow the child to play with equipment used in the treatment. Let the child use a stethoscope, reflex hammer, tongue blade, and dolls with appropriate attachments for the anticipated procedure. Be truthful about pain.

   b. Plan structured sessions for the child aged 2–7 years using dolls and other play equipment to teach him or her about the planned treatment and to clarify his or her misconceptions (Fig. 12-2). This age group is capable of understanding the inside of the body, and should be encouraged to ask questions. Drawing on a body outline can help determine the child's understanding of the illness.

   c. Seven- to 13-year-olds are science-oriented. They may feel a doll is immature. This age group has the ability to reason, to make generalizations, and to understand the concept of time. Be alert, however, to misconceptions about the illness.

RATIONALE/EXPECTED OUTCOME (EO)

EO: The child and family will be provided with information to lessen anxiety.

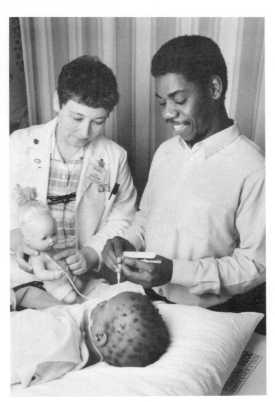

Figure 12-2.

PROCEDURE

RATIONALE/EXPECTED OUTCOME (EO)

    d. The adolescent can incorporate medical terminology into his or her vocabulary. This age group is preoccupied with physical changes and with not looking different from their peers. They want to be in control of their care but may be embarrassed to ask questions.

    e. Describe the postoperative experience according to the child's need to know and readiness to learn. Do not overwhelm the child with threatening details or too much information at one time. Provide small amounts of information at a time, with frequent reinforcement.

    f. Give the younger child explanations the evening before surgery; the older child, who has a more complicated concept of time, may be prepared gradually at several different sessions.

    g. Teach the child those things that can be done to hasten recovery, such as deep breathing, coughing, and turning.

EO: Demonstration of postoperative procedures promotes cooperation by the child and the family.

4. Discuss the activity schedule with the child and family:
   a. Time of surgery
   b. Need for NPO orders
   c. Approximate length of surgery
   d. Anticipated admission to a critical care unit
   e. Anticipated postoperative and posthospitalization activity

5. Discuss preoperative discomfort such as medications and treatments. Discuss postoperative discomfort and the relief available with medication.

6. Provide opportunity for child and parent to express concerns.

EO: The child and parents will verbalize a minimal amount of anxiety.

7. Record specific teaching information so other team members can reinforce the same information.

8. Monitor temperature, pulse, respirations, and blood pressure. Any abnormal vital signs need to be reported to the physician.

9. Give nothing by mouth for the period prescribed prior to surgery.

10. Make certain that all preoperative procedures have been completed, such as enemas, baths, irrigations, and preoperative medications.

11. Bathe the child and give or help with mouth care.

12. Dress the child in a clean hospital gown.

13. Observe for loose teeth, dental appliances, or contact lenses. Remove jewelry. Remove nail polish.

14. Ensure that a consent form for the surgical procedure and anesthesia has been correctly signed and witnessed.

A signed informed consent will help protect the hospital and personnel from legal action.

15. Ensure that all laboratory reports, radiology reports, and the results of any other tests are included in the chart.

These reports may show signs of infection, bleeding tendencies, anemia, or other results that would contraindicate surgery.

PROCEDURE	**RATIONALE/EXPECTED OUTCOME (EO)**

16. Make certain that the child's identification and allergy wristband is securely attached.

> This will prevent faulty identification of the child in the operating room.

17. Give preoperative medications if ordered by physician.

18. Have a familiar person accompany the child to the operating room. Never leave the child unattended during transport or in the operating area. Allow the parent to carry the child. If the child is in a crib or cart, ensure that the side rails are up and secure. Allow the child to take a familiar object (a blanket or toy) to the operating room.

> Orientation of the child by a familiar person tends to provide a sense of security in a strange situation.

Postoperative

19. Restraint or constant attention may be necessary to prevent dislodging of IV lines, dressings, drains, or chest tubes.

> When emerging from anesthesia, children become restless or experience emergence excitement.

20. Place oxygen and suction near the bed and use as necessary or as ordered.

> *EO: The child demonstrates no pulmonary complications.*

21. Vital signs and blood pressure are taken as often as necessary, depending on the child's condition: Usually every 15 minutes for 1 hour; every 30 minutes for the next hour; then hourly until stable.

> Lowered temperature, increased pulse rate, or decreased blood pressure may indicate shock.

22. Keep child warm. Note skin color when vital signs are taken.

> Pale, cool, clammy skin indicates shock. Flushing, increased pulse rate, drying of the mouth, and reduced bronchial secretions are normal actions of atropine.

23. Assess presence and character of breath sounds, equal chest excursions, and signs of respiratory distress (retractions, grunting, nasal flaring) with vital signs.

> Tracheal intubation may cause laryngeal edema, resulting in respiratory distress. Depressed respirations may be caused by drugs used during surgery.
>
> *EO: The child breathes in a normal respiratory pattern, and has equal chest expansion and no retractions.*

24. Monitor arterial blood gases (ABGs) as ordered for indications of hypoxia. Place pulse oximeter on child and monitor.

25. Medicate for pain as necessary to ensure adequate tidal volume.

> Postoperative pain and decreased energy levels may cause the child to hypoventilate.

26. Have child take a deep breath, turn, and cough. Splint operative site (chest or abdomen) with pillow or hand before doing these procedures to minimize discomfort.

27. Monitor vital signs every 4 hours and as necessary once stable. Watch for systemic indications of infection (elevated temperature, decreased blood pressure, increased pulse, and respiration).

> *EO: The child will have a postoperative course uncomplicated by wound or skin infection.*

28. Maintain aseptic technique when handling IV lines, suctioning, or changing dressings.

29. Inspect surgical wound, IV lines, chest tube, or other tube sites for redness, swelling, or drainage every 1–2 hours. Encircle drainage on the dressing with a pen and time. Reinforce dressings if bleeding is present. Keep dressing dry—diaper child below incision site if possible.

> The surgical wound as well as the placement of lines and tubes all present potential sources of infection.

PROCEDURE

30. Provide vascular catheter insertion site care—maintain an occlusive dressing; change dressings as ordered.

31. Assess the child's neurologic function as soon as possible after return from surgery (Fig. 12-3)
    a. Check pupil size and response to light. Pupil dilation is normal if receiving sympathomimetic agents (dopamine) or vagolytic agents (atropine).
    b. Check movement and strength of all extremities.
    c. Note muscle tone and withdrawal.
    d. Note level of orientation.

RATIONALE/EXPECTED OUTCOME (EO)

The child may develop neurologic impairment as a result of hypoxia, acidosis, poor systemic perfusion, thromboembolism, or electrolyte imbalance.

EO: The child will demonstrate appropriate movement of extremities, appropriate response to questions, and appropriate pupil response.

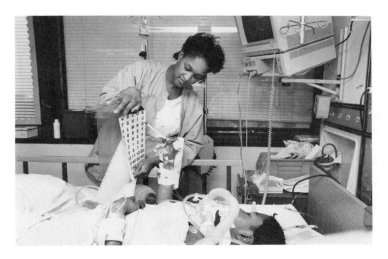

Figure 12-3.

32. Monitor for signs of increased cranial pressure:
    a. Irritability or lethargy
    b. Pupil dilation or constriction and decreased response to light
    c. Bradycardia
    d. Changes in respiratory pattern
    e. Increased systolic blood pressure with widening pulse pressure
    f. Fullness of fontanelle
    (See Unit 8 for detailed information on ICP.)

33. Calculate maintenance caloric and fluid requirements (Tables 12-1 and 12-2).

EO: The child will maintain normal intracranial pressure.

If the child is unable to take oral maintenance calories within 24–48 hours after surgery, alternative methods of alimentation need to be discussed.

EO: The child will maintain adequate nutrition through oral, tube, or parenteral routes.

Table 12-1. Calorie Requirements in Children

Age	Daily Requirements
High risk neonate	120–150 calories/kg
Normal neonate	100–120 calories/kg
1–2 years	90–100 calories/kg
2–6 years	80–90 calories/kg
7–9 years	70–80 calories/kg

(continued)

Table 12-1. *(continued)*

Age	Daily Requirements
10–12 years	50–60 calories/kg

Note: Ill children (those with fever or pain, or who have undergone surgery) may require extra calories above the maintenance value, and comatose or physically impaired children may require fewer calories because of a lack of exercise.

(From Hazinski, M. (1984). *Nursing care of the critically ill child.* St. Louis: C.V. Mosby Company, with permission).

Table 12-2. Fluid Requirements for Children

Child's Weight	Kilogram Body Weight Formula
Newborns (0–72 hours)	60–100 ml/kg
0–10 kg	100 mL/kg (may increase up to 150 mL/kg if renal or cardiac function adequate)
11–20 kg	1000 mL for first 10 kg, plus 50 mL/kg for each kg over 10 kg
21–30 kg	1500 mL for the first 20 kg, plus 20 mL/kg for each kg over 20 kg

(From Hazinski, M. (1984). *Nursing care of the critically ill child.* St. Louis: C.V. Mosby Company, with permission).

PROCEDURE

34. Assess bowel sounds, bowel patterns, and frequency of bowel movements. Encourage clear fluids when bowel sounds return, and progress as tolerated if vomiting and nausea are absent. Provide opportunities for activity. Give laxatives or enemas if nursing strategies are not effective.

35. Monitor serum electrolyte balance. Report abnormalities to the physician. The physician may order the following medications:
    - If *metabolic acidosis*, sodium bicarbonate may be given (1–4 m Eq/kg/dose Max. 8 m Eq/kg/24 hrs)
    - If *hypoglycemia*, glucose may be given (D50 0.5–1.0 mL/kg/dose; D25 1–2 mL/kg/dose)
    - If *hypocalcemia*, calcium may be given (10% calcium chloride, 20–50 mg/kg; 10% calcium gluconate, 100–200 mg/kg)
    - If *hypokalemia*, potassium chloride may be given (IV: 3 m Eq/kg/24 hr; oral: 2–4 m Eq/kg/24 hr)
    - If *hyperkalemia*, give 1 gm resin of sodium polystyrene sulfonate/kg/rectal dose given in 4 divided doses
    Regular insulin 0.2 u/kg with 200–400 mg/kg glucose (D25 W) IV.

36. Measure the child's fluid output. Output includes urine and nasogastric, ileostomy, colostomy, and chest tube drainage.

37. Monitor for evidence of urinary tract infection, including burning sensation with urination, hematuria, and cloudy or odorous urine.

RATIONALE/EXPECTED OUTCOME (EO)

Inadequate activity, decreased and lack of bowel peristalsis lead to constipation.

EO: The child will maintain normal bowel patterns.

Children may develop postoperative electrolyte imbalances related to the use of diuretics, stress response, and fluid and blood administration.

EO: The child will demonstrate normal serum electrolytes. The child will not demonstrate signs or complications of electrolyte imbalance.

Output should range from 0.5–1.0 mL/kg/hr in the child. Urine volume >2 mL/kg/hr and a specific gravity <1.010 suggest hydration in the neonate.

EO: The child will demonstrate a urine output of 0.5–2.0 mL/kg/hr when fluid intake is adequate.

PROCEDURE	RATIONALE/EXPECTED OUTCOME (EO)
38. Test urine for the presence of blood and protein. Specific gravity should be measured every 4 hours.	If urine is positive for blood and is rusty in color, spin a urine sample in a centrifuge: —If blood precipitates, then blood is due to trauma. —If urine remains rusty, then RBC fragments are a result of intravascular hemolysis. *EO: The child will maintain a normal serum BUN and creatinine.*

Patient/Family Education: Home Care Considerations

1. Provide the child and parent with information necessary to provide care at home:
   a. Techniques for special treatments (dressing changes, postural drainage)
   b. Dose, route, administration techniques, effects and side effects of medications
   c. Times and intervals of follow-up appointments
   d. Indications for contacting the physician.

2. Initiate referrals to support services:
   a. Physical or occupational therapy
   b. Social services
   c. Home nursing care
   d. Equipment vendors.

References

Durst, L.M. (1990). Preoperative teaching videotape: The effect on children's behavior. *AORN J, 52*(3), 576–579, 581–582, 584.

Idriss, F.S. (1982). *In* Postoperative management of the pediatric surgical patient. *Critical care for surgical patients.* New York: Macmillan Publishing Co., Inc.

Luegenbiehl, D.L., Brophy, G.H., Artigue, G.S., et al. (1990). Standardized assessment of blood loss. *Maternal Child Nursing, 15*(4), 241–244.

Moushey, R., Siracore, M.L., & Diomede, B. (1988). A perioperative teaching program: A collaborative process for children and their families. *Journal of Pediatric Nursing, 3*(1), 40–45.

Smallwood, S.B. (1988). Preparing children for surgery: Learning through play. *AORN J, 47*(1), 177–178, 180–181, 183.

Spicher, C.M., & Yund, C. (1989). Effects of preadmission preparation on compliance with home care instructions. *Journal of Pediatric Nursing, 4*(4), 255–262.

Pain Assessment

13

Definition/Purpose

As defined by the International Association for the Study of Pain in 1979, "Pain is an unpleasant sensory and emotional experience associated with actual or potential tissue damage or described in terms of such damage." The first implication of this definition is that pain is both a sensory and an emotional experience which may or may not bear a relationship to the sensation or injury that produced it, but may be altered by emotional factors. Secondly, pain is a subjective phenomenon. Subjective experiences are best evaluated by self-report, which presents a difficulty for preverbal children. Thirdly, this definition states that if pain is reported even in the absence of tissue damage, such an experience should be accepted as pain.

The difficulty of obtaining an objective, accurate measure of pain in pediatric patients is evident by the number of methods currently available. Most are not acceptable to all age groups and none are universally acceptable. Factors affecting pain assessment in children include:

1. Limited vocabulary
2. Few previous experiences with pain
3. Limited ability to understand pain-related questions and provide verbal self-report
4. Limited behavioral expressions in young children
5. Lack of research on pain-related physiology and behavior in pediatric patients.

Cognitive Measure of Pain

Cognitive or self-reported measures of pain are important because they attempt to evaluate the intensity and the nature of the experience felt by the child. This method is limited in infants and toddlers, who are nonverbal, and in older children, who will respond with a biased answer depending on who is asking the question. Simple scales (see Appendix 5) designed for use with children (painful faces, color of pain, hurt thermometer) quantitate the intensity of pain but do not assess the other characteristics of the pain experience. Most of these scales can be applied to children above the age of 7. They are not applicable to infants or sedated, retarded, or nonverbal children.

Behavioral Measures of Pain

Changes in behavior associated with painful circumstances can be labeled by some as stress or distress rather than pain. Behavioral changes associated with pain may be classified therefore as simple motor responses, facial expressions, crying, and complex behavioral changes. These measures are applicable to any age, can be observed in an unobtrusive fashion, and are reproducible. These responses, however, may have different subjective contents for different children, and many behaviors, such as crying, reflect pain in certain situations and anxiety or fear in others.

Physiologic Measures of Pain

Significant changes in cardiovascular parameters, transcutaneous oxygen, and palmar sweating have been noted in infants and children undergoing painful procedures. Heart rate and blood pressure are markedly increased during and after painful procedures. Some researchers may say that these changes are related to the duration of the stimulus and the individual temperament of the child; however, the heart rate and blood pressure have been shown to decrease with the administration of local anesthesia. Large fluctuations of the transcutaneous PO_2 occur during surgical procedures, and such changes can be prevented by giving local anesthesia. Palmar sweating has also been validated as a physiologic measure of the emotional state of term neonates and is related to the state of arousal and crying.

Hormonal and metabolic changes have been measured in infants and children undergoing surgery. Plasma renin activity was increased after painful procedures and returned to basal levels in 60 minutes.

It becomes apparent that there is no single standard for assessing pain. Clinicians make use of all three types of data. Because pain is amplified by stress, fear, and anxiety, efforts are directed toward relaxation and reduction of anxiety as well as the use of a variety of drugs.

Standard of Care

1. Assess the child at least every 3 hours for the degree of pain experienced. When administering pain medications, assess the degree of pain before and at least one hour after administration of the medication.

2. If the child is 7 years or older, use a numerical scale with 0 being no pain and 3 being the most severe pain; if the child is younger than 7 years, use colors:

   0 = Yellow = No pain

   1 = Blue   = Small amount of pain/discomfort

   2 = Orange = Moderate amount of pain/discomfort

   3 = Red   = Severe amount of pain/discomfort

   Younger children may use a face scale or full/empty glass scale (see Appendix 5).

3. Document on a flow sheet the child's perception of the degree of pain experienced.

4. Document your perception of the degree of pain experienced by the child on a flow sheet.

5. Assess and document the child's activity when experiencing pain and with pain relief (for example, when ambulating, in bed, sleeping, watching television, making facial expressions).

6. Assess and document activities that might provide distraction from pain, such as television, music, visitors, arts and crafts.

7. Document methods that help the child to relax (for example, music, reading, warm packs, imaging, focusing, massage).

8. Administer analgesic appropriate for degree of pain. Pain medications should be administered around the clock. Narcotics are most effective when administered every 3 hours. Non-narcotics may be given every 4 hours in addition to narcotics. When giving non-narcotics separately, administer every 4 hours.

9. The route of administration should be oral, intravenous push, or patient-controlled analgesia (PCA). Intramuscular injections should be avoided unless absolutely necessary or if the patient cannot be convinced otherwise. (For PCA administration, see PCA procedure.)

10. Monitor vital signs every 4 hours with attention to respiratory status and heart rate.

11. Monitor the child's level of consciousness. (Report changes in sensorium.)

12. Provide comfort measures and emotional support.

Assessment

1. Assess the child's pain profile: History of pain, including frequency of pain experiences; length of time pain is experienced; disease (if any) with which specific pain is associated (such as sickle cell disease); how the child manages pain at home; and what relieves the pain.
2. Assess the physical findings for changes in vital signs, dilated pupils, flushed or moist skin, loss of appetite, guarding of a body part, pulling of a body part, flexing of knees for abdominal pain, grinding of teeth, rigid posture, or psychosomatic complaints.
3. Assess the child's ability to cope with pain. Coping patterns may vary and can be associated with developmental age, history of pain, and cultural differences.
4. Assess for secondary complications related to pain (for example, pneumonia).
5. Assess for allergies.

Nursing Diagnoses

The following is a list of possible diagnoses and could apply, depending on the child's age, clinical situation, and physical condition:

Pain

Ineffective individual coping

Impaired physical mobility

Anxiety

Fear

Fatigue

Self-esteem disturbance

Planning

When planning to assess and deal with pain the following may be gathered:

Warm packs/heating pad/TENS unit (Transcutaneous Electrical Nerve Stimulator)

Pillows

Medications

PCA pump (see Chapter 28)

Pain flowsheet (see Appendix 5)

(Equipment will vary with the interventions.)

Interventions

PROCEDURE

1. Assess the developmental level of the child. Talk with the child about pain and pain relief measures. Listen to the parents' concerns. Explain the rationale for pain control with the child and parents.

RATIONALE/EXPECTED OUTCOME (EO)

Communication and teaching will need to be at a level which the child can or is willing to understand. Pain affects children's ability to cope with illness and thus interferes with their ability to reach their developmental potential.

EO: The child will be able to state the choice of pain management. The child will participate and cooperate with pain management.

PROCEDURE	**RATIONALE/EXPECTED OUTCOME (EO)**
2. Review orders. Ask for adjustments as necessary.	Pain management should seek to provide adequate pain relief. The nurse serves as a patient's advocate. *EO: The child will receive adequate pain management. The child will be given the appropriate amount of medication.*
3. Assess level of pain prior to administration of analgesic by use of a pain rating scale.	This allows the child and nurse to identify and rate the pain. It will allow for comparison and feedback for appropriate medication doses. *EO: The child will be able to articulate the degree of pain experienced.*
4. Administer analgesic around the clock at consistent intervals.	Analgesics administered on a consistent schedule allow for adequate blood levels of analgesia, thereby eliminating or minimizing pain. *EO: The child will receive appropriate, consistent relief of pain.*
5. Assess the level of pain by use of the pain rating scale 30 minutes after analgesic is administered.	To identify the child's perceived response to analgesia. *EO: The child's rating of pain will be less than before administration of the analgesic.*
6. Monitor the child's vital signs with attention to respirations and heart rate 30 minutes after administration of the medication.	Respiratory embarrassment, altered cardiac status, and changes in sensorium can be associated with narcotics. *EO: The child will be monitored for side effects of the drugs administered.*
7. Document on a flow sheet the medication administered, route of administration, child's vital signs, activity, interventions, rating of pain, and the nurse's rating of pain.	This tool provides a comprehensive picture of the child's pain experience and interventions, and allows for evaluation.
8. Chart summary of pain management and evaluation of outcome using appropriate nursing diagnoses.	*EO: The child will have all interventions in regard to pain management documented in the medical record.*

Patient/Family Education: Home Care Considerations

1. Review with the child and family the pain management program (general guidelines):
   a. Pain management in the home could include use of plain acetaminophen (10–15 mg/kg/dose) for intermittent pain every 4 hours as needed.
   b. If pain is consistent and uncomfortable, acetaminophen with codeine may be used every 4 hours around the clock. Nonsteroidal anti-inflammatory drugs may also be useful for acute and chronic pain.
   c. If pain is unrelieved with pain medication or after 8–12 hours, the family should notify the physician.
2. Review with child and family signs and symptoms of side effects of pain medication, which include respiratory embarrassment, alteration in cardiac status, and changes in level of consciousness.
3. Review with child and family methods of providing diversional activity and methods of relaxation that will support comfort measures.
4. Provide emotional support for child and family. Encourage them to communicate concerns and frustrations.
5. Make appointment for follow-up care.

References

Adams, J. (1989). Pain assessment: The special challenge of assessing pain in children. *Dimensions in Oncology Nursing, 3*(3), 25–31.

Baker, C., & Wong, D. (1987). Q.U.E.S.T.: a process pain assessment in children. *Orthopedic Nursing, 6*(1), 11–20.

Blass, E. M., & Hoffmeyer, M. A. (1991). Sucrose as an analgesic for newborn infants. *Pediatrics, 87*(2), 215–218.

Broome, M. E., & Slack, J. F. (1990). Influences on nurses' management of pain in children. *Maternal Child Nursing, 15*(3), 158–166.

Cook, J.D. (1986). Music as an intervention in oncology settings. *Cancer Nursing, 9*(1), 23–28.

Donovan, M. (1982). Cancer pain: You can help. *Nursing Clinics of North America, 17*(4), 712–727.

Eland, J.M. (1988). Pharmacologic management of acute and chronic pediatric pain. *Issues in Comprehensive Pediatric Nursing, 11*(2/3), 93–111.

Elander, G., Lindberg, T., & Quarnstrom, B. (1991). Pain relief in infants after major surgery. *Journal of Pediatric Surgery, 26*(2), 128–131.

Favaloro, R., & Touzel, B. (1990). A comparison of adolescents' and nurses' postoperative pain ratings and perceptions. *Pediatric Nursing, 16*(4), 414–416.

Gregory, G.A. (1989). *Pediatric anesthesia.* New York: Churchill Livingstone.

Kinney, T., & Ware, R. (1988). Advances in the management of sickle cell disease. *Pediatric Consult. 7*(3), 1–7.

McCaffery, M. (1980). Relieving pain with non-invasive techniques. *Nursing, 10,* 55–57.

McGuire, D. (1984). The measurement of clinical pain. *Nursing Research, 33*(3), 152–156.

Morrison, R., & Vedro, D. (1989). Pain management in the child with sickle cell disease. *Pediatric Nursing, 15*(6), 595–599.

Price, S. (1990). Pain: Its experience, assessment and management in children. *Nursing Times, 89*(9), 42–45.

Schechter, N., Berrien, F., & Katz, S. (1988). The use of patient-controlled analgesic in adolescents with sickle cell pain crisis: A preliminary report. *Journal of Pain and Symptom Management, 3*(2), 109–113.

Schechter, U. L., Bernstein, B. A., Bick, A., et al. (1991). Individual differences in children's response to pain: Role of temperament and parental characteristics. *Pediatrics, 87*(2), 171–177.

Stevens, B. (1990). Development and testing of a pediatric pain management sheet. *Pediatric Nursing, 16*(6), 543–548.

Stewart, M. (1977). *Measurement of clinical pain.* Boston: Little, Brown and Company.

Taylor, A., Skelton, J., & Butcher, J. (1984). Duration of pain condition and physical pathology as determinants of nurses' assessments of patients in pain. *Nursing Research, 33*(1), 4–8.

Vichinsky, E., Johnson, R., & Lubin B. (1982). Multi-disciplinary approach to pain management in sickle cell disease. *American Journal of Pediatric Hematology/Oncology, 4*(3), 328–333.

Wallace, M. (1989). Temperament: A variable in children's pain management. *Pediatric Nursing, 15*(2), 118–121.

Whipple, B. (1987). Methods of pain control: Review of research and literature. *Image, 19*(3), 142–146.

Assessment of Suspected Child Abuse and Neglect

14

Definition/Purpose

Child abuse is the nonaccidental injury or neglect of a child by a caretaker. It includes physical and emotional neglect, sexual abuse, and physical or psychological attack.

Assessment for suspected abuse or neglect involves the evaluation of a child's physical, developmental, and psychosocial status to determine if abuse or neglect is occurring. Protection of the child is the primary purpose of this assessment.

Care must be taken, however, not to misdiagnose cases as child abuse or neglect when the child may be suffering from a genetic disease, such as osteogenesis imperfecta, or a bleeding disorder. Carefully compiled nursing histories should include genetic, social, nutritional, and medical information. Falsely accused families deserve compassionate understanding.

Standard of Care

1. Perform a physical assessment on all children presented for health care attention.
2. Report suspicions to the proper authority or to a child protection agency.

Assessment

1. Assess the child's physical findings, including past history and current condition (Table 14-1).

Table 14-1. Signs of Child Abuse or Neglect

Physical Abuse

Ecchymoses/hematomas
Abrasions/contusions/lacerations
Bites
Curvilinear/arcuate lesions
Ligature marks
Burns
Traumatic alopecia

Sexual Abuse

Syphilis
Ecchymoses in genital or perineal area
Genital irritation/discharge
Genital herpes
Genital or perianal warts
Genital or perianal mollusucum contagiosum

Emotional Abuse

Self-mutilation
Nutritional hair loss/skin abnormalities
Feces and dirt in skin folds
Long-standing skin conditions

---

2. Assess parent–child behaviors, relationship, and social interactions.
3. Assess parents' knowledge of a child's normal growth and development.
4. Assess parents' coping mechanisms, especially with regard to family situation, crisis management, and outside support network.
5. Assess parents' child care arrangements.

Nursing Diagnoses

The following is a list of possible diagnoses and could apply, depending on the child's age, clinical situation, and physical condition:

Pain

High risk for injury

Impaired skin integrity

Altered parenting

Fear

Anxiety

Altered growth and development

Ineffective family coping

Altered nutrition: less than body requirements

Fluid volume deficit

Self-esteem disturbance

Planning

To assess a child, the following equipment must be gathered:

Stethoscope

Sphygmomanometer

Penlight

Thermometer

Sterile specimen containers and swabs

Scale

Measuring tape

Interventions

PROCEDURE	**RATIONALE/EXPECTED OUTCOME (EO)**
1. Observe child's general condition, including clothes, hygiene, and interactions with parent and staff.	Feces/dirt in the skin folds or under the nails show a failure to provide for the child's basic needs. Multiple rat or dog bites may indicate that the child has been left alone for long periods of time. Self-mutilation (sucking, scratching, head banging, rubbing, or biting) may be traced back to emotional abuse.
	EO: Disturbances in self-concept will be recognized, and interventions planned.
2. Explain the physical exam in a developmentally appropriate manner. Explain each step as it occurs.	*EO: The child will cooperate with the examination, facilitating accurate assessment.*
3. Gather equipment. Let the child see and handle equipment.	Handling unfamiliar items helps to allay fears.
	EO: The child's fears will be reduced.

PROCEDURE

4. Wash your hands.
5. Take vital signs and measure height and weight on appropriate scale (see Vital Signs Measurements).

6. Measure head circumference and abdominal circumference, if applicable.

7. Evaluate level of consciousness; for example, alertness, speech, and orientation (in the child 2 years and older), developmental level, and pain (see Pain Assessment).

8. With room lights out, observe pupillary reaction to penlight.
9. Inspect sclera, conjunctiva, and retina for hemorrhages.

10. Inspect and palpate orbits for swelling, hematomas.
11. Inspect all body skin for signs of obvious injury such as burns, fractures, bruises, and edema (Fig. 14-1). Look for pattern injuries and scars including teeth, wire hanger, comb or buckle marks, scratches, cigar or cigarette-size burn scars (Fig. 14-2).

RATIONALE/EXPECTED OUTCOME (EO)

Vital signs, height, and weight indicate overall condition and nutritional status.

EO: The child will be correctly diagnosed.

Head and abdominal circumference, especially in infants, may indicate unseen injury or alternative diagnoses, such as hydrocephalus or malabsorption.

These results may indicate head injury, infection, or social deprivation. Pain reactions may be altered in the abused child.

Room must be darkened for accurate assessment.

Retina hemorrhages (flame-shaped optic fundi) are always significant and may result from choking or shaking.

EO: The child's neurologic status will be adequately assessed and maintained.

Many old injuries, especially "patterned" scars, are highly suspicious indicators of physical abuse. Bruises in various stages of healing suggest repeated beatings.

EO: The child's injuries will be treated.

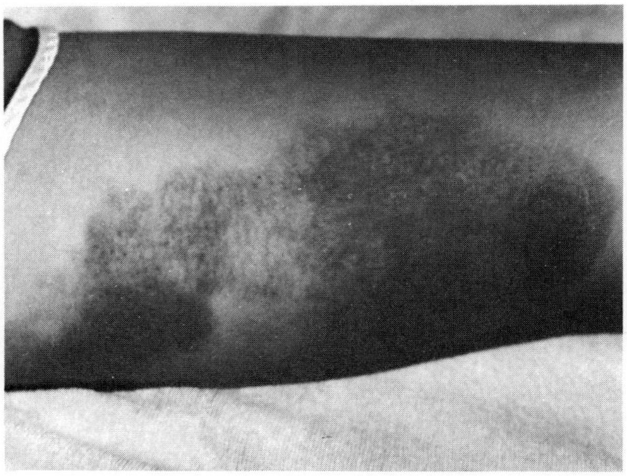

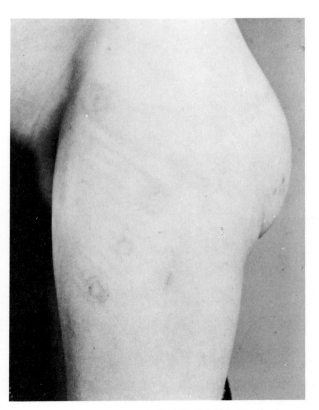

Figure 14-1. (From Pillitteri, A. (1987). Child Health Nursing. Boston: Little, Brown, p. 1338.)

Figure 14-2. (From Pillitteri, A. (1987). Child Health Nursing. Boston: Little, Brown, p. 1337.)

PROCEDURE

RATIONALE/EXPECTED OUTCOME (EO)

12. Evaluate for dehydration, especially skin condition and turgor, mucous membranes, and the anterior fontanelle (in infants). (See Assessment of Hydrational Status.)

Dehydration may be a sign of neglect or underlying illness; failure to thrive may be cause to suspect infection, AIDS, or malabsorption.

EO: The child will be hydrated.

13. Evaluate extremities for symmetry of size and strength and range of motion.

Old fractures, especially in infants, may never have been treated, resulting in musculoskeletal defects.

14. Inspect genitalia for bleeding, swelling, bruises, foul discharge, and enlarged vaginal or anal openings.

These findings invite strong suspicion of sexual abuse.

15. Obtain urine, vaginal, or anal cultures as necessary (see Obtaining Urine Specimens).

EO: Infections will be identified and treated.

16. Inspect and palpate abdomen. Evaluate for distension, rigidity, tenderness, and discoloration.

These findings may indicate abdominal trauma; bruising may not be visible.

EO: Injuries to deep viscera will be identified.

17. Observe parental behavior. Look for apathy, overconcern, conflicting stories or evidence, belligerence, hostility, or fear.

18. Interview parent regarding family situation, support network, knowledge of growth and development, crisis management.

A parent in crisis, with little support and lack of self-esteem may become abusive.

EO: Parenting abilities will be enhanced with appropriate intervention and support.

19. Ask about circumstances surrounding child's injuries or illness.

Parent may state exactly how injury or illness occurred.

EO: The family will acknowledge abusive activities.

20. Arrange or obtain radiologic and laboratory screenings, such as full body x-rays, electrolytes, and toxicology screening.

These are necessary for accurate diagnosis and treatment.

21. Document all findings, and inform the physician or social worker.

An informed, objective description facilitates correct diagnosis.

EO: The child will be protected from further injury.

22. Notify in-house abuse team, or local child protection agency.

23. If possible, admit child. In the event of parent's refusal, allow them to leave and call local authorities immediately.

The family may deny the abuse, may be unaware that the child's injuries result from abuse, or may feel the need to protect the abuser.

24. If the child is in imminent danger, obtain administrative support for an emergency custodial hearing.

In emergency situations, the health care team may treat patients without consent.

25. Explain reason for admission to parent; explain necessity of reporting to child protection agency.

Parents may or may not be revealed as abusive or neglectful. Their parental rights need to be respected.

EO: The parent will recognize abuse and their own high-risk behaviors.

Patient/Family Education: Home Care Considerations

1. Provide parent/family with information concerning child's injury, treatment, and prognosis.
2. Provide parent/family with referrals to social work and child protection agency.
3. Instruct parent/family about normal child growth and development:
   a. Physical milestones/achievements
   b. Nutrition
   c. Discipline/limit setting
   d. Emotional needs

4. Provide nonjudgmental support and role-modeling.
5. Help parents explore their feelings; assist in defining stressors and help develop methods of managing them in order to avoid abusing the child.
6. Encourage professional counseling; provide hot-line numbers:

Parents Anonymous:	800-421-0353
	800-421-8253
Abuse Hotline:	800-25-ABUSE
	800-252-2873

References

Christensen, M.L., Schommer, B.L., & Velasquez, J. (1984). Child abuse. *Journal of Maternal/Child Nursing* (Special Feature), *9*(2), 107–117.

Helberg, J.L. (1983). Documentation in child abuse. *American Journal of Nursing, 83*(2), 236–239.

Jurgrau, A. (1990). How to spot child abuse. *RN, 10,* 26–32.

Leatherland, J. (1986). Do you know child abuse when you see it? *RN, 49*(11), 28–30.

Lewin, L. (1990). Establishing a therapeutic relationship with an abused child. *Pediatric Nursing, 16*(3), 263–267.

Mittleman, R.E., Mittleman, H.S., & Wetli, C.V. (1987). What child abuse really looks like. *American Journal of Nursing, 87*(9)/1185A–1186B, 1188D, 1188F.

Ryan, M.T. (1984). Identifying the sexually abused child. *Pediatric Nursing, 10*(6), 419–421.

Wong, D. (1987). False allegations of child abuse: The other side of the tragedy. *Pediatric Nursing, 13*(5), 329–333.

Cultural Assessment

15

Definition/Purpose

Cultural assessment identifies patterns of shared beliefs, values, and customs that influence health behaviors. Values are ideals and beliefs created by a particular culture that give meaning to the lives of its participants. Each culture's value system, or highest held beliefs, make it unique.

To better understand a culture, it is important to explore these elements:

1. Religion. In some cultures religion plays an important role in altering attitudes and lifestyles. Illness may be viewed as punishment for a violation of religious codes.

2. Communication. Styles of communication vary among cultures. Cultural groups differ in the way that information is understood. If information is perceived differently or inaccurately, then the desired response will not occur.

3. Education and life views. Depending on the culture, some groups focus on the here and now, whereas others plan life around the future. Formal education dominates the more literate cultures, while other cultures use informal learning styles that focus on social order and traditional skills.

4. Family practices. Family roles vary from culture to culture. Child rearing, discipline, birth control, and the child's role in the family differ among cultural groups.

5. Health and illness beliefs. The way individuals define health and illness creates the values by which they respond to a given experience. In some cultures, preventive medicine (such as immunization) has limited importance. Culture influences, defines, and gives meaning to the illness experience.

Cultural information enables nurses to provide meaningful interventions, teaching, discharge planning, and prescribed treatment regimes. It must be emphasized that this type of assessment will take a number of sessions.

Standard of Care

1. Perform a cultural assessment on all children presented for health care.
2. Incorporate information learned from the assessment into the child's care, discharge planning, and patient and family teaching.

Assessment

1. Assess for congenital, hereditary, and chronic illnesses.
2. Assess family structure, patterns of interaction, socioeconomic status, and usual pattern of coping with illness.
3. Assess family's belief systems.
4. Assess patterns of daily living.

Nursing Diagnoses

The following is a list of possible diagnoses and could apply, depending on the child's age, clinical situation, and physical condition:

Noncompliance with medical treatment

Pain

Fear

Anxiety

Altered nutrition: more than body requirements

Altered nutrition: less than body requirements

Planning

Gather assessment tools or forms.

Interventions

PROCEDURE	RATIONALE/EXPECTED OUTCOME (EO)
1. Obtain family history of congenital anomalies and chronic illnesses.	The most effective way to identify factors that influence behavior and care is to do a cultural assessment.
2. Examine the child for congenital anomalies.	Certain congenital anomalies and chronic illnesses are more common in some racial and cultural groups: • Sickle cell anemia—More common in people with African or Mediterranean backgrounds. • Tay–Sachs disease—Individuals of Eastern European Jewish descent may carry a gene for this hereditary disease. • Lactase deficiency—90% of African-Americans, Asians, and Native Americans have this deficiency. • Thalassemia—Most commonly found in people of Mediterranean, Asian (especially Chinese), and African origin. • G6PD deficiency—Affects 10% of the black population.
3. Determine how parents care for the child with congenital anomalies or chronic illness at home. Care practices devised by parents may work best for their child.	Continued care by parents maintains their skills and knowledge.
4. Allow parents to continue to provide certain aspects of care.	Some cultures prefer to have personal care such as bathing and feeding done by family members. *EO: The child's family will be active participants in the child's care.*
5. Determine native language, fluency with spoken and written English, and, if necessary, who is the usual or most reliable translator.	A common language facilitates performing an assessment, delivering care, and providing patient and family teaching. Language can often be a barrier to receiving adequate health care. *EO: The family and health care provider will communicate effectively with one another.*
6. If a family member cannot act as a translator, obtain a hospital translator. Many cities have emergency "translator banks" or phone numbers.	
7. Observe nonverbal communication between child and other family members, and between family and	Your ability to develop a relationship with the child and family depends on interpreting nonverbal communica-

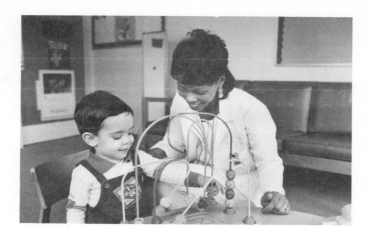

Figure 15-1.

PROCEDURE	**RATIONALE/EXPECTED OUTCOME (EO)**

health care providers: When do they use silence? How much eye contact to they maintain? (Fig. 15-1).

tion and respecting taboos governing touching, privacy, and closeness.

EO: Child and family will not express undue distress due to cultural differences in communication.

8. Determine the appropriate physical distance for family members or health care providers. How do they touch?

9. Respect the family's style of nonverbal communication.

10. Do not violate taboos of touching, privacy, or closeness.

The significance of touch as a healing gesture is well known. However, the touch of a stranger in some cultures is not acceptable.

11. Explain the purpose of all procedures and treatments, especially when certain taboos will need to be broken in order to provide care.

To ignore or contradict the family's background may result in refusal of care or noncompliance with therapy.

EO: The child and family will understand the purpose of a particular procedure or test.

EO: The child's and family's attitudes and beliefs will be respected by the healthcare members.

12. Determine if family identifies with a distinct cultural, racial, national, or religious group. Display an accepting, nonjudgmental attitude about the family's beliefs.

13. Address distinctive aspects of the child's and family's culture, including their racial, national, or religious identification.

Addressing the family's cultural needs makes hospitalization less distressing.

EO: The child's support systems and ways of coping are maintained.

14. Negotiate care or procedures that are acceptable to both the parents and health care providers. If at all possible, do not force the child to participate in care that is in conflict with his or her values.

15. If requested by the family, obtain appropriate clergy. Allow the family's clergy to attend them during hospitalization.

16. Avoid stereotyping.

Strong cultural identity may elicit stereotyped responses from health care providers.

17. Determine family's structure, including who lives in the house, who are the wage earners, who visits the child in the hospital, and who takes care of the child at home.

Understanding the family's structure enables the nurse to target interventions to the appropriate person to help the family to maintain a community of support. Children and other family members feel more comfortable and

PROCEDURE	**RATIONALE/EXPECTED OUTCOME (EO)**

secure when they continue their usual child care practices.

EO: The family's parenting practices will be maintained and supported.

18. Determine who provides emotional and physical support for the family during crisis.

19. Determine who makes decisions, and how decisions are made. Take into consideration the cultural role of the family member who makes most of the important decisions.

To disregard this fact or proceed with care that is not approved by the family can result in conflict.

20. Determine how hospitalization or illness will interfere with the usual way the child is cared for.

21. Be flexible when interpreting visiting guidelines.

22. Encourage siblings to visit.

In some cultures, having a large extended family present during an illness is important.

23. Provide overnight facilities for family members.

24. Determine the family's religious orientation, and determine how important their religion is to them.

Religious and superstitious practices provide safety, comfort, and a sense of wholeness; they contribute to restoring health and preventing further illness.

EO: Family members will express hope and value in their own belief system.

25. Determine how hospitalization will interfere with the family's usual religious practices.

26. Determine which superstitions the family follows. How will hospitalization interfere with their superstitions?

27. Allow the family to continue to practice religious and superstitious customs that are not detrimental to the child's care.

28. Explain medical and nursing practices and their expected outcomes.

29. Determine what the child usually eats.

Food may have a symbolic role in restoring health.

EO: The child will maintain adequate nutrition.

30. Determine which foods are forbidden. Which foods are believed to bring health?

EO: The child's dietary practices will be accommodated as much as possible.

31. Are mealtimes prescribed, or chosen by the child?

Children may refuse to eat food that is unfamiliar to them.

32. Determine special rituals for food preparation. Provide desired foods.

33. If necessary, encourage the family to bring food from home.

If the child is not on a dietary restriction, family members can bring home-prepared foods into the hospital.

34. Teach the child and family about therapeutic diets that can be maintained within the framework of their culture.

35. Determine what family believes will restore health. Who usually helps to restore health? What health-restoring treatments did the child receive at home? Will the treatment the child is receiving in the hospital restore health?

When treatment is consistent with the family's beliefs concerning the cause of illness and appropriate treatment, compliance with treatment will increase.

EO: Family members will take an active role in treatment decisions.

PROCEDURE	**RATIONALE/EXPECTED OUTCOME (EO)**
36. Explain disease and treatments in terms of the family's cultural view.	
37. If treatments are not within the family's belief system, seek help from clergy or other respected members of the family's cultural community. Take into consideration the cultural role of the family member who makes the most important decisions.	Special consideration should be given to informal as well as formal support groups within the family and the community who may offer assistance.
38. Determine how the family is oriented towards time. Determine which is most important to them: past, present, or future.	Medical treatment is usually oriented towards the future. These treatments have little meaning to past- or present-oriented cultures.
39. Determine how punctual the family is, and what being punctual means to them.	Punctuality may have a symbolic meaning.
40. If it is impossible to restore health, determine the death ritual to be followed.	*EO: The family's death rituals will be respected.*
41. If the family refuses treatment, identify legal avenues that may be necessary to authorize continued treatment.	
42. Allow the family access to the body after death. When a newborn dies, take photographs of the infant.	The parents may want these pictures later.

Patient/Family Education: Home Care Considerations

1. Provide instructions in a language and a format (verbal or written) that the family understands.
2. Explain treatments and cause of illness from the family's (not the health care provider's) perspective.
3. Address the concerns of the significant decision makers and care providers in the family.
4. Provide nonjudgmental support and respect for the family's beliefs.
5. Help parents explore feelings concerning illness, hospitalization, and treatment.

References

Boyle, J.S., & Andrews, M. (1989). *Transcultural concepts in nursing care.* Glenview, IL: Scott Foresman and Company.

Brink, P.J. (1984). Value orientations as a cultural assessment tool in cultural diversity. *Nursing Research, 33*(4), 198–203.

Fong, C.M. (1985). Ethnicity and nursing practice. *Topics in Clinical Nursing, 7*(3), 1–10.

Lawson, L. V. (1990). Culturally sensitive support for grieving parents. *Maternal Child Nursing, 15*(2), 76–79.

Neiderhauser, V. (1989). Health care of the immigrant children: Incorporating culture into practice. *Pediatric Nursing, 15* (6), 569–574.

Orque, M.S., Bloch, B., & Monrroy, L.S. (1983). *Ethnic nursing are: A multicultural approach.* St. Louis, MO: C. V. Mosby.

Rothschild, H., ed. (1980). *Biocultural aspects of disease.* New York: Academic Press.

Tripp-Reimer, T., Brink, P.J., & Saunder, J.M. (1984). Cultural assessment: Content and process. *Nursing Outlook, 32* (2), 78–82.

General Nursing Care Procedures

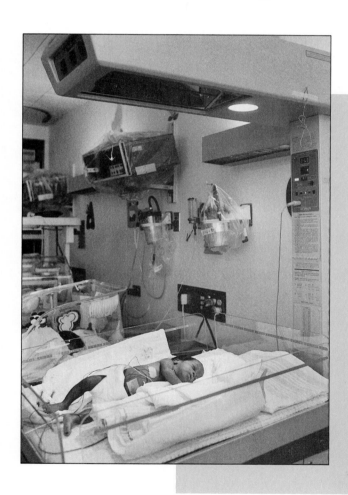

Unit III

Baby Bath

16

Definition/Purpose

Bathing the neonate removes bacteria, body wastes, and environmental contaminants from the skin. It also provides an opportunity for careful inspection of the infant along with promoting cleanliness and comfort.

Standards of Care

1. A sponge bath is given to the neonate until 2 weeks of age. Bathing in a basin or small tub is allowed for stable infants who are older than 2 weeks and whose umbilical cords have healed and dried.
2. Any type of bathing is contraindicated until the neonate's temperature is between 36.5–37°C (97.8–98.6°F).
3. Baths should not be given immediately after feeding due to the risk of regurgitation and aspiration caused by excessive manipulation.

Assessment

1. Assess the pertinent maternal history and the neonate's physical findings for weight, length, vital signs, general appearance, condition of cord, reflexes and responses to stimuli, muscle tone, activity pattern, and behaviors.
2. Assess psychosocial and developmental factors such as parents' preparation for the neonate and their available support systems.
3. Assess the family's knowledge of the physical care needs of the neonate, their anticipated lifestyle changes, and their willingness to learn.

Nursing Diagnoses

The following is a list of possible diagnoses and could apply, depending on the child's age, clinical situation, and physical condition:

High risk for altered body temperature

Hypothermia

High risk for injury

High risk for impaired skin integrity

Planning

When planning to bathe the neonate, the following equipment must be gathered:

Basin with warm water (40.6°C or 105°F)

Mild soap

Cotton balls

Soft washcloth

Diaper

Dry clean clothing

Blanket

Nonsterile gloves

Alcohol pad (if umbilical cord care is indicated)

Comb

Baby lotion

Towel

- If soap is used, it should be used sparingly because it tends to dry the neonate's skin.
- Cotton-tipped applicators are not to be used for cleaning. The applicators can break when the baby moves, causing injury to the mucous membranes of the nose or to the eardrum.
- Powders are to be avoided because the infant may inhale the powder. Powders also tend to cake with moisture and can cause skin irritation.

Interventions

PROCEDURE	**RATIONALE/EXPECTED OUTCOME (EO)**
1. Wash the child from head to feet. Dry washed areas with a towel, giving added emphasis to skin folds.	The bath will move from an area that is cleaner to an area that is dirtier.
2. Moisten a cotton ball with water and wipe eyes from inner canthus to outer canthus. Repeat with a clean cotton ball on the other eye.	This will remove any accumulated eye discharge and prevent irritation of the lacrimal duct.
	EO: The child will remain free from injury during the bath.
3. Wet washcloth and wring. Gently wash one side of the face from forehead to chin, going around the nose and mouth. Repeat on other side of the face. Do not use soap on the face.	Soap will irritate the eyes.
4. Dry infant's face with towel.	
5. To cleanse the baby's scalp, pick up baby securely by sliding hand under the baby until the head is well supported in the palm of the hand. Cover ears with thumb and middle finger (Fig. 16-1). Hold baby's head over the basin. Soap and rinse head and dry with towel.	This will prevent water from entering the ears.

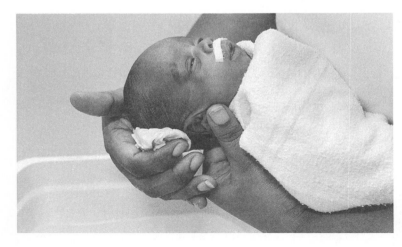

Figure 16-1.

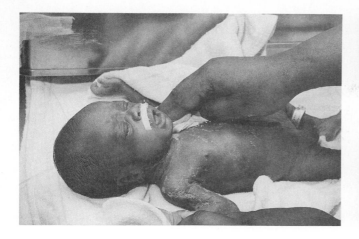

Figure 16-2.

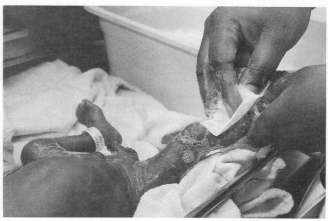

Figure 16-3.

PROCEDURE

6. Continue washing ears and neck, giving particular attention to the skin folds of the neck, behind the ears, and the external part of the ears. Wipe washed areas repeatedly to rinse off soap.

7. Remove infant's shirt. Wash trunk and arms (Fig. 16-2). Wash between fingers. Turn infant on side to wash back.

8. Cover infant with a blanket. Rinse and wring washcloth, then wipe away soap. Repeat to ensure removal of soap.

9. Dry area with towel. Cover trunk after drying.

10. Remove diaper, exposing lower half of body. Keep upper half of body covered with blanket.

11. Lightly soap washcloth, wipe over abdomen and around umbilical cord. Work down each leg to the foot, using long stroking motions (Fig. 16-3). Wash between toes. Clean around umbilical cord with alcohol swab or sterile applicator.

12. Rinse washcloth and wipe soap off body, paying particular attention to skin creases.

13. Wash genitalia with cotton balls. Spread apart the female's labia and clean between folds, using a front-to-back motion. Use each cotton ball for one stroke only.

14. The male genitalia should be washed with cotton balls from penis to anus. Do not retract the foreskin of the penis.

15. Next wash the anus and between the gluteal fold and buttocks.

16. Dry lower half of body. Rediaper. Redress and position the infant in the isolette or bassinet.

RATIONALE/EXPECTED OUTCOME (EO)

Soap remaining on the skin can cause drying and chafing of the skin.

EO: The child's skin will remain intact without drying or chafing.

Keep infant covered to prevent heat loss or hypothermia.

EO: The infant will be bathed and maintain a normal temperature.

This prevents the vaginal and urethral areas from being contaminated.

The normal foreskin is adherent to the glans at birth and is not fully retractable in 90% of males until 3 years of age. Retraction of the foreskin may lead to incomplete return of the foreskin to its normal location and paraphimosis. The foreskin then becomes edematous and requires manual reduction with sedation.

PROCEDURE

RATIONALE/EXPECTED OUTCOME (EO)

17. Document any abnormalities in the skin surface in the medical record.
    • Desquamation—peeling of the skin during the first 2–4 weeks of life.
    • Milia—tiny, white papillae occurring on the nose and chin that are caused by obstruction of the sebaceous glands; these disappear in 1–2 weeks.
    • Jaundice—yellow discoloration of the skin that appears between the third and seventh day of life.
    • Telangiectatic nevi ("stork bites")—flat, red localized areas of capillary dilation forming a variety of angiomas, most notably on the upper eyelids; these disappear usually by 2 years of age.
    • Forceps marks—marks left on part of the body where the blades exerted pressure.

18. Document the infant's tolerance of the bath process.

EO: The child's response to the bath technique will be recorded in the medical record.

Patient/Family Education: Home Care Considerations

1. Demonstrate bathing techniques and have the parent or other responsible adult give the bath before discharge.

2. Instruct the family to observe and assess the infant's condition during the bath.

References

Reeder, S., & Martin, L. (1992). *Maternity nursing: Family, newborn and women's health care.* (17th ed.). Philadelphia: J. B. Lippincott Company.

Rosdahl, C. (1991). *Textbook of basic nursing.* (5th ed.). Philadelphia: J. B. Lippincott Company.

Umbilical Cord Care

17

Definition/Purpose

After ligation at delivery, the umbilical stump undergoes necrosis as a result of interruption of its blood supply. Bacterial colonization follows soon after birth. Organisms may invade the umbilical cord stump and surrounding tissue. The initial infection is cellulitis, but peritonitis, liver abscess, and sepsis may follow. Care of the cord is done to control bleeding, prevent infection, and promote healing.

Standard of Care

1. Assess stump with every diaper change for bleeding or discharge at the base.
2. Fold diaper below the level of the umbilical stump to prevent pressure and irritation.
3. Apply alcohol to the base of the cord with every diaper change.
4. Monitor vital signs every 4 hours with attention to an elevation in temperature.
5. Provide home instruction to parents for proper care of the cord stump before infant's discharge.

Assessment

1. Assess the pertinent maternal and delivery history, including gestational age, rupture of membranes, fetal tolerance of labor, and length of labor.
2. Assess the physical findings, including the infant's general appearance and the condition of the cord.
3. Assess the parents' knowledge of the infant's needs and their willingness to learn how to attend them.

Cord Appearance

Normal	Abnormal	Significance
3 vessels (2 arteries and 1 vein)	2 vessels (1 artery and 1 vein)	Possible internal congenital anomalies
Bluish-white, gelatinous structure	Meconium stained	Distress in utero
	Red with discharge	Infection
	Thick cord	Large for gestational age
	Small cord	Small for gestational age
Abdominal musculature strong	Abdominal musculature weak	Mass hernia of the cord through which viscera, intestines and other organs enter (omphalocele, gastroschisis)

Nursing Diagnoses

The following is a list of possible diagnoses and could apply, depending on the child's age, clinical situation, and physical condition:

Impaired skin integrity

High risk for infection

Planning

The following equipment needs to be gathered for umbilical cord care:

Clamp remover

Nonsterile gloves

1 alcohol wipe or cotton ball soaked in alcohol

1 clean diaper

Interventions

PROCEDURE	**RATIONALE/EXPECTED OUTCOME (EO)**
1. Gather necessary equipment.	
2. Wash hands.	
3. Position infant supine.	Allows for complete exposure of umbilicus.
4. Remove soiled diaper away from the umbilicus.	Harmful bacteria should not come in contact with the umbilical area.
5. Put on gloves.	*EO: The infant's umbilicus will not become infected.*
6. Inspect the cord closely during the first 24 hours and then daily for any abnormalities. Notify the physician of any abnormalities.	The base of the cord should be dry and clean. Bleeding may be due to injury to the cord. If the base of the cord is moist, a urachus, which in fetal life connects the bladder with the umbilicus, may still be patent and draining urine. If the base is moist, red, warm, or foul-smelling, infection may be present.
7. Cleanse area at base of stump in a circular motion with alcohol wipe or cotton ball (Fig. 17-1).	Friction decreases the number of pathogens on skin. The circular motion moves pathogens away from any open areas at the base of the cord. Alcohol accelerates the drying of the cord.

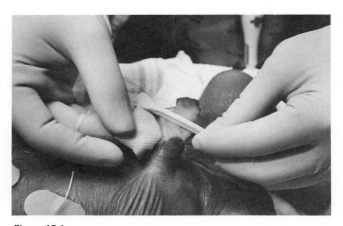

Figure 17-1.

PROCEDURE	**RATIONALE/EXPECTED OUTCOME (EO)**
	EO: The infant's cord will dry and fall off in 6–14 days without evidence of infection.
8. Remove cord clamp after 24 hours.	To prevent stress and irritation on the drying stump.
	EO: The infant's umbilical stump will not begin to bleed.
9. Replace diaper. Fold down front below area of umbilicus and secure.	Decreases friction and irritation on the umbilical stump. Allows air to circulate to promote drying.
	EO: The infant will not develop irritation at the base of the cord.
10. Position infant upright or side-lying while sleeping.	Avoiding the prone position will decrease stress on the cord and prevent it from becoming irritated or falling off prematurely.
	EO: The infant's cord will not fall off prematurely.
11. Document the condition of the cord in the medical record.	During the first day of life the cord begins to dry and shrink. It changes in color from a dull yellow–brown to black and sloughs off by 6–10 days after birth.

Patient/Family Education: Home Care Considerations

1. Instruct family to perform cord care with every diaper change.
2. Identify signs and symptoms of infection (for example, swelling, odor, or green discharge from base of cord; elevated axillary temperature) and what the parents should do if infection occurs.
3. Remind parents not to pull the cord.
4. Discuss ways to hold and dress the infant to maximize circulation and prevent irritation of the area.
5. Remind parents not to give a tub bath until the cord is off and the area is dry (approximately 6–14 days).

Reference

Reeder, S.J., & Martin, L.L. (1992). *Maternity nursing: Family, newborn and women's healthcare.* (17th ed.). Philadelphia, PA: J.B. Lippincott Company.

Intake and Output Measurements

18

Definition/Purpose

Normally, fluid enters the body through three sources: oral liquids, water in foods, and water formed by oxidation of foods. Electrolytes are present in both food and liquids. The chief functions of electrolytes include regulation of acid–base balance and water distribution, transmission of nerve impulses, and clotting of blood. Within a normal diet, an excess of essential electrolytes is taken in and the unused electrolytes are excreted.

Fluids leave the body by several routes. One way is through the skin. The amount of water lost by diffusion through the skin is obligatory; that is, it will be lost regardless of intake. Water is also lost through the skin by perspiration. The amount of water lost will vary depending on the temperature of the body and the environment. Another route by which fluids leave the body is through expired air. The amount of water lost from the lungs will vary with the rate and depth of respirations. Large quantities of fluid are secreted into the gastrointestinal tract. Almost all of this fluid is reabsorbed, except in the conditions of diarrhea and vomiting. Lastly, the kidney is the major organ that regulates fluid and electrolytes.

Illness is usually accompanied by some disturbance of body fluids. As the nurse, you have the responsibility for making observations that will serve as a basis for decision making. One of these observations is the child's intake and output.

Intake is defined as any fluid taken into the body via an oral, intravenous, or feeding tube route. *Output* is defined as any fluid excreted from the body in the form of stool, urine, vomitus, or wound drainage. These measurements, along with insensible losses (water lost from the skin through evaporation, from the lungs through exhalation, and from the skin through perspiration), aid the physician in the calculation of fluid replacement.

Standard of Care

1. Intake and output recordings need to be made on the following types of children:
   a. Cardiac patients, especially those in cardiac failure
   b. Children receiving intravenous fluids
   c. Renal patients
   d. Postoperative patients
   e. Children with the diagnosis of failure to thrive
   f. Children with drainage from tubes or wounds
   g. Children with indwelling urinary catheters
   h. Children with diagnoses related to fluid status (for example, vomiting, or gastroenteritis)
   i. Children with diabetes or diabetes insipidus
   j. Children taking medications that affect fluid balance (for example, Lasix, corticosteroids, or potassium).
2. Intake and output entries need to be timed when recorded on the appropriate sheet.

Assessment

1. Assess the history and physical findings for the current course of the illness, others

sick at home, normal weight of the child, home care regarding diet and fluids, normal bowel pattern, vital signs, level of hydration, level of consciousness, and verbalizations of discomfort or pain.

2. Assess the child's and parents' psychosocial or developmental concerns, with emphasis on the family's daily routine and their past experience in the hospital environment, and on accurate recording of intake and output.

Nursing Diagnoses

The following is a list of possible diagnoses and could apply, depending on the child's age, clinical situation, and physical condition:

High risk for infection

Anxiety

Fluid volume excess

Fluid volume deficit

Alteration in tissue perfusion

Planning

To accurately measure and record the intake and output of a child, the following equipment is needed:

Nonsterile gloves

Graduated measurement container

Scale (for diaper weight)

Intake/output bedside chart (see example)

Measuring cup, syringe, graduated baby bottle (to measure intake).

Interventions

PROCEDURE

1. Explain to the child and parents the need to accurately record all intake and output. Explain what will be measured and how they can help in the process.

2. Intake will include, but not be limited to:
   • Intravenous intake measured every 1–2 hours
   • Blood/blood product intake measured every 1–2 hours
   • All oral fluid intake
   • All enteral fluid intake.

3. Output will include but not be limited to:
   • Urine output
   • Stool output
   • Vomitus output
   • Wound or tube drainage.

4. Record intake and output in milliliters (mL).

5. Total intake and output at the end of each shift and at the end of 24 hours.

6. Measure intake of intravenous fluid with the help of

RATIONALE/EXPECTED OUTCOME (EO)

The parents or child will tend to cooperate if they understand what is expected of them.

EO: The parents or child will understand their role in helping to achieve an accurate intake and output record.

Record all intake and output as comparable amounts.

EO: The child will have intake and output measured accurately and in terms that personnel will understand.

PROCEDURE   **RATIONALE/EXPECTED OUTCOME (EO)**

an infusion pump and microdrip chamber (Fig. 18-1). Ask family member to keep track of oral intake if unlimited or give child a measured amount of fluid and record as consumed. Fluid may be measured in a syringe, medicine cup, or in predetermined amounts: (1 frozen pop = 45 mL).

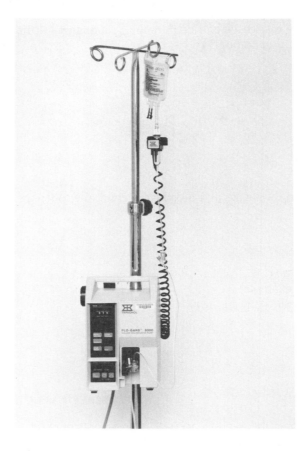

Figure 18-1.

7. To measure output, put on gloves.

Bodily drainage needs to be handled in accordance with universal precaution guidelines.

8. Pour material to be measured into a graduated measuring cylinder. Read the measurement from eye level.

9. Discard material in appropriate container for waste, and rinse cylinder according to policy.

10. Remove gloves and wash hands.

11. Record time and amount of output on bedside sheet and document its appearance and other characteristics in the medical record.

12. Output of urine and stool for incontinent children must be determined by diaper weight.

EO: The incontinent child will have output measured and recorded accurately every shift and totaled for 24 hours.

13. Balance scale at zero. Place a clean diaper on the scale. Record weight on front of the clean diaper. Then, when soiled, reweigh diaper and subtract the clean diaper weight from the soiled weight.

Note that the clean diaper used to zero the scale must be of the same size and type as the soiled diaper.
The difference in weight between clean and soiled diaper will equal output: (1 oz = 30 mL).

PROCEDURE

14. Record output on bedside sheet, noting whether the measurement was urine only, stool only, or both: (1 gm = 1 mL).

RATIONALE/EXPECTED OUTCOME (EO)

The weight of the fluid measured in grams is the same as the volume of fluid measured in milliliters (mL).

Patient/Family Education: Home Care Considerations

1. If the family needs to continue to monitor the child's intake and output after discharge, instruct them on what needs to be recorded and how they can accomplish this at home.

2. If the family needs to alert the physician for signs of fluid overload or depletion, list these symptoms for the family:

    Overload—Edema, increased weight, difficulty breathing (especially when lying down), weakness, fatigue, or increased blood pressure

    Depletion—Poor skin turgor, depressed fontanelle, sunken eyes, decreased weight, rapid pulse, dry mucous membranes, decreased urine output, concentrated urine, decreased fluid intake, increased body temperature, weakness, lethargy, or confusion.

References

Metheny, N. (1980). *Nurses' handbook of fluid balance.* Philadelphia: J.B. Lippincott Co.

Moss, J.R., & Craft, M. J. (1990). Accurate assessment of infant emesis volume. *Pediatric Nursing, 16*(5), 455–457.

Taylor, C., Lillis, C., & LeMone, P. (1989). *Fundamentals of nursing; The art and science of nursing care.* Philadelphia, J.B. Lippincott Company.

Safety

19

Definition/Purpose

Accidents are a leading cause of death among infants and children. Hospitalized children may be accident-prone because they lack understanding of the dangers inherent in the hospital environment. It is the responsibility of healthcare workers to have an understanding of the developmental level at which each child is operating and to plan for safety accordingly.

Standard of Care

1. Safety factors will be incorporated into every child's care plan to prevent accidents in the hospital and as a practical demonstration to parents of how accidents common to children can be prevented.
2. Issues related to safety will be incorporated into discharge teaching in the form of direct instruction and audiovisual and written materials.
3. The reasons for certain restrictions, especially the use of restraints, will be explained to the child and family before these restrictions are applied.

Assessment

1. Assess the pertinent history of the child and family for findings of accident-prone behavior (such as trauma-related hospitalizations and multiple trips to the emergency room).
2. Assess the physical findings for marks or bruises on the body, old surgical scars, or healed bone fractures (detectable by x-ray).
3. Assess the developmental level at which the child is functioning.
4. Assess the family's knowledge of safety issues and their willingness to learn.

Nursing Diagnoses

The following is a list of possible diagnoses and could apply, depending on the child's age, clinical situation, and physical condition:

High risk for aspiration

Altered growth and development

High risk for injury

Impaired mobility

Impaired skin integrity

Pain

Planning

When planning to ensure a child's safety, properly functioning, age-appropriate equipment must be available. Most safety hazards are observed by the care giver.

Interventions

| **PROCEDURE** | **RATIONALE/EXPECTED OUTCOME (EO)** |

Transporting Children

1. Infants can be transported to other areas in their cribs or bassinets. Baby carriages and strollers with a seat belt may also be used.

An infant or young child should not be carried off the unit because of the danger of the nurse falling.

EO: The child will be transported off the unit in a safe manner determined by his or her age, condition, and destination.

2. Children can be transported to other areas on gurneys or in wheelchairs equipped with a seat belt. Gurneys must have side rails. A wagon may also be used for this purpose.

Environmental Factors

3. Floors are cleared of fluid or other objects that might contribute to falls.
4. Showers and tubs should have a nonskid surface.
5. Electrical equipment must be maintained in good working order. Equipment with broken plugs or exposed wires must be taken out of service until repaired.
6. Instruments and solutions must be kept in cabinets or on shelves where ambulatory children cannot reach them.

Children may mistake solutions and medicine for food or candy, and may ingest them.

7. Utility and treatment room doors must be kept closed and off limits to children.
8. Medicine cabinets must be locked when not in use.
9. Medicine must not be left on a bedside table.
10. Electrical outlets must be covered.

This will prevent burns that occur when children insert their fingers into the outlet or insert objects that will conduct electricity.

EO: The child's environment will be examined by the care giver and maintained in a safe manner.

Cribs and Beds

11. The catches on the sides of a crib must be in good condition and hold the rail up. The wheels on cribs must be in the locked position.

Children may use the side rails to pull themselves up, and could fall out of bed if the rails do not hold in the upright position.

12. Side rails must always be up when the child is in bed (Fig. 19-1). When giving care to the child in bed, keep one hand on him or her to prevent a fall.

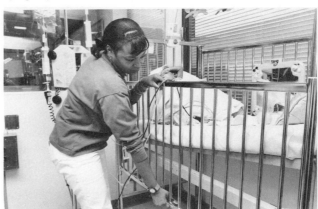

Figure 19-1.

PROCEDURE	**RATIONALE/EXPECTED OUTCOME (EO)**

13. The crib bars must be close enough together that a child's head cannot be caught between them ($<2\frac{3}{8}$ inches).

14. A net or bubble top can be added to the crib (Fig. 19-2).

The child may crawl over the side rail.

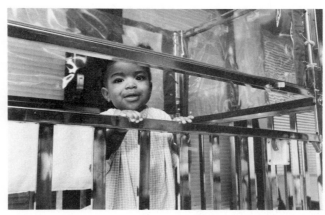

Figure 19-2.

15. Bumper pads can be used.

The child will be prevented from getting caught between the mattress and the crib sides and from hitting a part of his or her body on the rails.

16. Hi–Lo beds should remain in the low position.

Toilet-trained children will be able to climb out of bed safely to go to the bathroom.

EO: The child's hospital bed will be a safe place for the child to rest.

Toys

17. Toys must be allergy-free, washable, and unbreakable, and should not have small removable parts.

These parts can be aspirated, swallowed, or inserted in ears and nose.

18. Friction toys cannot be allowed under an oxygen tent.

Sparks in a high-oxygen environment can cause combustion.

19. Avoid toys with long strings.

Children can strangle on the string.

Food

20. Bottles must never be propped, nor should feeding be forced.

There is a danger of aspiration which may cause pulmonary infiltrates or sudden death.

21. Avoid foods that can be aspirated (for example, hot dogs, popcorn, peanuts, peas, corn, beans, raisins, and raw apple).

EO: The child will not aspirate on foods known to cause problems.

Restraints

22. Jacket restraint—Can be used to help children remain flat in bed or to prevent the child from falling out of a high chair or wheelchair. The jacket is put on using the strings in the back.

The major danger of this type of restraint is strangulation through pressure of the jacket that has slipped out of place and encircles the child's neck.

23. Mummy restraint—A blanket is used to wrap the baby up, with only the head exposed. The infant is placed on the blanket, and one side of the blanket is pulled firmly over the shoulder. The remainder of that side is tucked under the opposite side of the child's body. The procedure is then repeated on the other side.

This is used to immobilize the infant's arms and legs for a brief period of time.

PROCEDURE

24. Elbow restraint—This restraint is made from a double piece of muslin with pockets sewn in for tongue blades. The tongue blades should reach from the axilla to the wrist, so the elbow cannot be bent when the restraint is applied around the arm and the string is tied.

25. Extremity (clove hitch) restraint—This restraint is made from a piece of gauze placed in a figure eight. The circles are placed around the extremity and tied to the bed frame. Remove the restraint every 2 hours and observe the fingers and toes of the restrained extremity from coldness and discoloration. Stimulate the child while the restraint is removed.

Other Safety Concerns

26. Children must be properly identified with an identification band on an extremity (Fig. 19-3).

RATIONALE/EXPECTED OUTCOME (EO)

This is used to hold the elbow in an extended position so that the infant cannot reach the face. The major danger of this type of restraint is impaired circulation to the hand.

This is used to immobilize one or more extremities.

Observe the restrained extremity for coldness and discoloration, which would indicate a lack of circulation and too tight restraint.

EO: The child will suffer no injury from the restraint and will be positioned in a comfortable manner.

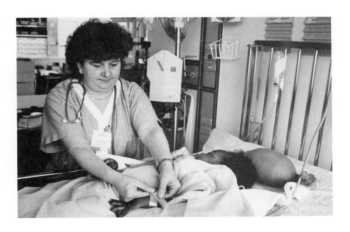

Figure 19-3.

27. Hospital clothing must fit properly.

28. Isolation techniques must be carried out on all children with infectious illnesses.

29. Adequate handwashing facilities must be available.

Clothing that is too small is uncomfortable. Pajama legs that are too long may cause the child to fall.
Slippers that are too large may fall off.

This ensures the safety of other children from becoming exposed to infectious diseases.

EO: The child will be free from nosocomial infections and injury while in the hospital.

Patient/Family Education: Home Care Considerations

1. Make parents aware that children will explore every part of their environment and tell them what precautions can be taken to prevent accidents. The following are some suggestions that can be discussed with the parent during various well-child visits:

Newborn

1. Encourage the use of car seats. Make parents aware of car seat laws.

2. Promote crib safety—
    • Pull all crib sides up when the baby is unattended.
    • Use crib bumpers.
    • Avoid mobiles or toys with long strings or pins.
    • Make sure that the distance between crib bars is less than 2⅜ inches.
3. Do not use plastic bags to cover mattresses.
4. Do not leave a plastic bag or pillow within the infant's reach.
5. Set water heater thermostat at less than 48.8°C (120° F).
6. Do not leave the infant on a bed or other surface from which he or she may fall.

2–4 Weeks

1. Encourage the family to purchase smoke detectors.
2. Place a washcloth at the bottom of the bathtub to keep the infant from slipping.
3. Never leave the infant alone in a car.
4. Never jiggle or shake the infant's head vigorously.
5. Do not place a string or necklace around the infant's neck (especially to hold a pacifier).

2 Months

1. Do not place an infant seat on anything but the floor when the seat is used outside the car.
2. Do not hold the infant when drinking a hot liquid or when smoking.
3. Use a playpen for the infant after 3 months of age.
4. Select toys that are unbreakable, contain no small detachable parts or sharp edges, and are too large to swallow.
5. Keep garbage in a lidded container.

4 Months

1. Discourage the purchase of a walker.
2. Be conscious of buttons that can pull off clothes, toys, or furnishings.
3. Guard against ingestion of harmful objects. Keep baby powders, cleaners, and small objects out of reach.
4. The high chair should have a wide base to keep it stable. It should also have a seat belt and a tray that latches on both sides.

6 Months

1. Never leave the baby unattended in a tub of water. Ignore telephone calls and doorbells while bathing the child.
2. Keep plastic bags and latex balloons out of reach.
3. Insert plastic plugs in outlets.
4. Use safety gates on stairs.
5. Avoid using appliances with dangling electrical cords.
6. Keep a supply of syrup of ipecac. Teach the parents the correct dose of ipecac and emphasize that if a poisoning occurs, they should call the Poison Control Center before administering anything. (Under 12 months—15 mL of syrup of ipecac plus 100 mL of water. Give second dose in 20 minutes if no vomiting occurs.) Over 12 months—30 mL of syrup of ipecac plus 200 mL of water. Give second dose in 20 minutes if no vomiting occurs.
7. Lighted pipes, cigarettes, and cigars can burn the child. Keep them out of reach.

9 Months

1. Upgrade infant car seat to a toddler seat when child weighs 20 pounds.
2. Install screens on windows to prevent child from falling out.
3. Keep sharp objects (such as knives, tools, or razor blades) and other hazardous objects (such as coins, beads, or glass) in a secure place.
4. Avoid foods that can be aspirated (for example, hot dogs, peanuts, popcorn, frozen peas, corn, beans, raisins, and raw apple).
5. Do not store toxic substances in empty bottles or jars.
6. Keep washer and dryer closed so child cannot crawl inside.

12 Months

1. Lock up poisons and medicines.
2. Confine outside play to within fences or gates.
3. Do not permit child near the lawn mower, running machinery, or a car that is backing up.
4. Keep all plants out of the baby's reach. (A number of houseplants are poisonous if eaten.)

15 Months

1. The crib mattress should be lowered since the child may climb out of bed.
2. Place safety caps on medicine.
3. Turn pan handles toward the back of the stove.
4. Keep the child away from hot stoves, space heaters, wall heaters, irons, and fireplaces.
5. Never leave the child unsupervised in or near a swimming pool, a full bathtub, a bucket of water, or a ditch. Keep the toilet lid down.

18–24 Months

1. Never leave the child unattended at home or in a car.
2. Lock up disc batteries, toys, or other objects that can cut or be swallowed.

3 Years

1. The child under 4 years old may use a regular car seat belt if he or she weighs 40 pounds, and is 40 inches tall.
2. Store knives and firearms out of reach.
3. Teach the child the danger of chasing a ball into the street.
4. Advise the child to be careful around strange dogs.
5. Talk to the child about not following strangers and not accepting touching that they do not like by others.

4 Years

1. Teach the child what to do in case of fire.
2. Teach the child his or her name, address, and telephone number in case they are lost.

References

Marlow, D. (1988). *Textbook of pediatric nursing*. Philadelphia: W.B. Saunders Company.

Scipien, G. M., Bernard, M. U., Chard, M. A., et al. (1986). *Comprehensive pediatric nursing*. New York: McGraw-Hill Book Company.

Temperature Stabilization

20

Definition/Purpose

Temperature stabilization employs various interventions designed to achieve and maintain a child's body temperature within normal limits, 36.5–37.5°C (97.8–99.6°F). Stabilizing the body temperature within this range will prevent the complications and sequelae related to hypothermia and hyperthermia, including seizures, electrolyte imbalance, cardiac dysrhythmias, and shock.

Standard of Care

1. Temperatures are measured on admission and at least every 8 hours unless otherwise indicated.
2. Temperatures <36.5°C (97.8°F) or >37.5°C (99.6°F) require assessment at least every 2 hours.
3. Notification of physicians should occur for any new onset of hypo- or hyperthermia, as well as temperatures that are unresponsive to already prescribed interventions.

Assessment

1. Assess child for history of recent illness or exposure, especially infectious illness and childhood diseases.
2. Assess vital signs along with temperature.
3. Assess age and weight. Assess for weight change and dietary history, especially in the newborn and low-birth-weight infant. Each degree Celsius of temperature elevation increases the basal metabolic rate by 12%.
4. Assess skin for temperature and hydration.
5. Assess neurologic status. Injury to or disease of the hypothalamus or the pituitary can produce an alteration in the regulation of body temperature.

Nursing Diagnoses

The following is a list of possible diagnoses and could apply, depending on the child's age, clinical situation, and physical condition:

Ineffective thermoregulation

Hypothermia

Hyperthermia

Fluid volume deficit

Impaired gas exchange

Altered nutrition, less than body requirements

Impaired verbal communication

Altered thought process

High risk for infection

High risk for injury

Planning

In planning to care for a child who is hyper- or hypothermic, the following equipment must be gathered:

Thermometer

For Hypothermia

Blankets

Head covers

Booties

Overbed warmer

Warming lights

Heated/humidified O_2

IV fluids

Heated peritoneal dialysate

For Hyperthermia

Wash basin

Tepid water

Cloths

Cooling mattress

Oral fluids

IV fluids

Antipyretics

Interventions

PROCEDURE	RATIONALE/EXPECTED OUTCOME (EO)
1. Prepare the child or parent in a way appropriate to child's developmental level.	Prior knowledge will allay fears and encourage cooperation.
2. Obtain equipment for temperature measurement, considering age and diagnosis (see Temperature Assessment).	Temperature should be obtained using the safest and most accurate method. *EO: The child will remain injury-free during the temperature determination.*
3. Obtain subsequent measurements using the same method and instrument, unless otherwise indicated. Document any change in method or instrument.	A change in method (axillary versus oral) may indicate a false increase or decrease in actual temperature. *EO: True alterations in temperature will be recognized and treated if necessary.*

For Hypothermia

4. Evaluate for potential causes: • Lack of clothing or covers • Cold environment • Diagnosis-related • Dehydration • Hypoglycemia	Heat transfer between the child and the environment is altered by air humidity, air temperature, rate of movement of air, thickness of the body, and the degree of dilation and blood flow through the skin blood vessels. *EO: Hypothermia will be controlled with prompt diagnosis and intervention.*

PROCEDURE   **RATIONALE/EXPECTED OUTCOME (EO)**

- Sepsis
- Wet covers
- Ventilation with cold, dry oxygen
- Starvation.

5. Provide adequate or extra clothing and blankets. Cover the child's head and feet (Fig. 20-1).

Covering the head will significantly decrease heat loss.

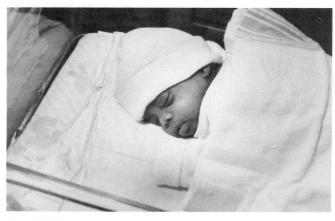

Figure 20-1.

6. Notify physician if there is evidence of dehydration, hypoglycemia, or diagnosis-related temperature drop. Report lack of response to nursing interventions.

In the newborn or infant, hypoglycemia or hypothermia may be an early sign of sepsis.

EO: Infant will have adequate nutrition and hydration.

7. Provide infant with over-bed warmer or place in heated isolette (Figs. 20-2 and 20-3) (may require physician's order). Monitor infant's temperature, as well as all other vital signs, every 2 hours. Monitor equipment temperature and function.

Rewarming a cold-stressed infant may lead to electrolyte and cardiac disturbances requiring close observation.

EO: The infant will be warmed without adverse effects.

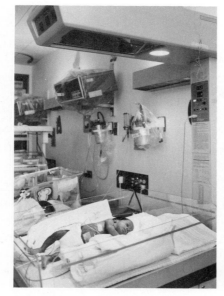

Figure 20-2.

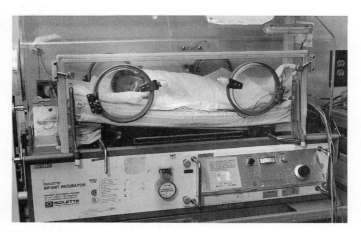

Figure 20-3.

PROCEDURE

8. Unresponsive or severe hypothermia may require the provision of heated IV fluids or heated peritoneal dialysis fluid and close observation.

9. Place the profoundly hypothermic patient on a cardiorespiratory monitor.

For Hyperthermia

10. Evaluate for potential causes:
    • Diagnosis-related (malignant hyperthermia, heat stroke, or exhaustion)
    • Overdressed/covered
    • Heated environment
    • Dehydration
    • Infection
    • Blood transfusion.

11. Remove excess coverings.

12. Control environment:
    • Decrease heat.
    • Decrease heating devices.
    • Control sunlight.

13. Encourage oral fluids if tolerated.

14. Maintain IV fluid therapy.

15. Provide medications, (for example, antibiotics and antipyretics) if ordered, and monitor response.

16. For children with infections, consider appropriate isolation (see Infection Control).

17. Notify physician of hyperthermia unresponsive to provided interventions.

RATIONALE/EXPECTED OUTCOME (EO)

Profound hypothermia can cause ischemia and tissue destruction in the vital organs if not promptly treated and reversed.

EO: The child's vital organs will not be injured.

Cardiac arrythmias may be present. Note that cardiac drugs have little effect until body temperature is near normal.

EO: Progressive hyperthermia and potential injury will be averted with prompt diagnosis and intervention.

Decreasing covers will increase cooling via evaporation and convection.

Sunlight can significantly raise room temperature.

There is an increase in fluid loss due to evaporation from the skin and respiratory loss in the febrile patient.

EO: The child will be adequately hydrated.

Hyperthermia is often indicative of infectious processes requiring further intervention.

EO: The child's temperature will be normal and infections will be treated.

Pediatric patients may need to be isolated prior to definitive diagnosis in order to prevent contagious transmission.

Further evaluation and treatment may be required. Fulminant malignant hyperthermia is characterized by muscle stiffness, fever, metabolic and respiratory acidosis, irregular tachycardia, unstable blood pressure, hyperventilation, hyperkalemia, and hypercalcemia. The mortality rate is high (10%). Treatment includes cessation of triggering agents, drugs to correct electrolyte imbalance, and vigorous external and internal cooling.

EO: Complications of hyperthermia will be prevented.

PROCEDURE

RATIONALE/EXPECTED OUTCOME (EO)

18. A high temperature or intractable hyperthermia may require the provision of tepid sponge baths or the placement of a cooling mattress (Fig. 20-4). Monitor the child's response and avoid chilling.

Chilling causes shivering, which increases heat production.

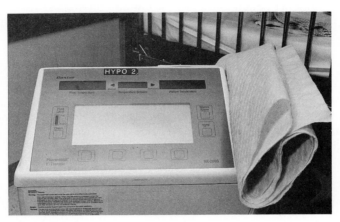

Figure 20-4.

Patient/Family Education: Home Care Considerations

1. Explain temperature measurement and the necessity for serial measurements.
2. Explain procedures, extra equipment, and the rationale for maintaining a normal temperature.
3. Instruct patient on:
   a. Methods of temperature measurement
   b. Reading a thermometer
   c. Normal range of temperature
   d. Clothing appropriate to the environment
   e. Medication dosage and methods of administration, including antipyretics and antibiotics. Parents need to be reminded that antipyretics should not include aspirin, due to its link with Reye's syndrome.
   f. When to call physician or hospital.

References

DeLapp, T.D. (1983). Accidental hypothermia. *American Journal of Nursing, 83*(1), 63–67.

Gregory, G.A. (1989). *Pediatric anesthesia.* New York: Churchill Livingstone.

Morgan, T.O. (1989). Caring for hypothermic patient. *Nursing '89,* January, 64T–V.

Monitoring: Cardiac and Respiratory

21

Definition/Purpose

Monitoring is the observation of the cardiac and respiratory systems for normal or abnormal conditions. Monitoring is done by a mechanical device that provides visual and auditory warnings when abnormal functions of the cardiac or respiratory systems occur. A cardiac monitor will assess heart and respiratory functions. It may or may not have a visual display. It can monitor heart function in any signal lead. A respiratory monitor will assess only respiratory function. It usually does not have a visual display.

Standard of Care

1. Monitor any child with a history of
   a. Congenital heart disease
   b. Compromised cardiac output
   c. Apnea or family history of SIDS
   d. Tracheostomy
   e. Seizure (febrile) or seizure disorder
   f. Neurological deficit
   g. Severe fluid and electrolyte imbalances
   h. Supplemental oxygen or mechanical ventilation
   i. Medication administration that may interfere with or alter cardiac or respiratory function.
2. Monitor vital signs independently of the machine every 4 hours.
3. Monitor the unit function, cables, electrodes, and alarm limits every 8 hours.
4. Change electrodes every 48 hours, or as necessary.
5. Place child and monitor in a central location to be seen and heard easily.

Assessment

1. Assess the past and present medical history of the child with emphasis on cardiac or respiratory diseases. Assess the need for noninvasive versus invasive monitoring.
2. Assess the child's physical findings such as color, pulses, level of consciousness, breath sounds, and use of accessory muscles.
3. Assess the child's developmental level, coping mechanisms, previous experience in a medical environment, and previous experience with external monitoring devices.

Nursing Diagnoses

The following is a list of possible diagnoses and could apply, depending on the child's age, clinical situation, and physical condition:

Ineffective airway clearance

Ineffective breathing pattern

Decreased cardiac output

Fluid volume excess

Fluid volume deficit

Impaired gas exchange

Altered tissue perfusion, cerebral and cardiopulmonary

Planning

When planning to place a child on a monitor, gather the following equipment:

Alcohol wipes

4 electrode patches (select appropriate size based on anterior chest size)

Monitor with 4 lead wires (cardiopulmonary or apnea)

Interventions

PROCEDURE	**RATIONALE/EXPECTED OUTCOME (EO)**
1. Prepare the child in a developmentally appropriate manner.	The child and parent will tend to cooperate with the procedure if they understand what to expect. *EO: The child and parent will describe application of the monitor correctly. The child will cooperate with application of the monitor, as developmentally appropriate.*
2. Gather necessary equipment.	

3. Apply electrodes as follows:
  a. Determine appropriate areas to place electrodes on anterior chest wall:
    1) Positive (+): left side of chest, lowest palpable rib, midclavicular
    2) Negative (−): right shoulder below clavicular hollow
    3) Ground (G): left shoulder below clavicular hollow
    4) Respiratory: right side of chest, lowest palpable rib, midclavicular.
	Proper placement will ensure a clear and accurate reading of the cardiopulmonary systems. Placement in this manner will ensure an accurate reading in lead II.
	
	EO: The child will have a properly applied monitoring device.

b. Wipe areas of electrode placement with alcohol and let dry thoroughly.	Cleansing the skin with alcohol will remove dirt, skin oil, lotions, and powder and allow the electrodes to adhere completely. *EO: The child will not experience skin breakdown. The child's electrodes will adhere completely to the skin.*
c. Peel backing from electrodes and place on predetermined areas. Note that some snap-on lead wires need to be attached to the electrodes prior to placement.	

4. Attach lead wires as follows (Fig. 21-1):
  a. White—right arm
  b. Black—left arm
  c. Green—right leg
  d. Red—left leg
	Following the American Heart Association guidelines for lead attachments will ensure consistent and accurate EKG readings in lead II and detect chest excursion for respiratory monitoring.
	
	EO: The child will have accurate monitoring of the EKG in lead II and accurate respiratory monitoring.

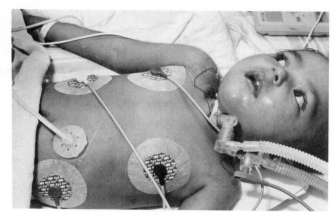

Figure 21-1.

PROCEDURE

5. Set machine as follows:
   a. Turn machine on with alarms silenced.
   b. Set alarm limits
      1) Cardiac—15 bpm above and below resting heart rate.
      2) Respiratory—15 bpm above and below resting respiratory rate.
      3) Apneic delay—(with apnea monitor only) 15 seconds.
   c. Set machine to lead II (if applicable).
   d. Turn alarms on.

6. Respond to all alarms immediately by:
   a. Assessing the child for any cardiopulmonary changes

   b. Resetting the alarms.

7. Document application of the monitor, skin integrity under the electrodes, alarm limits, and any triggered alarms in the medical record.

RATIONALE/EXPECTED OUTCOME (EO)

Setting of alarm limits above and below the child's resting heart and respiratory rates allows for changes due to increases or decreases in activity level.

EO: The child will have monitor alarms limits set accurately for heart and respiratory rates.

Any reading above 15 seconds is no longer considered a functional apneic episode.

EO: The child will not experience apnea longer than 15 seconds.

Immediate response and assessment will prevent the child from having decreased cardiac output or periods of hypoxia.

EO: The child will not experience any prolonged periods of apnea or decrease heart rate.

EO: The child will receive immediate emergency care in the event of a decreased heart rate or respiratory rate.

EO: The procedure and any alarms will be documented in the medical record for future reference.

Patient/Family Education: Home Care Considerations

1. Instruct parents on:
   a. Proper application of monitor belt or electrodes to child's chest
   b. How to use the monitor (alarms, reset button)
   c. When the child is to wear the monitor.

2. Instruct parent(s) and two additional caregivers on emergency measures to be started in the event of a cardiac or pulmonary system failure.

3. Assist the family in adapting to a child requiring home monitoring:
   a. Normal integration
   b. Growth and development
   c. Discipline (as necessary)
   d. Activities of daily living.

4. Instruct parents on safety measures related to the equipment: remove the child from the monitor when bathing; do not attempt to repair or modify the monitor; position cords and wires so that no one will trip on them, and plug monitor into a three-pronged grounded outlet).

5. Assist the family in notifying the local police, fire departments, and utility companies that there is a monitored child in the home.

References

Brown, S.L. (1987). Cardiopulmonary assessment and care of the pediatric patient: Are the little ones different? *Journal of Post Anesthesia Nursing, 2*(2), 98–103.

Nathanson, I., O'Donnell, M., & Commins, M. F. (1989). Cardiorespiratory patterns during alarms in infants using apnea/bradycardia monitors. *American Journal of Diseases in Childhood,* April, 476–480.

Phillips, S. (1989). Monitoring vital sign changes in children. *Nursing '89, 19*(10), 48–49.

Infection Control: Isolation

22

Definition/Purpose

Isolation precautions are designed to prevent the spread of disease among patients, families, and personnel. The isolation precautions recommended are based on the concept that agent and host factors are difficult to control; thus attention to infection control should be directed at transmission.

Microorganisms are transmitted by more than one route. The differences in infectivity and the mode of transmission form the basis for the differences in isolation precautions. There are four routes of transmission—contact, vehicle, airborne, and vectorborne.

Contact transmission can be divided into three subgroups—direct contact, indirect contact, and droplet contact. *Direct contact* involves physical transfer between a host and an infected person. Direct contact can occur between a patient and hospital personnel or between two patients. *Indirect contact* involves personal contact of a host with contaminated objects such as bed linens, clothing, instruments, or dressings. *Droplet contact* involves infectious agents coming in contact with the conjunctivae, nose, or mouth of a host as a result of talking, sneezing, or coughing by an infected person who has a clinical disease or is a carrier of the organism. This type of transmission is considered "contact" transmission rather than airborne, since droplets travel no more than 3 feet.

The vehicle route of disease transmission applies to these contaminated items:

1. Food, as in salmonellosis
2. Water, as in legionellosis
3. Blood, as in hepatitis B or non-A, non-B hepatitis
4. Drugs, as in bacteremia from infusion of contaminated products.

Airborne transmission occurs by dissemination of dust particles in the air containing the infectious agent or by droplet nuclei suspended in the air for a long period of time. Organisms carried in this manner are dispersed by air currents before being inhaled by or deposited on the host.

Vectorborne transmission occurs when a vector such as a mosquito transmits a disease-producing agent such as malaria.

The hospital is responsible for ensuring that patients are placed on appropriate isolation precautions. All personnel are responsible for complying with isolation precautions and teaching by example.

Seven isolation categories will be described here:

- Universal precautions
- Strict isolation
- Respiratory isolation
- Enteric isolation
- Contact precautions (drainage or secretions precautions)
- Blood and other body fluid precautions
- Respiratory syncytial virus (RSV) precautions.

Universal Precautions

Since medical history and examination cannot reliably identify all persons infected with

HBV, HIV, or other blood-borne pathogens, blood and body fluid precautions should be used for all patients. The purpose of universal precautions is threefold:

1. To minimize the health care worker's contact with blood and body fluids
2. To minimize the likelihood of transmitting organisms present in blood and body fluids to the health care worker and to the patient
3. To minimize the risk of nosocomial infections to the patient population.

Body fluids subject to universal precautions are:

1. Blood
2. Any body fluid containing visible blood
3. Semen
4. Vaginal secretions
5. Tissues/tissue fluids
6. Cerebrospinal fluid
7. Synovial fluid
8. Pleural fluid
9. Peritoneal fluid
10. Pericardial fluid
11. Amniotic fluid.

Universal precautions do not apply to feces, nasal secretions, sputum, sweat, tears, urine, or vomitus unless they contain visible blood. Lastly, it must be remembered that universal precautions are meant to complement routine infection control practice in health care facilities. The individual judgment of the healthcare worker must be depended upon in specific clinical situations.

Strict Isolation

This isolation category is designed to prevent transmission of highly contagious or virulent infections that may be spread by both air and contact.

Diseases requiring strict isolation include:

1. Congenital rubella syndrome
2. Diphtheria
3. Herpes zoster
4. Viral hemorrhagic fevers (for example, Lassa fever and Marburg virus disease)
5. Pneumonic plague
6. Rabies
7. Smallpox
8. Varicella (chickenpox).

Respiratory Isolation

This isolation category is designed to prevent transmission of infectious diseases over short distances via the air (droplet transmission).

Diseases requiring respiratory isolation include:

1. Epiglottitis
2. Erythema infectiosum (fifth disease)
3. Measles
4. Meningitis
5. Meningococcemia
6. Mumps
7. Pertussis (whooping cough)

8. Rubella (disease or exposure)

9. Varicella exposure within the previous 21 days

10. Tuberculosis.

Enteric Isolation

This isolation category is designed to prevent infections that are transmitted by direct or indirect contact with feces. Most infections in this category cause gastrointestinal symptoms, but some do not.

Diseases requiring enteric isolation include:

1. Cholera

2. Amebic dysentery

3. Poliomyelitis

4. Necrotizing enterocolitis

5. Hepatitis, viral, type A

6. Enteroviral infections

7. Gastroenteritis caused by
   - *Campylobacter*
   - *Escherichia coli*
   - *Shigella*
   - *Salmonella*

8. Coxsackievirus

9. Typhoid fever (Salmonella typhi).

Contact Precautions (wound and skin precautions)

This isolation category is designed to prevent infections that are transmitted by direct or indirect contact with purulent material or drainage from an infected body site. Diseases included in this category are those that result in the production of infective purulent material, drainage, or secretions, unless that disease is included in another isolation category that requires more rigorous precautions.

Diseases requiring contact precautions include:

1. Anthrax

2. Abscess (where drainage can be contained in a dressing)

3. Minor burns

4. Cellulitis

5. Gas gangrene

6. Herpes simplex, primary, recurrent, localized

7. Scarlet fever

8. Skin infections (minor or limited)

9. Scalded skin syndrome (Ritter's disease)

10. Impetigo

Blood and Body Fluid Precautions

This isolation category is designed to prevent infections that are transmitted by direct or indirect contact with infective blood or body fluids. For some diseases in this category, such as malaria, only blood is infective; for other diseases, such as hepatitis B, both blood and body fluids are infective.

Diseases requiring blood and body fluid precautions include:

1. AIDS

2. Syphilis (congenital and untreated; primary and secondary with skin and mucous membrane lesions)

3. Gas gangrene
4. Hepatitis B; non A, non B hepatitis
5. Wounds (any wound infected with multi-resistant bacteria)
6. Scabies
7. Babesiosis
8. Malaria
9. Rat bite fever
10. Tuberculosis (renal or draining sinus tracts).

Protective Isolation

This isolation category is designed to prevent infections in children being admitted to the hospital for bone marrow transplantation. A commonly used tool for protective isolation is the laminar air flow room. This room continuously recirculates and filters air to maintain a sterile environment. Visitors and health team members need to wash their hands and don masks, gloves, gowns, and booties before entering the room. The child receives a sterile, low-bacteria diet and antibiotics to sterilize the gastrointestinal tract.

Respiratory Syncytial Virus (RSV) Precautions

This isolation category is designed to prevent transmission of highly communicable viral respiratory diseases that can be spread by both contact and airborne routes. These diseases are spread primarily by close or direct contact with either the patient or articles that have come in contact with the patient's secretions.

 Diseases requiring RSV precautions include:

1. Viral pneumonia caused by:
   - RSV
   - Adenovirus
   - Coronavirus
   - Influenza virus
   - Rhinovirus.
2. Acute respiratory infections in infants and children of all ages including:
   - Bronchiolitis
   - Bronchitis
   - Common colds
   - Croup
   - Influenza.

Standard of Care

1. *Hand washing.* Hands should be washed before and after every patient contact. Personnel should always wash their hands even when gloves are used. When caring for patients infected with virulent organisms, personnel should consider using antiseptics for hand washing, because they will inhibit many microorganisms that may not be removed by normal handwashing.
2. *Private room.* A private room is indicated for patients with infections caused by virulent organisms. It reduces the possibility of transmission by separating infected or colonized patients from susceptible patients and reminds personnel to wash their hands before leaving the room. A private room should contain bathing and toilet facilities. In a few instances (such as chicken pox), the private room needs special ventilation, which results in a negative air pressure in the room in relation to the anteroom or hall when the room door is closed. The ventilation air, which should result in 6 air changes per hour, should be discharged outdoors or receive filtration before being recirculated to other rooms.

3. *Roommates for patients on isolation.* Patients infected by the same microorganisms may share a room. Infants and young children with the same respiratory syndrome may share a room. Cohorting patients in this manner is useful during community outbreaks when there is a shortage of private rooms. If an infected patient shares a room with a noninfected patient, it is imperative that personnel and visitors (including parents) take measures to prevent the spread of the infection.

4. *Masks.* Masks prevent transmission of infectious agents through the air and protect the wearer from inhaling both particle aerosols that travel 3 feet or less and small particle aerosols that remain suspended in the air. Masks should be used only once because they are ineffective when moist. Masks should cover both the nose and the mouth.

5. *Gowns.* Gowns are recommended if soiling of clothes with infective materials is likely (for example, holding an infant who has infectious diarrhea). Gowns are worn only once and are not to be worn outside the patient's room.

6. *Gloves.* Gloves must be worn by the healthcare worker when there is potential for contact with any of the following body fluids: blood or any body fluid containing visible blood, semen, vaginal secretions, tissues, cerebrospinal fluid, synovial fluid, pleural fluid, peritoneal fluid, pericardial fluid, and amniotic fluid. Gloves must be worn when handling any articles contaminated with these fluids and when cleaning up these fluids from the environment. No-touch technique (the ability to perform a procedure without gloves and without contaminating hands) is acceptable for some activities, such as changing diapers. Gloves must be changed and hands washed between patients. Gloves are to be removed for nonpatient care activities unless contamination with body fluids is expected. Intact latex and intact vinyl gloves are equally effective barriers. The type of glove selected should be appropriate for the task to be performed. Used gloves should be discarded in an appropriate receptacle.

7. *Needles and syringes.* To prevent needle-stick injuries, used needles, syringes, and scalpels should not be recapped, but placed in the nearest designated puncture-resistant container.

8. *Thermometers.* Disposable glass thermometers are available and should be used for patients on isolation precautions. The thermometer may be sent home with the child on discharge.

9. *Food trays.* Dishes and utensils used by patients in isolation will be bagged in a red plastic bag, tied shut, and removed from the patient's room by the nurse.

10. *Linen.* Soiled linen should be handled as little as possible and with a minimum of agitation to prevent microbial contamination of the air and of persons handling the linen. Linen must be bagged in a single yellow bag or double-bagged in a hot-water soluble bag and then a yellow bag. The nurse will remove the linen bags from the patient's room and place them in a designated location.

11. *Toys, books, and magazines.* Any of these articles soiled with infective material should be disinfected or destroyed.

12. *Specimens.* All specimens for laboratory examination from patients on isolation must be placed in a container with a tight-fitting lid, labeled with an isolation sticker, and bagged in a clear plastic bag.

13. *Transporting of patients.* Patients in isolation should be taken out of their isolation area only for medically indicated reasons. Appropriate barriers to prevent disease transmission should be provided for the entire period the patient is out of the isolated room. The area to which the patient is to be taken should be notified of the patient's pending arrival and techniques to be applied to prevent the spread of infections.

14. *Postmortem handling of bodies.* Personnel should use the same precautions to protect themselves during postmortem handling of bodies that they would use if

the patient were still alive. Masks, however, are not necessary unless aerosols are expected to be generated. Autopsy personnel should be notified about the patient's disease so that appropriate precautions can be maintained (Table 22-1).

Table 22-1. Summary of Precautions

Isolation Type	Private Room	Mask/Gown	Gloves	Dishes	Linen	Garbage	Comments
Strict	Yes—usually special ventilation required	Yes/Yes	Yes	Yes	Yes	Yes	Toys must be decontaminated before reuse.
Respiratory	Yes	Yes/No	No	No	No	Yes	No special consideration for toys.
Enteric	Patients with same organism may share a room.	No/No*	Yes	Yes	Yes	Yes	Clean grossly contaminated toys with an antimicrobial agent.
Contact	No	No/No*	Yes	Yes	Yes	Yes	Clean grossly contaminated toys with an antimicrobial agent.
Blood or Body	Yes—if patient's hygiene is poor.	No/No*	Yes	Yes	Yes	Yes	Clean grossly contaminated toys with an antimicrobial agent.
RSV	Yes—cohorting is suggested during outbreaks.	Yes/No*	Yes	No	No	Yes	Toys must be decontaminated before reuse.
Protective	Yes	Yes (including shoe covers).	Yes	Yes	Yes	Yes	Games and toys must be decontaminated prior to being taken into the room.

* If soiling with secretions is likely, a gown is required.

Assessment

1. Assess the pertinent history for recent exposure to communicable disease, recent travel, and immunization status of child and family.
2. Assess the physical findings in relation to vital signs, respiratory and gastrointestinal symptoms, neurologic compromise, and skin disorders.
3. Assess the family's knowledge of the disease, their acceptance of treatment, and their willingness to learn the care needed by their child.
4. Assess psychosocial and developmental factors that would influence the child in isolation (for example, age, coping mechanisms, daily habits, and activities).

Nursing Diagnoses

The following is a list of possible diagnoses and could apply, depending on the child's age, clinical situation, and physical condition:

Anxiety

Fear

Ineffective individual coping

Ineffective family coping, compromised

Ineffective family coping, disabling

Altered family process

Social isolation

Sensory/perceptual alterations: visual, auditory, tactile, olfactory

Planning

When planning to set up an area for isolation, the following equipment must be obtained:

Outside Room

Isolation cart (for masks and gowns) (Fig. 22-1)

Appropriate isolation sign for door of room (Fig. 22-2)

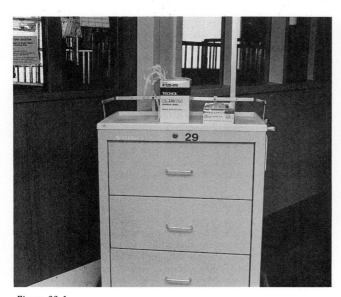

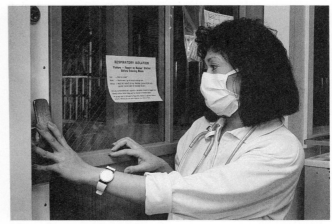

Figure 22-2.

Figure 22-1.

Inside Room

Examination gloves

Red and yellow bags

Thermometer kit

Container for needle disposal (Fig. 22-3)

Fluid measurement container.

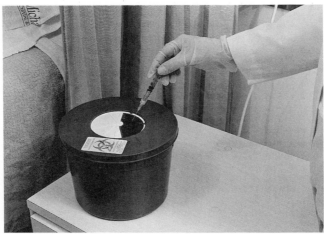

Figure 22-3.

Interventions

PROCEDURE	**RATIONALE/EXPECTED OUTCOME (EO)**
1. Obtain necessary equipment to prepare the room for isolation.	*EO: The child will not pose a threat to the health of others.*
2. Place the appropriate equipment inside and outside the room.	
3. Explain to the child or parents the rationale for isolation—inform them of those body secretions or excretions that contain the infecting organism and demonstrate techniques to contain the organism and prevent transmission.	Information and discussion concerning the transmission of the disease to friends, siblings, or adult family members will help alleviate fear and anxiety. *EO: The child or parent will have decreased apprehension about the disease and the isolation procedure.*
4. Explain the expected duration of isolation.	The child will be isolated from individuals at risk and may become bored or restless from the restrictions imposed. *EO: The child will be entertained without being socially isolated.*
5. Provide age-appropriate quiet activities (for example, artwork, records, TV, or board games).	
6. Provide for continuation of school through the hospital teacher.	
7. Encourage phone calls from friends and family.	
8. Encourage a limited number of family members, depending on the reason for the isolation, to visit and provide a social time for the child.	

Patient/Family Education: Home Care Considerations

1. Review with the family the description of the disease, methods of control, action needed for the child's health and education and their contacts and community (report these to the health department)
2. Urge immediate medical care for exposed children, particularly those who have not been immunized or who are immunocompromised.
3. Provide guidelines for the child's return to day care or school.

References

Children's Memorial Hospital. (1985). *Guidelines for infection control.* Chicago: Children's Memorial Hospital.

Michael Reese Hospital and Medical Center. (1988). *Policy manual.* Chicago: Michael Reese Hospital and Medical Center.

Michael Reese Hospital and Medical Center. (1988). Pediatric guidelines for infection control of human immunodeficiency virus in hospitals, medical offices, schools and other settings. *Pediatrics,* November. 801–807.

Plotkin, S. A., Evans H. E., Fast, N. C., et al. (1988). Task force on pediatric AIDS—Pediatric guidelines for infection control of HIV in hospitals, medical offices, schools and other settings. *Pediatrics, 85*(5), 801–807.

U.S. Department of Health and Human Services/Public Health Service. (1988). *Morbidity and Mortality Weekly Report 37* (24). Rockville, MD: Centers for Disease Control.

Weinstein, S.A., Gontz, N. M., Pelletier, C., et al. (1989). Bacterial surface contamination of patients' linen: Isolation precautions versus standard care. *American Journal of Infection Control, 17*(5), 264–267.

Medication Administration Procedures

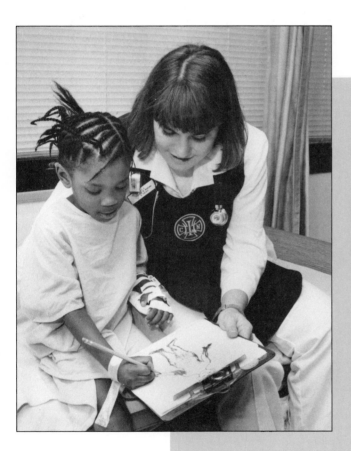

Unit IV

Medication Administration

23

Definition/Purpose

To safely and accurately administer medication to a child, taking into account weight, surface area, and the ability of the child to absorb, metabolize, and excrete the medication.

Standard of Care

To avoid medication errors, always follow these five steps in preparing and administering medications to pediatric patients:

1. *Right child.* Always check the identification band of the child before administering the medication. Never assume that the child in the bed is the child assigned to that bed. Children sometimes switch beds. If the identification band is missing, the nurse needs to identify the child by asking a parent, caretaker, or the child (if he or she is old enough), and then replace the band immediately.

2. *Right drug.* Check the label on the medication. If the label is not clear, or is suspicious or confusing, do not give the medication. Call the pharmacist and have the drug relabeled. Check the drug's expiration date; do not administer outdated drugs. Check the consistency and color of the drug and be aware of the signs of deterioration.

3. *Right dose.* If in doubt about how much medication is an appropriate dose, check a reference before administering it. Check your institution's policy for which medications need to be double-checked by two people (for example, insulin and digoxin). When reducing a standard dose to a smaller dose, take time to calculate the dosage. Always clarify poorly written orders. Decimal points in orders may result in serious errors if overlooked or interpreted incorrectly. The use of unapproved abbreviations also causes confusion. Lastly, check drug references before mixing any medications to determine the compatibility of the drugs.

4. *Right route.* Some drugs are never given by certain routes because the route would hinder the action of the drug. Always question a confusing or inappropriate order.

5. *Right time.* Always make a note of when the medication is to be given. Check the amount of the drug in stock so that the desired dose is available at the proper administration time.

Follow these nine rules in guiding your medication administration to the pediatric patient:

1. Never give a child a choice of whether or not to receive medicine. The medication is ordered and is necessary for recovery; therefore, there is no choice to be made.

2. However, do give choices that allow the child some control over the situation, such as the kind of juice, the number of bandages, or the injection site.

3. Never lie. Do not tell a child that a shot will not hurt.

4. Keep explanations simple and brief. Use words that the child will comprehend.

5. Assure the child that it is all right to be afraid and that it is okay to cry.

6. Do not talk in front of the child as if the child were not there. Include the child in the conversation when talking to parents.

7. Be positive in approaching the child. Be firm and assertive when explaining to the child what will happen.

8. Keep the time between explanation and execution to a minimum. The younger the child, the shorter the time should be. Keep the explanation simple. Preparations such as setting up injections, solutions, or instrument trays should be done out of the child's sight.

9. Obtain parental cooperation. Parents may be able to calm a frightened child, persuade the child to take the medication, and achieve cooperation for care.

Assessment

1. Assess the child or family for any previous experience with medications or hospitalizations.

2. Assess the child's level of consciousness; pulmonary, cardiovascular, and gastrointestinal functions; muscle strength and mass.

3. Assess the child's developmental level and usual coping mechanisms (Table 23–1).

4. Assess the child for allergies to medications.

Table 23-1. Developmental Considerations

Age	Behaviors	Nursing Actions
Birth–3 months	1. Reaches randomly toward mouth and has a strong reflex to grasp objects	1. The infant's hands must be held to prevent spilling of medications.
	2. Poor head control	2. The infant's head must be supported while medications are being given.
	3. Tongue movement may force medication out of mouth	3. A syringe or dropper should be placed along the side of the mouth.
	4. Sucks as a reflex with stimulation	4. Use this natural sucking desire by placing oral medications into a nipple and administering in that manner.
	5. Stops sucking when full	5. Administer medications before feeding when infant is hungry. Be aware that some medications' absorption will be affected by food.
	6. Infant responds to tactile stimulation	6. The likelihood that the medication is taken will increase if the infant is held in a feeding position.
3–12 months	7. Begins to develop fine muscle control and advances from sitting to crawling	7. Medication must be kept out of reach to avoid accidental ingestion.
	8. Tongue may protrude when swallowing	8. Administer medication with a syringe.
	9. Responds to tactile stimuli	9. Physical comfort (holding) given after a medication will be helpful.
12–30 months	10. Advances from independent walking to running without falling	10. Allow the toddler to choose position for taking a medication.
	11. Advances from messy self-feeding to proficient feeding with minimal spilling	11. Allow the toddler to take medicine from a cup or spoon.

(continued)

Table 23-1. (*continued*)

Age	Behaviors	Nursing Actions
	12. Has voluntary tongue control. Begins to drink from a cup.	12. Disguise medication in a small amount of food to decrease incidence of spitting out medication.
	13. Develops second molars	13. Chewable tablets may be an alternative.
	14. Exhibits independence and self-assertiveness	14. Allow as much freedom as possible. Use games to gain confidence. Use a consistent firm approach. Give immediate praise for cooperation.
	15. Responds to sense of time and simple direction	15. Given directions to "Drink this now" and "Open your mouth".
	16. Responds to and participates in routines of daily living	16. Involve the parents and include the toddler in medicine routines.
	17. Expresses feelings easily	17. Allow for expression through play.
30 months–6 years	18. Knows full name	18. Ask the child his or her name before giving the medicine.
	19. Is easily influenced by others when responding to new foods or tastes	19. Approach the child in a calm positive manner when giving medications.
	20. Has a good sense of time and a tolerance of frustration	20. Use correct immediate rewards for the young child and delayed gratification for the older child.
	21. Enjoys making decisions	21. Give choices when possible.
	22. Has many fantasies. Has fear of mutilation	22. Give simple explanations. Stress that the medication is not being given because the child is bad.
	23. Is more coordinated	23. Can hold cup and may be able to master pill-taking.
	24. Begins to lose teeth	24. Chewable tablets may be inappropriate because of loose teeth.
6–12 years	25. Strives for independence	25. Give acceptable choices. Respect the need for regression during hospitalization.
	26. Has concern for bodily mutilation	26. Give reassurance that medication given, especially injectables, will not cause harm. Reinforce that medications should only be taken when given by nurse or parent.
	27. Can tell time	27. Include the child in daily schedule of medication. Make the child a poster of medications and time due so he or she can be involved in care.
	28. Is concerned with body image and privacy	28. Provide private area for administration of medication, especially injections.
	29. Peer support and interaction are important	29. Allow child to share experiences with others.
12+ years	30. Strives for independence	30. Write a contract with the adolescent, spelling out expectations for self-medication.
	31. Is able to understand abstract theories	31. Explain why medications are given and how they work.

(*continued*)

Table 23-1. (*continued*)

Age	Behaviors	Nursing Actions
	32. Decisions are influenced by peers	32. Encourage teens to talk with their peers in a support group. Work with teens to plan medication schedule around their activities. Differentiate pill-taking from drug-taking.
	33. Questions authority figures	33. Be honest and provide medication information in writing.
	34. Is concerned with sex and sexuality	34. Explain relationship between illness, medications, and sexuality. For example, emphasize that "This medication will not react with your birth control pills."

Nursing Diagnoses

The following is a list of possible diagnoses and could apply, depending on the child's age, clinical situation, and physical condition:

Fear

Anxiety

High risk for injury

Pain

Powerlessness

Self-esteem disturbance

Planning

When planning to administer a medication, assemble the appropriate equipment:

Medicine dropper

Syringe (with or without needle)

Nipple

Medicine cup and spoon

Finger cot

Alcohol

Adhesive bandage

Lubricant

Interventions

PROCEDURE

RATIONALE/EXPECTED OUTCOME (EO)

Oral Medications

1. *Dropper.* Wash hands. Hold the infant in the cradle position and stabilize the head against your body.

The infant should be held on the nurse's or parent's lap to provide security and comfort. If infant cannot be held,

PROCEDURE

Hold infant's arm with your free arm. Press on the infant's chin to open mouth. Squirt the medication to the back and side of the mouth in small amounts.

2. *Syringe.* Hold the infant or toddler in the cradle position, supporting the head and holding the arms. Place the syringe to the back and side of the mouth and give the medication slowly, allowing the child to swallow.

3. *Nipple.* Hold the infant in the cradle position, squirting the medication from the syringe into the nipple. Pour the medication from a cup into the nipple. Allow the infant to suck the medication from the nipple. Follow the medication with 2–3 mL of water (Fig. 23-1).

RATIONALE/EXPECTED OUTCOME (EO)

lift the baby's head off the mattress and cradle in your hand.

EO: The child will receive an accurate dose of the medication in the least frightening method for the child.

Give the infant or toddler 3–4 squirts per 5 mL of medication.

EO: The safe administration of the medication will allay the fears of both child and parent.

Do not add medication to the infant's formula, since the infant may not take the entire feeding. Avoid giving medications with essential foods such as milk, cereal, or juice so the infant does not associate food with medication and refuse to take it in the future. Nonessential foods such as applesauce or Jello can be used in small amounts.

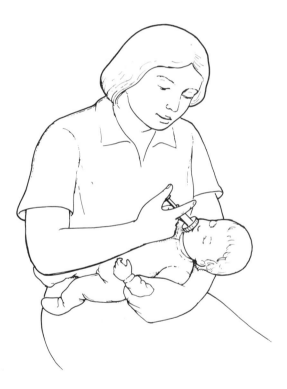

Figure 23-1.

4. *Medicine cup.* A cup can be used for the older infant, toddler, preschooler, school-age child, and adolescent. For the younger patient, a parent or the child may hold the cup. Stay with the child until the entire dose is swallowed.

A spoon is an effective alternative to the medicine cup. Disguise a disagreeable taste in a small amount of food like applesauce. Syrup is also good for mixing medications that do not dissolve in water. Dilute alcohol-based elixirs with water before administering.

EO: The child has a sense of power and control over medication administration.

PROCEDURE

5. *Chewable tablets.* Tablets may be chewed by the child or crushed and given in a fruit syrup or applesauce. Check with the pharmacist to see if crushing the tablet will affect drug absorption or action. Do not give a child a tablet if he or she resists, as the child could easily aspirate.

6. *Capsules.* Older children may enjoy swallowing a capsule. Place the capsule on the back of the tongue and have them swallow a lot of fluid. Stay with the child until all the medicine is swallowed. Some capsules may also be opened and the contents sprinkled on a spoonful of food. Check with the pharmacist to see which capsules can be opened.

Nose Drops. Hold the infant in the cradle position, stabilizing the head with your arm, and tilting it back slightly. Squeeze the drops into each nostril as you try to comfort and hold the infant in this position for at least 1 minute. (Place a toddler's head over a pillow.) Squeeze the drops into each nostril. The school-age child and adolescent may give themselves their own medication since they can sniff the medication into the nasal passages.

Ear Drops. Position infants and toddlers on their sides. The pinna of the ear is to be pulled down and back. Instill warm drops into the external canal and gently massage the area anterior to the ear (Fig. 23-2).

RATIONALE/EXPECTED OUTCOME (EO)

An increasing number of medications are designed to release the active ingredient over a period of time. Disrupting the formulation of these products can affect the rate of absorption and potentiate the risk of toxic side effects.

Because infants are nose-breathers and nasal congestion inhibits sucking, nose drops should be given 20–30 minutes before feeding. Keeping the infant in a backward tilt will allow the drug to coat the nasal surface. Avoid placing the toddler over the edge of the bed, as it will frighten him or her. The lowered position is necessary, as the infant and toddler cannot sniff the medication into the nasal passages.

Warm drops avoid causing pain of the tympanic membrane. The gentle massaging facilitates entry of the drops.

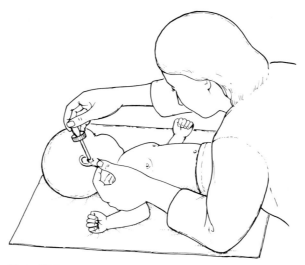

Figure 23-2.

For children over 3 years, pull the pinna upwards and back. After the instillation, the child should maintain the position for 5–10 minutes. A cotton pledget placed into the ear canal can prevent the medication from leaking out; however, it must be loose enough to allow discharge to drain from the ear canal.

The anatomy of the ear changes, necessitating the difference in instillation.
This will ensure that the medication remains in contact with the ear canal.

PROCEDURE

Eye Drops or Ointment. Place the child in a supine position, restraining him or her as necessary to safely instill the medication. (You may need help from another person.) Pull the lower eyelid down and out to form a cup. Drop the solution into cup. The medicine will enter the conjunctiva. Close the eye gently and attempt to keep it closed for a few moments (Fig. 23-3).

RATIONALE/EXPECTED OUTCOME (EO)

Toddlers will resist anyone or anything coming near their faces.
This facilitates bathing the eye with the medication.

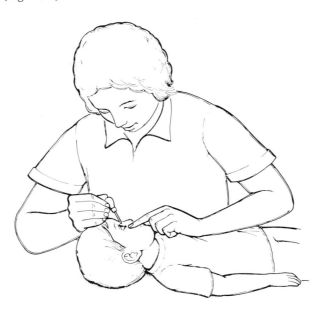

Figure 23-3.

Ointments are applied along the inner canthus in an outward direction. Avoid touching the tip of the dropper or ointment tube to the body part.

Rectal Medications. Place the child in a side-lying or prone position. Lubricate the suppository with a water soluble gel. Using a finger cot, gently insert the suppository into the rectum. Do not insert your finger more than $\frac{1}{2}$ inch. The buttocks should be held tightly together for 5–10 minutes.

Multidose bottles or tubes of medication easily support the growth of bacteria from contaminated dropper tips.

The administration of rectal medication may be resisted by children, even if they are accustomed to having their temperature taken rectally.

This will prevent quick expulsion of the medication, which gives the drug inadequate time to absorb. Concern for privacy is significant during the school-age and adolescent years. Provide privacy and assess whether the child wants the parents present.

Intramuscular Injections

Choosing the Site

Factors that must be considered:
1. Amount of muscle mass
2. Type of medication to be given
3. Amount and character of the medication. The volume of solution should be no more than 1.0 mL for infants and small children and 2.0 mL in the older child.
4. Number of injections to be given during the course of treatment
5. Ability of the child to assume the necessary position.
Always dispose of needles in a puncture-proof container.

PROCEDURE

1. *Vastus Lateralis.* This main muscle in the thigh is used most often for IM injections in all age groups, but especially in infants. Locate the trochanter of the femur and the knee, and divide the area into thirds. Give the injection into the middle third, grasping the thigh and compressing the muscle. Direct the needle perpendicular to the skin or at a 45° angle toward the knee (Fig. 23-4*A* and 23-4*B*).

RATIONALE/EXPECTED OUTCOME (EO)

Assess the child's muscle mass before choosing a needle:

- Infant—Use either a 25-gauge, $\frac{5}{8}$-inch needle or a 23-gauge, 1-inch needle.
- Toddler, school-age, or adolescent—a 22-gauge, 1–1½-inch needle is acceptable.

EO: The child will safely have an intramuscular drug administered.

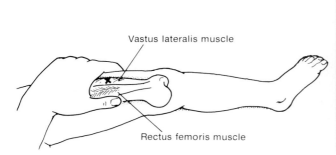

Figure 23-4A.

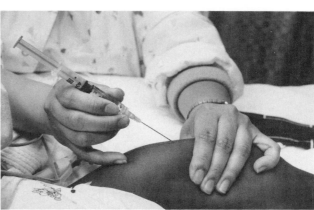

Figure 23-4B.

2. *Ventrogluteal.* Place your index finger on the anterior-superior iliac spine and your second finger at the iliac crest (Fig. 23-5). Inject the medication be-

These muscles contain no important nerves.

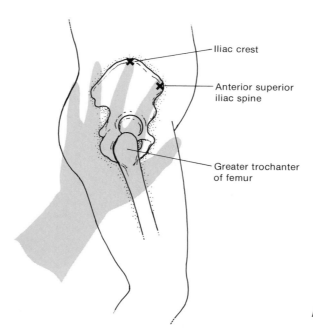

Figure 23-5.

PROCEDURE

RATIONALE/EXPECTED OUTCOME (EO)

low the iliac crest at a 90° angle inside the triangle formed by these landmarks. Limit the amount of medication injected into one site:

- Infant—$\frac{1}{2}$–$\frac{3}{4}$ mL
- Toddler—1 mL
- School-age child or adolescent—$1\frac{1}{2}$–3 mL.

Avoid giving injections to children in their beds or in the playroom since they should consider these safe places. If possible, take the child to the treatment room for painful procedures. Cover the puncture site with an adhesive bandage to prevent small children from thinking their insides are leaking out.

3. *Gluteal region.* The posterior gluteal muscle is not recommended as an injection site until the child has been walking for at least 1 year. Place the child supine and encourage a toe-in position (Fig. 23-6).

   Palpate the posterior-superior iliac spine and the head of the greater trochanter of the femur. Give the injection superior and lateral to an imaginary line between these landmarks. Direct the needle in a straight back-to-front course (Fig. 23-7).

EO: The child engages in constructive activities that channel his or her emotions.

Walking helps develop the gluteal muscle.
The toe-in position relaxes the muscle.

EO: The child learns and uses muscle relaxation techniques.

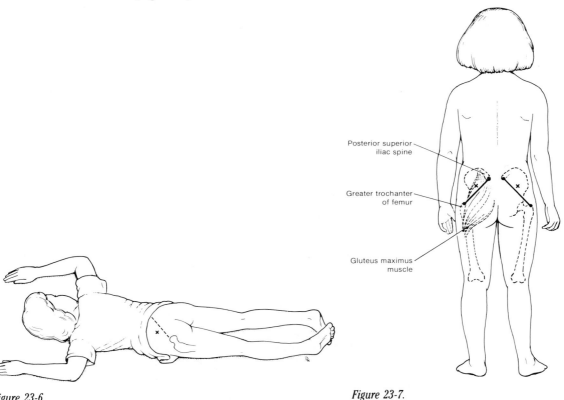

Posterior superior
iliac spine

Greater trochanter
of femur

Gluteus maximus
muscle

Figure 23-6.

Figure 23-7.

4. *Deltoid.* The deltoid muscle is shallow and can only accommodate a small amount of fluid (1.0 mL). Position the child in any position that is convenient for the child and the person who will help hold the

Repeated injections in this area are painful. This is an excellent site for an on-time immunization.
Do not use for infants.
Rotate all injection sites if possible.

PROCEDURE   **RATIONALE/EXPECTED OUTCOME (EO)**

child. The child's entire arm and shoulder should be exposed. Give the injection in the densest part of the muscle, above the armpit and below the acromion. Grasp the muscle mass and compress, inserting the needle slightly upward toward the shoulder (Fig. 23-8).

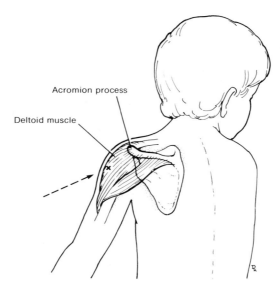

Acromion process

Deltoid muscle

Figure 23-8.

Intradermal Injections. The medial surface of the forearm is the most common site for administration. These injections are made into the upper layers of the skin (as in TB skin tests and allergy tests). A needle should be inserted bevel-up at a 15° angle. A 25-gauge, $\frac{5}{8}$-inch needle should be used. No more than 0.1 mL should be injected. A small bleb should form (Fig. 23-9).

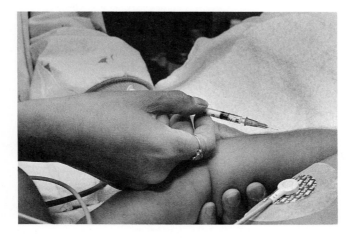

Figure 23-9.

Subcutaneous Injections. Subcutaneous injections are made just below the skin. All IM injection sites can be used, as well as interscapular, abdominal wall, and subscapular areas. Drugs given this way (for example, epinephrine, heparin, insulin) are absorbed slowly.

The advantages of subcutaneous injections include the presence of many sites and the unlikelihood of damaging nerves or blood vessels. The disadvantage is the limited kinds of drugs and the limited volumes of them that can be injected.

PROCEDURE

Hold the tissue to form a cushion, insert the needle in a dart-like fashion, and release the tissue. Aspirate and then inject the medicine. Withdraw the needle quickly and massage the site with dry gauze. A 26-gauge, ⅜-inch needle or 25-gauge, ⅝-inch needle should be used. No more than 0.5 mL of medication should be given to a small child or 1.0 mL to the preschooler and adolescent (Fig. 23-10).

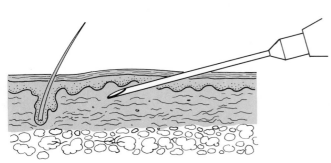

Figure 23-10A.

RATIONALE/EXPECTED OUTCOME (EO)

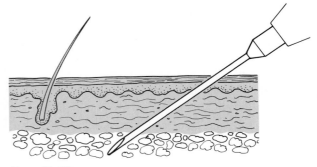

Figure 23-10B.

Z-Track. After drawing up the ordered medication and 0.2 to 0.3 mL of air, replace the needle with a new one. Pull the skin laterally away from the intended injection site. After cleaning the site, insert the needle and inject the medication slowly. When you have completed the injection, wait 10 seconds before you withdraw the needle (Fig. 23-11).

This will ensure proper entry into muscle tissue.

EO: The child will receive the medication with the least irritation and discoloration.

This will prevent seepage of the medication from the site.

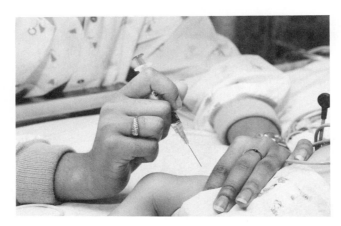

Figure 23-11.

Withdraw the needle and allow the retracted skin to resume its normal position. Do not massage the site.

This will seal off the needle track.
The medication could be forced into the subcutaneous tissue and cause irritation if massaged.

Patient/Family Education: Home Care Considerations

1. The parent or child will be informed of the name of the medication given to the child and why it is necessary to the medical treatment.
2. The parent will know how to provide comfort measures for the distressed infant or child:
   a. Provide human contact.

b. Provide vestibular stimulation—Rocking in supine position or being held upright over the shoulder.

c. Provide a pacifier, especially for the infant who is NPO.

d. Record parent's voice so that it can be played back in parent's absence.

e. Allow the child to play with syringes with the needles removed to reduce stress and provide an outlet for anger.

3. If the child is being discharged on medication the parent will need to know the following:

a. Nature of the drug

b. Purpose for which the drug is given

c. Amount of drug to be given

d. Frequency with which drug will be given (the next dose to be given following discharge)

e. Length of time for drug to be administered

f. How the drug is to be administered

g. Anticipated effects of the drug

h. Signs that might indicate an adverse reaction to the drug, and whom to contact.

4. The parent will be given a demonstration of how to administer the medication and will return the demonstration.

References

Beecroft, P., & Redick, S. (1989). Possible complications of intramuscular injections on the pediatric unit. *Pediatric Nursing, 15*(4), 333–336.

Howry, L.B., & Bindler, R.M. (1981). *Pediatric medications*. Philadelphia: J.B. Lippincott Company.

Keen, M.F. (1986). Comparison of intramuscular injection techniques to reduce site discomfort and lesions. *Nursing Research, 35*(4), 207–210.

Litteral, J. (1990). What are the clinically important drug–nutrient interactions? *Pediatric Nursing, 16*(6), 594–596.

Mitchell, J.F., & Pavlicki, K.S. (1990). Oral dose forms that should not be crushed: 1990 revision. *Hospital Pharmacy, 25,* 329–335, Pawlicki, K. S. *25*

Petrillo, J., & Sanger, S. (1980). *Emotional care of hospitalized children* (2nd ed.). Philadelphia: J.B. Lippincott Company.

Stewart, C., & Stewart, L. (1984). *Pediatric medication: An emergency and critical care reference*. Rockville, MD: Aspen Systems Corporation.

Intravenous Medications

24

Definition/Purpose

Administering medications via the intravenous route has become common in the pediatric setting. Intravenous injections are the most effective way to elicit a quick response and are the only acceptable routes for administration of some drugs. They also provide less traumatic administration of medications to children. The following groups of children are prime candidates for IV medication administration:

- Children with poor absorption due to vomiting or diarrhea
- Children who require a high serum concentration of a drug in a short period of time (as in sepsis, increased intracranial pressure, and meningitis)
- Children with resistant infections who require IV medications over a long period of time.

The site selected for intravenous fluid and medication administration depends on accessibility and convenience. For infants, a superficial vein of the hand, foot, or wrist is usually easy to find and stabilize. Also, veins of the scalp have no valves; thus IVs can be inserted in either direction. For toddlers and older children, any accessible vein may be used.

Standard of Care

1. Properly dilute the medication using the package directions. Never use a different volume of diluent, since the powder will be displaced in a different proportion. For neonates, use sterile water or normal saline without preservatives.

2. Check the package for the type of solution in which the drug may be given, as this varies for different medications. Also check the amount of solution to be administered.

3. Check the length of time over which the drug may safely be given.

4. Consider the rate of infusion that the infant or child may tolerate. If the only accessible vein is small or fragile, you may want to infuse the drug at a slower rate. Be alert for drugs which must be given within a limited time frame in order to avoid disintegration.

5. Check the compatibility of all the drugs the child is receiving by the intravenous route.

6. Assess the cumulative effect of all the drugs the child is receiving. For example, two different drugs the child may be receiving may both have a tendency to cause renal failure. Make the appropriate assessments and notify the physician of problems.

7. Assess the IV site prior to infusion of the medication. The medication should not be given if there is any sign of IV infiltration.

8. Medication labels must be placed on the IV bag, buretrol, or tubing to indicate that the additions have been made.

9. Follow any IV medications with an appropriate flush solution to ensure that all the medication has been infused.

10. Use an IV pump whenever possible to ensure a constant rate of drug infusion.

Assessment

1. Assess for any previous problems with IVs and IV medications (for example, infiltrations and chemical burns).
2. Assess the location of the IV, the medication to be given, the hydrational status and weight of the child, and the appropriateness of the dose ordered.
3. Assess the child's coping mechanisms for painful procedures, according to age and developmental level and what comforts the child.
4. Assess the family's knowledge of IV therapy and medication administration via the intravenous route.
5. Assess whether child is allergic to medication.

Nursing Diagnoses

The following is a list of possible diagnoses and could apply, depending on the child's age, clinical situation, and physical condition:

Fear

Pain

Impaired skin integrity

Fluid volume excess

Planning

Assemble the following equipment in order to administer intravenous medications:

Medication to be administered

Appropriate dilution solution for medication

Needles

Syringes

Functioning IV line on an infusion pump

Alcohol swabs

Medication labels.

Interventions

PROCEDURE

1. Explain to the child or parent the need for IV medications and how they will be administered. Emphasis must be placed on the fact that some medication can be given by different IV methods.

2. **Retrograde Infusion**
   The medication is injected into a port or stopcock in the IV line. Clamp the IV tubing near the child to allow the medication to flow away from the child.

RATIONALE/EXPECTED OUTCOME (EO)

The parent needs to understand that different techniques may be used to administer the same drug and that each technique delivers the drug appropriately.

EO: The parent or child will express their fears and concerns to the staff.

This method is chosen for small infants or children who cannot tolerate a high IV infusion rate or excess fluid volume.

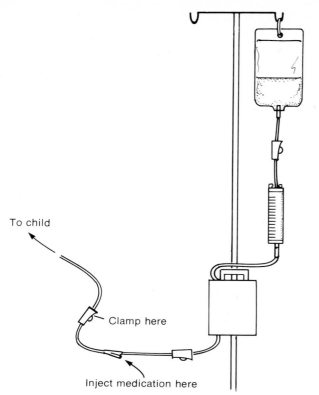

To child

Clamp here

Inject medication here

Figure 24-1.

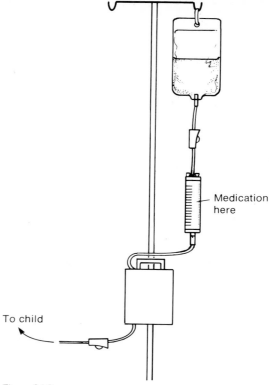

Medication here

To child

Figure 24-2.

PROCEDURE

When the clamp is released the medication will flow with the IV solution toward the child at the rate set on the pump (Fig. 24-1).

3. ***Controlled Volume Chamber Infusion***
   The medication is injected into the buretrol above the IV pump. Clamp the buretrol air vent before gently mixing the medication in the buretrol fluid. Unclamp the air vent when you are done mixing (Fig. 24-2).

4. ***IV Push***
   The medication is injected directly into a port or stopcock close to the IV insertion site. Clamp the IV tubing above the port or stopcock so the medication will be pushed toward the patient and not backward up the tubing. Check carefully the time during which the drug can be given. Constantly assess child during administration. A variation to IV push is the use of a syringe pump with concentrated medication inserted into the IV line at the medication port and set for a specific infusion rate.

5. ***Piggyback Infusions***
   The medication is mixed in a secondary IV bag. The secondary administration set is then inserted via a needle into a port of the primary IV solution.

RATIONALE/EXPECTED OUTCOME (EO)

EO: The child will maintain appropriate fluid volume for age, size, diagnosis, and status.

A disadvantage of this method is that it is not practical for use in infants and small children, whose IV rates are slow. Also, only one drug may be given at a time using this method.

EO: The child will be free from pain associated with continuous IV therapy and medication administration.

This method is often used in emergency situations when the medication should not be excessively diluted or when peak drug levels are desirable. It is also used for postoperative pain control.

EO: The child's skin will remain free of irritation from the medication administered.

PROCEDURE	RATIONALE/EXPECTED OUTCOME (EO)
The piggyback solution may be placed on a pump, or it can be dripped to gravity (Fig. 24-3).	If the piggyback bag is left to gravity, it must be at a higher level than the primary IV solution.

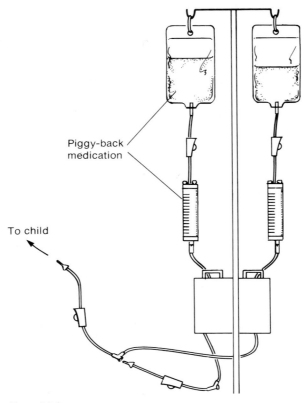

Piggy-back medication

To child

Figure 24-3.

Patient/Family Education: Home Care Considerations

1. Prepare the child and family for the IV therapy according to their level of understanding. Some children may need reassurance that the IV procedure is safe and has no connection to illegal "street" drugs. Be honest in describing any physical sensations that the child may feel when the medication infuses.

2. If the child will require intravenous medication at home, the medication can be administered via a central venous line or via a peripheral route using sterile technique. The family must be instructed on how to administer the medication safely and what adverse reactions to watch for.

References

Axton, S.E., & Fugate, T. (1987). A protocol for pediatric IV medication. *American Journal of Nursing, 87*(7), 943–946D.

DeMonaco, J.J. (1988). IV drug therapy: New technologies for consideration. *Journal of Intravenous Nursing, 11*(5), 316–320.

Hardgrove, C. (1987). Administration of IV medications in the NICU: The development of a procedure. *Neonatal Network, 6*(2), 41–58.

Howry, L.B. (1981). *Pediatric medications.* Philadelphia: J.B. Lippincott.

Lunn, J.K., & Wilson, A. (1986). Retrograde medication administration: A predictable and simple system for pediatric drug delivery. *Focus on Critical Care, 13*(6), 59–63.

Stewart, C., & Stewart, L. (1984). *Pediatric medications: An emergency and critical care reference.* Rockville, M.D.: Aspen Systems Corporation.

Topical Medications

25

Definition/Purpose

Topical medication treatment is the application of an active ingredient directly to an affected area. Most skin disorders will respond to topical therapy.

A variety of agents and methods are available for treatment of dermatologic problems. They are applied via a pharmacologically inert vehicle that contributes to the therapy with physical properties that protect, soothe, or cleanse. When choosing an agent, the following must be considered:

1. Choice of the active ingredient
2. Proper vehicle
3. Cosmetic effect
4. Cost
5. Instructions needed for its use.

In addition, there are several basic concepts that need to be kept in mind when using topical therapy:

1. Overtreatment should be avoided. Broken or inflamed skin is more absorbent than intact skin; thus, less medication may be needed if the child's skin is broken or inflamed.
2. Chemicals that are nonirritating to intact skin may be quite irritating to inflamed skin.
3. The dermatitic skin is more apt to develop allergic contact-type sensitization to substances applied.

The most frequently used topical treatments for skin disorders are:

1. Wet dressings
2. Soaks
3. Lotions and shake solutions
4. Baths
5. Creams or ointments
6. Pastes
7. Powders
8. Occlusive dressings
9. Soaps and shampoos
10. Sunscreening agents
11. Glucocorticoid therapy
12. Other: chemical cautery, cryosurgery, or ultraviolet therapy.

Standard of Care

1. As with all medications, never leave these topical medications within reach of a child. Place all medications in a locked cabinet.

2. Never leave a child alone with a basin, bucket, or tub of soak solution. Children can drown in a small amount of fluid or may ingest the solution.

3. The nurse will wear gloves to protect the child and the nurse from flora in open lesions on the skin.

4. The nurse will wear gloves for protection from the active ingredients in the therapy.

5. The nurse will determine if the child is allergic to the medication or its ingredients (such as iodine).

Assessment

1. Assess the pertinent history and physical findings in relation to history of onset; the presenting symptoms such as itching, pain and fever; the type of lesion and its configuration and distribution, and any associated characteristics such as moisture or swelling.

2. Assess developmental concerns such as age, coping mechanisms, body image status, loss of control, self-imposed isolation from peers and family, and compliance with health care treatments.

3. Assess the family's perception of the child's illness and their readiness and willingness to support the child and learn the home care needed for treatment.

Nursing Diagnoses

The following is a list of possible diagnoses and could apply, depending on the child's age, clinical situation, and physical condition:

Pain

Body image disturbance

High risk for infection

Impaired skin integrity

Altered nutrition, less than body requirements

Ineffective individual coping

High risk for altered body temperature

Fear

Planning

When planning to apply a topical medication, the following should be assembled:

Kerlix

Tape

Stockinette

Sterile gloves

Soak solution or lotion

Basin

Appropriate diversional toys

Thermometer

Tongue depressor

Thin plastic film

Mineral oil

Gloves.

Interventions

PROCEDURE

1. Explain to the child or parent the need for the application of topical medication, the expected duration of treatment, the actual application technique, and how the child and family can assist in the treatment.

2. *Wet Dressings.* The open wet dressings cool the skin by evaporation, relieve itching and inflammation, and cleanse the area by loosening and removing debris. Wet-to-dry dressings are common in burn care and help remove eschar when the dry dressing is removed. Any of a variety of solutions can be used.
   a. Gather equipment.
   b. Put on sterile gloves.
   c. Immerse Kerlix in desired solution (at room temperature).
   d. Wring out Kerlix roll slightly (Fig. 25-1A).
   e. Apply to affected area in a flat, smooth manner. Do not restrict motion of the joints. Allow elbows and knees to bend (Fig. 25-1B).

RATIONALE/EXPECTED OUTCOME (EO)

Inadequate preparation could lead to misconceptions and noncompliance with the treatment plan.

EO: The child or family verbalizes fears and feelings; they ask questions and comply with and participate in treatments.

EO: The child will have adequate would healing with maintenance of healthy skin.

Preserve the movement of the joint to prevent contractures and stiffening from occurring.

EO: The child will maintain function of body parts.

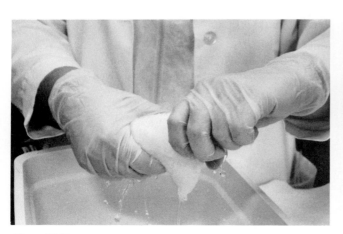

Figure 25-1A.

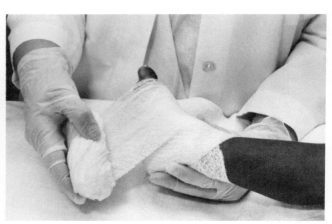

Figure 25-1B.

f. Hold dressings in place with stockinette and leave uncovered.
g. When evaporation begins to dry Kerlix, remove Kerlix, rewet, and reapply a new dressing. Do not pour solution directly on dressings while they are on the child.
h. Fresh solution at room temperature is applied at 2–3 hour intervals and remains on for 30–90 minutes.
i. Guard the child against chilling during the treatment. No more than $\frac{1}{3}$ of the body should be covered at one time.
   • Eliminate drafts in the room.
   • Regulate the room temperature for patient comfort.

Not removing the dressings prevents the nurse from observing the reaction of the skin to the treatment and can cause maceration of the skin due to excess moisture and increased concentration of the solution.

EO: The child will maintain a temperature within normal limits.

PROCEDURE	**RATIONALE/EXPECTED OUTCOME (EO)**

  • Keep bed linen dry.
  • Dry skin after the treatment.
 j. Record the skin's reaction to the treatment in the medical record.
3. *Soaks.* Soaks are used to remove crusts and for mild astringent action using similar solutions employed for wet dressings. Soaks may be used for younger children who are uncooperative in the use of wet dressings.
  a. Gather equipment.
  b. Pour room temperature solution into appropriate size basin.
  c. Immerse the body part into the basin for the prescribed amount of time (usually 30 minutes) (Fig. 25-2).

To gain cooperation of infants or toddlers, put colored toys at the bottom of the basin; preschoolers may be challenged to hold a floating item beneath the fluid surface or pretend to wash dishes, cars, or dolls.

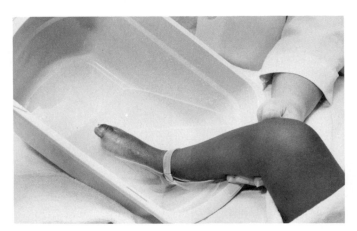

Figure 25-2.

  d. Dry the skin after the treatment and record the child's reaction to the treatment.
  e. **Never leave a child alone with a basin, bucket, or tub of solution.**

Children can drown in a small amount of fluid or drink the soak solution.

EO: The child will receive the treatment in a safe manner.

4. *Lotions.* Lotions are preparations of powder suspended in solution that are used for the purpose of lubricating, cooling, drying, or relieving itching.
  a. Shake the container until the solution is thoroughly mixed.
  b. Put on gloves.
  c. Place a small amount of lotion in one hand and spread it with the inner aspect of the other hand.
  d. Using long smooth strokes, apply the lotion to the body part (Fig. 25-3).
  e. Lotion is not applied to oozing surfaces.
  f. Lotions are not usually washed off between applications, but may be removed by soaking.

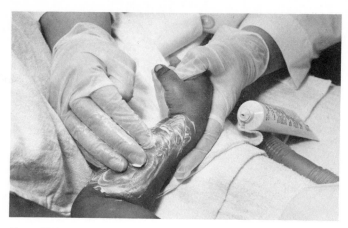

Figure 25-3.

PROCEDURE

5. *Baths.* These are useful in the treatment of widespread dermatitis by evenly distributing the antipruritic and anti-inflammatory effects of the solution.
   a. Scrub the tub thoroughly with a cleaning agent and rinse.
   b. Partially fill the tub with water. (Water should be between 96–100°F.)
   c. Add the medication and stir.
   d. The duration of treatment is usually 15–30 minutes.
   e. **Never leave the child alone in the tub.**
   f. Allow the child to play with toys in the bath.

   g. After removing the child from the bath, pat the skin dry with a towel rather than rubbing it dry.
6. *Creams and ointments.* These are used for lubrication, as a vehicle for medication, and for protection. They contain cold cream or oil.
   a. Assist the child in removing clothing over the area to be treated.
   b. Place a small amount of cream or ointment in one hand and spread it with the palm of the other hand.
   c. Use long smooth strokes to apply. Follow the direction of the hair growth when applying.
   d. The usual treatment schedule includes 2–3 applications of ointment a day.
7. *Pastes.* These are powders mixed with an ointment base. They are more porous and less occlusive than ointments. Pastes absorb moisture and produce a drying effect. Medications incorporated into pastes are released more slowly than from creams and ointments.
   a. Assist the child in removing clothing over area to be treated.

RATIONALE/EXPECTED OUTCOME (EO)

Children have the potential to drown, ingest the solution, fall, or turn on the hot water and burn themselves if left unattended.
Rubbing produces friction, which may irritate the skin condition being treated.

Medicated creams and ointments stain clothing.

Uneven, heavy application cakes and causes irritation; removal of heavily applied ointments requires vigorous rubbing that damages the skin.
Ointment in the follicles causes itching and blockage of ducts.

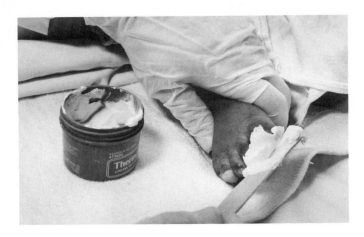

Figure 25-4.

PROCEDURE	**RATIONALE/EXPECTED OUTCOME (EO)**

PROCEDURE

    b. Obtain a tongue blade and liberally scoop out the paste and apply to skin surface (Fig. 25-4).

    c. Cover the treated area with loose-fitting clothes, diapers, or mittens.

    d. Pastes must be removed from the skin with mineral oil.

8. *Powders.* Powder application is controversial. It is effective for soothing, absorbing moisture, and protecting the skin by reducing friction, but may also be inhaled. The chief use is prophylactic.

    a. Expose skin surface to be treated.

    b. Sprinkle powder in the palm of the hand and apply to skin surface in a fine film.

9. *Occlusive dressings.* These are used in association with steroids. They are used in the treatment of chronic dermatoses. They promote moisture retention, nonvaporization of the medication, and maceration of the epidermis, all of which increases the penetration of the medication.

    a. Expose skin surface to be treated.

    b. A thin application of cream or ointment is applied to the skin.

    c. Cover the cream or ointment with a thin, transparent, pliable plastic film; anchor with adhesive tape.

    d. Keep the occlusive dressing in place for 8–10 hours, usually overnight.

    e. Observe the child for signs of adverse reactions to the medication (for example, nausea and vomiting).

    f. After removal of the dressing, observe the skin surface for signs of infection (for example, drainage, foul smell, increased pain, or swelling).

10. *Soaps and Shampoos.* Germicidal soaps and shampoos are useful for skin infections. Bacterial agents in the soap include hexachlorophene or povidone-iodine, which eliminate *Staphylococcus aureus*.

RATIONALE/EXPECTED OUTCOME (EO)

Pastes will not disappear into the skin as creams and ointments will.

This will help keep the medication in contact with the skin.

This will prevent caking or lumping of large amounts of powder when wet and will keep excess powder from being inhaled.

The child will have increased penetration of the medication due to the occlusive nature of the dressing.

The danger of bacterial and candidal infection increases with the retention of moisture under the plastic.

EO: The child is free from wound infection by discharge.

PROCEDURE	**RATIONALE/EXPECTED OUTCOME (EO)**
a. Wet the hair.	
b. Lather twice and rinse three times after each application of suds.	
c. Dry with a towel.	
d. If the scalp has areas of denuded skin and a hexachlorophene-based soap is used, watch for signs of CNS involvement (for example, restlessness, lethargy, or seizures).	Large amounts of hexachlorophene absorbed through the skin can cause nervous system symptoms.
11. *Sunscreening agents.* These chemicals absorb certain wavelengths of light and provide protection to the cutaneous surface when applied to the skin.	Sunburn is an acute erythema caused by overexposure to the rays of the sun. The use of chemical sunscreens minimizes the absorption of ultraviolet (UV) rays by the skin. The sun protection factor (SPF) rating ranges from 2–15. A high SPF rating denotes more protection or increased resistance to burning and tanning.
a. Place a small amount of the agent in one hand and spread it with the palm of the other hand.	
b. Apply a thin film to the light-exposed areas every 3–4 hours.	
12. Determine level of discomfort, considering extent of dermatologic problem, areas involved, age, and developmental level.	Pain receptors will respond to manipulation during treatments resulting in pain. *EO: The child will maintain an adequate level of comfort.*
13. Assess the level of discomfort using a 1–10 scale or color scale. (See Pain Assessment.)	*EO: The child verbalizes or exhibits behaviors that demonstrate decreased pain.*
14. Administer sedation or pain medication approximately 30–60 minutes before treatments; chart the medication's effect.	Unrelieved pain increases anxiety, interferes with sleep, decreases appetite, and leads to depression.
15. Provide diversional activity to distract child from pain or itching.	
16. Maintain environmental temperature of 24.4–28.9°C (76–84°F).	This will ensure comfort and warmth during treatments.
17. Provide an environment conducive to eating; remove soiled dressings or solutions.	Children with dermatologic problems require increased caloric intake to maintain nutrition and promote healing.
18. Do not schedule painful procedures immediately before meals.	
19. Convey a positive attitude toward the child. Reinforce the positive aspects of the child's appearance—do not dwell on the skin condition.	Emotional needs surface as the child becomes aware of body changes and the need for long-term therapy.
20. Involve child in planning treatment schedule.	
21. Encourage child in efforts to deal with multiple problems associated with the disorder (for example, discomfort, rejection, discouragement, or self-revulsion).	Nursing approaches should foster self-control, self-expression, and independence to provide the child with hope and self-esteem. *EO: The child and family will cope effectively with the disorder. The child will verbalize feelings about changes in own body. The child and family will identify goals and plans for home care and state safety measures when appropriate.*
22. Monitor child's and family's level of understanding of treatment and home care.	

Patient/Family Education: Home Care Considerations

1. Discuss the impact of returning to the family or school and peer reaction to the skin disorder.

2. Explain and demonstrate the topical medication procedure; have the child and family return the demonstration.

3. Instruct on possible side effects of the medication.

4. Instruct on the signs and symptoms of a wound infection, such as increased temperature, foul-smelling odor or discharge, swelling, pain, or increased redness.

5. Instruct the family on comfort measures:
   - Reduce external stimuli that aggravate discomfort, such as rough clothing.
   - Increase the room temperature.
   - Increase the humidity in the room.

6. Advise the adolescent not to use cosmetic preparations of any kind. Explain that deodorants and shaving lotions are considered cosmetic and will irritate the skin.

7. To prevent the spread of infection and prevent secondary infections, teach the child and family careful hand washing procedures. Also teach the child not to touch the lesions.

8. Teach the family to protect the child's healthy skin by keeping it dry.

References

Adams, R.M. (1971). Principles and practice of topical therapy. *Pediatric Clinics of North America,* 18, 685–712.

Malseed, R., & Harrigan, G. S. (1989). *Textbook of pharmacology and nursing care.* Philadelphia: J. B. Lippincott Company.

Mathus, N.R. (1977). Topical therapy: Choosing and using the proper vehicle. *Nursing '77* 7(11), 8–10.

McHenry, L.M., & Salerno, E. (1989). *Pharmacology in nursing.* (17th ed.) St. Louis: CV Mosby Company.

Swonger, A., & Matejski, M. (1991). *Nursing pharmacology.* (2nd. ed.). Philadelphia: J. B. Lippincott Company.

Ribavirin Therapy in the Treatment of RSV (Respiratory Syncytial Virus)

26

Definition/Purpose

Ribavirin is an antiviral drug that has been approved by the FDA in an aerosolized form for the treatment of serious respiratory syncytial virus (RSV) infections in hospitalized children. It is different from other antiviral drugs in both its spectrum of activity and its mode of administration.

Respiratory syncytial virus (RSV) was first isolated in 1956 in chimpanzees. The first human strains were discovered in children with pneumonia. RSV is the most important cause of lower respiratory tract disease in infants and children. It usually appears in yearly winter-to-spring outbreaks and infects all children during their first 3 years of life. Transplacental passage of maternal antibody against RSV does not appear to protect the newborn. For this reason, the first infection of RSV is determined by viral exposure. The mortality in hospitalized infants who were previously healthy is low (less than 1%). In infants with underlying disorders, such as pulmonary disease (especially bronchopulmonary dysplasia), prematurity, congenital heart disease, and immunodeficiency disease or therapy causing immunosuppression at any age, mortality is higher.

RSV is transmitted through contact with infected secretions. The virus is not airborne, but it is communicable. Aerosolization may occur during coughing, sneezing, or suctioning. The period of viral shedding is usually 3–8 days, but it may be as long as 4 weeks in the young infant. The virus can live for up to 30 minutes on objects. Inoculation usually occurs via the hands. The incubation period is 2–8 days.

RSV can cause both upper and lower respiratory disease. Primary infections tend to be more severe. The illness begins with an upper respiratory infection. Symptoms like rhinorrhea and fever appear first. Otitis media and conjunctivitis have also been reported. After a few days, a cough may develop. The cough often is spasmodic and may induce vomiting. As the disease progresses, croup, bronchiolitis, bronchitis, and pneumonia may develop. At this stage, retractions, cyanosis, apnea, dyspnea, tachypnea, and wheezing are observed. Lower tract disease is more common in children under 12 months and those who have underlying disorders.

Accurate diagnosis is made by clinical presentation and laboratory data. Viral antigen testing can be done in conjunction with cultures. Antigen tests can be determined within 6 hours.

The treatment of mild uncomplicated RSV is supportive. Trials of ribavirin treatment in infants hospitalized with RSV of the lower respiratory tract began in 1981. In multiple clinical trials, a more rapid improvement in clinical symptoms, improved oxygen saturations, and reduction in viral shedding have been documented in ribavirin-treated children.

Health care workers who care for children receiving ribavirin therapy have raised questions regarding their own safety. Ribavirin is reported to be a teratogen in animals and is not approved for use during pregnancy. No clinical evidence of side effects has been documented in nurses or respiratory therapists giving 20–24 hours of care over 5 consecutive days to a child on therapy. Conservative practice includes maintaining optimal room ventilation; using a filter mask and changing it every 2–4 hours; using gown, gloves, and good hand washing techniques; and not assigning pregnant healthcare workers to care for these children.

Standard of Care

1. Isolation procedures for children with RSV infection are essential. Contact isolation is required. Treatment with ribavirin does not eliminate the need for careful isolation of these children.
2. Candidates for ribavirin therapy include:
   a. Infants at high risk for severe or complicated RSV infection (those with underlying disease)
   b. Infants hospitalized with RSV who are severely ill:
      - PaO_2 values <65 mm Hg
      - $PaCO_2$ values >50 mm Hg
   c. Infants who are hospitalized with lower respiratory disease that is not initially severe, but who may be at risk of a complicated course by virtue of age (<6 weeks), or in whom prolonged illness might be detrimental to a neurologic or metabolic disease.

Assessment

1. Assess the physical findings and pertinent history for fever, cough, nasal discharge, feeding difficulties, prior similar illnesses, illnesses of household contacts, dyspnea, tachypnea, cyanosis, wheezing, and abnormal blood gas values.
2. Assess for positive viral antigen values.
3. Assess developmental factors and family knowledge of the rationale for the treatment with ribavirin and the isolation procedure. Determine the family's prior experiences with respiratory illness and their readiness to learn.

Nursing Diagnoses

The following is a list of possible diagnoses and could apply, depending on the child's age, clinical situation, and physical condition:

Fluid volume deficit

Diversional activity deficit

Ineffective airway clearance

High risk for altered body temperature

Pain

Impaired gas exchange

Ineffective family coping, compromised

Planning

In planning to care for a child receiving ribavirin therapy, the following equipment must be gathered:

Equipment needed for contact isolation (See Infection control procedure)

Normal saline nose drops

Suction catheter

Suction trap

Familiar toys and blankets

Thermometer

Stethoscope

Refractometer

Cardiopulmonary monitor.

Interventions

PROCEDURE	RATIONALE/EXPECTED OUTCOME (EO)
1. Orient child and parents to hospital routines and procedures.	The child and parents will have decreased anxiety and a better understanding of the treatment if they have their questions answered.
2. Allow the child and parents to ask questions about the proposed treatment for RSV.	*EO: The family understands hospital routines and the treatment that has been proposed.*
3. Obtain a specimen for antigen testing. a. Instill normal saline into the nasal passage. b. Attach the suction catheter to suction trap and suction machine. c. Suction nasopharynx to obtain specimen. d. Label and send to laboratory in protective bag. (Along with contact precautions, safety goggles may be used for procedures that induce aerosolization, such as suctioning.)	The best technique for obtaining a specimen is through aspiration of nasal secretions. Nasopharyngeal swabs or tracheal aspirates are not effective in retrieving the virus. *EO: The child will have an adequate specimen collected for antigen testing.*
4. Monitor vital signs every 4 hours, or more often as condition warrants.	
5. Assess breath sounds, respiratory effort, and color every 2–4 hours.	Inflammation of the lower respiratory tract alters the flow of air into and out of the alveoli. *EO: The child will have impending airway obstruction detected and treated.*
6. Assess secretions for amount, character and color.	
7. Assess level of consciousness.	
8. Use a cardiopulmonary monitor to observe respiratory and cardiac patterns.	
9. Monitor blood gases and perform other blood work as ordered by the physician.	*EO: The child maintains normal ABGs.*
10. Administer medications as ordered by the physician (for example, bronchodilators or ribavirin). a. Ribavirin is administered via an oxygen hood or tent for an average of 3–5 days for 12–20 hours each day. 20 mgm of ribavirin/mL of water is placed in a small-particle generator connected to the hood or tent. b. Intubated children may also receive ribavirin; however, antibacterial filters must be added to the circuit of ventilator tubing and must be changed every 2–4 hours. The entire circuit is changed every 24 hours.	Ribavirin must be administered as an aerosol with particles small enough to reach the lower respiratory tract. High levels of ribavirin in the respiratory secretions are obtained by this method with little systemic absorption. Deposition of the drug in the delivery system occurs and depends on humidity, temperature, and electrostatic forces. Precipitation of the drug in ventilator tubing around the expiratory valve could obstruct the valve, resulting in high positive end-expiratory pressure. Thus, this method should only be attempted by well-trained therapists, physicians, and nurses. *EO: The child will have ribavirin therapy administered safely and with continuous monitoring of respiratory status.*
11. Administer oxygen as ordered.	
12. Observe child for shivering, lethargy, decreased temperature, or irritability.	An infant can become stressed due to the cool, wet environment of a hood or tent. A dry environment is necessary to avoid evaporative heat loss. *EO: The child's temperature is maintained within normal limits.*

PROCEDURE	**RATIONALE/EXPECTED OUTCOME (EO)**
13. Reposition child; change linen and pajamas frequently.	*EO: The child will be as comfortable as possible during the therapy.*
14. Weigh child daily on same scale at same time each day.	
15. Record intake and output every shift and total on 24-hour basis.	*EO: The child has adequate intake and output for age and weight.*
16. Calculate fluid requirements for weight, including insensible loss and fever requirements.	Insensible water loss from tachypnea and fever will deplete total body water.
17. Check specific gravity with each void (or less frequently).	*EO: The child has a specific gravity of 1.003–1.020.*
18. Monitor mucous membranes, skin turgor, color of skin, tearing salvation, state of fontanelle, and eyeballs.	*EO: The child will remain hydrated.*
19. Serve the child small feedings with frequent rest periods.	This will decrease respiratory effort and prevent aspiration. *EO: The child will have minimal distress during feeding.*
20. Hold the child in an upright position.	
21. Encourage parents to participate in their child's care.	*EO: The parents participate in the child's care.*
22. Allow a familiar toy in tent or near hood. Make sure the toy is safe in an oxygen-enriched environment.	*EO: The child is engaged in appropriate activities.*
23. Allow child to explore a tent or hood before being placed into one.	
24. Assign a volunteer or foster grandparent to spend time with the child. Encourage family members to spend time with the child.	The child in isolation is prevented from interacting with staff and other children. Opportunities to decrease stress due to hospitalization are decreased.

Patient/Family Education: Home Care Considerations

1. Teach parents about RSV and its treatment.
2. Teach parents about contact isolation and good hand washing to prevent spread of the virus.
3. Teach parents how to interact with their child in isolation (for example, diversional activity, toys that are safe in an oxygenated environment, and toys that can be cleaned).

References

Adams, D. A., & McFadden, E. A. (1990). Respiratory syncytial viral infection in infants; Nursing implications. *Critical Care Nurse, 10*(2), 43–52.

American Academy of Pediatrics. (1988). *Reports of the Committee on Infectious Disease.* Elk Grove Village, IL: Author, 352–354, 526–530.

Groothuis, J., Gutierrez, K. M., & Lauer, B. A. (1988). Respiratory syncytial virus infection in children with bronchopulmonary dysplasia. *Pediatrics, 82*(2), 199–203.

McIntosh, K. (1987). Respiratory syncytial virus infections in infants and children: Diagnosis and treatment. *Pediatrics in Review,* September, 191–196.

Nederhand, K., Solon, J., & Sweet, J. I., (1989). Respiratory syncytial virus: A nursing perspective. *Pediatric Nursing,* July/August, 342–345.

Prows, C. A. (1989). Ribivarin's risks in reproduction—How great are they? *Maternal Child Nursing, 14*(6), 400–404.

Rashotte, J. (1989). The seasonal invader . . . respiratory syncytial virus. *Canadian Nurse, 85*(10), 28–32.

Chemotherapy

27

Definition/Purpose

Chemotherapy (antineoplastic drug therapy) is used in the treatment of children with cancer to prevent or reduce the rate of recurrence or to treat metastasis. Cancer chemotherapy can consist of just one drug or of a group of drugs that work together (combination chemotherapy). A treatment plan that also includes surgery or radiation therapy is called combined modality treatment. In adjuvant chemotherapy, anticancer drugs are used after another treatment to destroy any cancer cells that may remain after surgery or radiation.

Antineoplastic drugs are classified as cell-cycle–specific or cell-cycle–nonspecific, depending upon where the cell's reproductive cycle they exert their effect. These drugs fall into six categories: alkylating agents, antimetabolites, antibiotics, hormones, vinca alkaloids, and miscellaneous. Knowledge regarding the mode of action and the cell cycle type have implications in terms of timing and sequence of drugs as well as side effects and toxicity.

Antineoplastic drugs may be administered in several ways. In some cases the drugs are given to achieve a systemic effect, whereas in others the drugs are used to obtain a local effect. The method of administration depends on the site of the cancer and the drug (or combination of drugs) to be used. Usual methods of administration include oral, intramuscular, intravenous, and intrathecal routes, as well as infusions into tumors and implants.

Standard of Care

1. Precautions for Medication Administration
   a. Disposable surgical *latex* gloves should be worn during all chemotherapy drug administration. Polyvinyl chloride (PVC) gloves are permeable to a variety of drugs and should not be worn to handle chemotherapy drugs (Fig. 27-1).

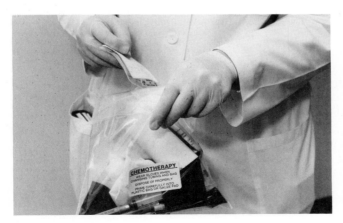

Figure 27-1.

   b. Gloves should be changed every 30 minutes when working steadily with these agents. Gloves should be changed immediately after overt contamination.
   c. Double-gloving is recommended for cleaning up spills.

    d. Syringes and intravenous sets with Luer-lock fittings should be used.

    e. When priming the intravenous site, the distal tip cover must be removed before priming. Priming should be performed into a sterile, alcohol-dampened gauze sponge.

2. Disposal Precautions

    a. Place contaminated materials in a leak-proof, puncture-proof container appropriately marked as hazardous waste (Fig. 27-2).

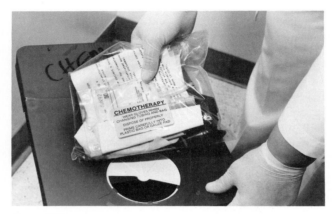

Figure 27-2.

    b. Chemotherapy drug waste should be transported according to institutional procedures for contaminated material.

3. Compounding Precautions

    a. All mixing of chemotherapy agents should be performed in a Class II biological safety cabinet.

    b. Hands must be washed before gloving and again after the gloves are removed.

    c. Care must be taken to avoid puncturing of gloves.

    d. Medication vials should be vented with a hydrophobic filter to eliminate internal pressure or vacuum.

    e. Before opening ampules, care should be taken to ensure that no liquid remains in the tip of the ampule. A sterile, alcohol-dampened gauze sponge should be wrapped around the neck of the ampule to reduce aerosolization.

4. Personnel Policy Recommendations

    a. All personnel working with chemotherapy agents must receive special training.

    b. Access to the compounding area must be limited to necessary authorized personnel only.

    c. Acute exposure episodes must be documented, and the persons involved must be referred for medical examination.

Assessment

1. Assess the pertinent history and physical findings for the type of cancer, signs and symptoms of primary or metastatic spread, resistance to infection, activity level, nutritional state (electrolyte balance), and disability related to the cancer.

2. Assess the child's height and weight; these measurements are used to calculate the correct dose of medication to be administered.

3. Assess psychosocial and developmental concerns related to expectations for the therapy, previous experiences with chemotherapy, support systems, cultural beliefs and habits, and the impact of body image on social interaction.

4. Assess the patient's and family's knowledge regarding the definition and need for

chemotherapy, their expectations for therapy, and their willingness and readiness to learn.

Nursing Diagnoses

The following is a list of possible diagnoses and could apply, depending on the child's age, clinical situation, and physical condition:

Anxiety

High risk for injury

Fluid volume deficit

High risk for infection

Body image disturbance

Diarrhea

Altered oral mucous membrane

Altered nutrition, less than body requirements

Planning

When planning to care for a child receiving chemotherapy, the following equipment is needed:

Latex gloves

Puncture-proof, leak-proof container

Alcohol pads

Thermometer

Blood pressure machine

Stethoscope

Intake/Output sheet

Sponge stick or soft toothbrush

Interventions

PROCEDURE	**RATIONALE/EXPECTED OUTCOME (EO)**
1. Explain each step in the treatment protocol with the child and family. Reinforce the reasons behind the treatment plan, the expected side effects, and interventions to alleviate side effects.	The diagnosis of cancer and its treatment brings about fear and anxiety. The ability to cope with the disease and treatment will be influenced by knowledge of the expected interventions. *EO: The child and family will indicate a reduction of fear and anxiety.* *EO: The child and family will understand the goals of the therapy.*
2. Observe child for bleeding: 　a. Blood in stool 　b. Bleeding from gums 　c. Bleeding from puncture sites 　d. Epistaxis 　e. Bruising	The child receiving chemotherapy may have bone marrow suppression leading to decreased platelet count and bleeding. *EO: The child is free from injury and bleeding.*
3. Monitor CBC and platelet count.	
4. Transfuse as ordered by the physician.	

PROCEDURE	**RATIONALE/EXPECTED OUTCOME (EO)**
5. Monitor vital signs, especially temperature. Avoid rectal temperature measurement.	The child receiving chemotherapy may have bone marrow suppression leading to decreased level of WBCs and an increased risk of infection.
6. Monitor white blood count (WBC) as ordered by the physician.	
7. Maintain the child in protective isolation when WBCs decrease.	Children with counts of 500/mm³ (absolute neutrophil count) need to have adequate protection against infection.
8. Assess sources of infection: a. Intravenous site b. Respiratory c. Urinary d. Oral e. Perineal f. Injection or surgical sites.	*EO: The child will be free from infection.*
9. Maintain a patent IV.	
10. Monitor intravenous infusion for infiltration. Have written protocol available for the management of extravasation.	Chemotherapy drugs are caustic to tissue. Infiltration will lead to tissue necrosis. *EO: The child will have the chemotherapy agents administered in a safe manner. If extravasation occurs, it will be treated promptly.*
11. To minimize nausea and vomiting, administer antiemetics (as ordered).	Chemotherapy drugs destroy the epithelial lining of the GI tract, causing nausea and vomiting. *EO: The child maintains adequate nutrition and hydration.*
12. Maintain adequate hydration before, during, and after therapy.	
13. Maintain accurate intake and output.	
14. Provide small frequent meals.	*EO: The child will have his or her nausea and vomiting recognized and treated.*
15. Monitor electrolytes as ordered by the physician.	
16. Weigh child once a week or more frequently as needed.	
17. Provide information about relaxation techniques.	
18. Assess oral mucosa daily: a. Throat b. Lips c. Tongue d. Gums e. Cheeks f. Palate	Chemotherapy causes stomatitis and mucositis. *EO: The child will be free from oral discomfort.*
19. Perform gentle oral hygiene after eating and every 4 hours, using a sponge stick or soft toothbrush.	
20. Have child eat soft bland food.	Irritated and ulcerated tissues are sensitive to temperature and pressure. The child may have difficulty chewing or swallowing hard, spicy food. *EO: The child maintains normal fluid and dietary intake.*
21. Use oral anesthetics for mouth pain (as ordered).	
22. Allow verbalization of feelings related to the loss of hair.	Chemotherapy destroys all rapidly dividing cells, thus the destruction of hair follicles.

PROCEDURE

23. Inform the child and family about expected initiation, degree, and duration of hair loss.
    a. Hair loss begins 1–2 weeks after initiation of chemotherapy.
    b. The amount of hair lost depends on the drugs administered.
    c. Hair will grow back after chemotherapy is terminated; however, it may be a different texture or color.

24. Identify head coverings such as hats and scarves.

25. Monitor character and frequency of stool. Assess child's usual bowel pattern.

26. Maintain adequate nutrition while adjusting diet for the likelihood of diarrhea or constipation:
    a. Avoid extremes of hot or cold food.
    b. Encourage oral fluids.
    c. Serve small frequent meals.
    d. Serve low-residue diet, high in protein and calories.
    e. Eliminate foods that irritate or stimulate the GI tract.
    f. Use stool softeners as needed.

27. Medicate with antidiarrheal agents as ordered.

28. Clean and dry perineal area after each bowel movement.

RATIONALE/EXPECTED OUTCOME (EO)

EO: The child verbalizes feelings about a changing body image.

EO: The child will manage problems related to hair loss.

Diarrhea is the result of the chemotherapy's affect on the bowel mucosa.

EO: The child's diet will be adjusted to decrease the likelihood of diarrhea.

EO: The child has normal bowel movements (normal frequency and consistency).

EO: The child will have intact perineal skin.

Patient/Family Education: Home Care Considerations

1. Discuss expected side effects of the drugs and the methods used to minimize these effects:
   a. Nausea or vomiting
      - Eat frequent, small meals.
      - Avoid liquids at mealtime to prevent filling the stomach with fluid. Drink liquids at least one hour before meals.
      - Eat foods at room temperature.
      - Avoid strong odors, especially food odors.
      - Avoid sweet and fried foods.
      - Eat dry foods like toast, cereal, or crackers. These may help ease nausea.
   b. Diarrhea or constipation
      - Try a clear liquid diet.
      - Drink plenty of fluids—apple juice, water, weak tea, or broth.
      - Eat small amounts of food, but eat frequently.
      - Avoid milk and milk products.
      - Increase foods high in potassium—bananas, oranges, and potatoes.
   c. Dryness or soreness of the mouth and throat (stomatitis)
      - Drink plenty of fluids.
      - Suck on ice chips.
      - Avoid salt and spicy foods.
      - Avoid highly acidic foods—tomatoes, oranges, and grapefruit.
      - Use a soft toothbrush and brush gently.

- Make a soothing mouthrinse with 1 teaspoon of baking soda in 1 cup of water. Avoid mouthwashes that contain salt or alcohol.
- Use lip balm.

d. Infection
- Avoid crowds as well as people who have contagious illnesses.
- Wash hands well before eating and after using the bathroom.
- Do not cut or tear cuticles.
- After each bowel movement, clean the rectal area gently but thoroughly.
- Report signs of infection to the doctor (avoid taking rectal temperatures):
  Fever (38.3°C [100.4°F]) lasting longer than 24 hours
  Chills
  Sweating
  Diarrhea
  Cough or sore throat
  Burning sensation while urinating
  Drainage, redness at a wound

e. Photosensitivity
- Avoid sun exposure for up to 2 days after administration of agents.
- Use sun screens with a protective factor of 15 or greater.

f. Hemorrhagic cystitis
- Encourage fluids
- Void at frequent intervals

2. Stress the importance of follow-up appointments to monitor blood counts and the disease process.

3. Encourage adequate rest and activity periods.

4. Provide a list of support groups:

   American Cancer Society
   90 Park Avenue
   New York, New York 10016

   Candelighters Childhood Cancer Foundation
   Suite 1011
   2025 I Street N.W.
   Washington, D.C. 20006

   Leukemia Society of America, Inc.
   733 Third Avenue
   New York, New York 10017

   Make-a-Wish Foundation of America
   Suite 205
   4601 N. 16th Street
   Phoenix, Arizona 85016

References

Beardslee, C., Miller, S., et al. (1982). Body-related concerns of children with cancer as compared with the concerns of other children. *Maternal-Child Nursing, 10*(6), 121–134.

Becker, T. (1981). *Cancer Chemotherapy: A Manual for Nurses.* Boston: Little Brown & Co.

Groenwald, Susan L. (1987). *Cancer Nursing.* Boston: Jones and Bartlett Publishers, Inc.

Hockenberry, M., Coody, D.K., & Bennett, B.S. (1990). Childhood cancers: Incidence, etiology, diagnosis, and treatment. *Pediatric Nursing, 16*(3), 239–246.

Lilley, L. (1990). Side effects associated with pediatric chemotherapy: Management and patient education issues. *Pediatric Nursing 16*(3), 252–255.

Mulne, A. et al (1985). Adverse effects of cancer therapy in children. *Pediatrics in Review,* June, 259–268.

Venninga, K. (1985). Improving nutrition in children with cancer. *Pediatric Nursing, 11*(1), 18–20.

Waskerwitz, M. (1984). Special nursing care for children receiving chemotherapy. *Journal of Association of Pediatric Oncology Nurses, 1*(1), 16–25.

Patient-Controlled Analgesia (PCA)

28

Definition/Purpose

Patient-controlled analgesia is an intravenously programmed infusion of narcotic analgesia that allows patients to participate in the management of their own pain. The patient controls pain by the self-administration of narcotics within a set limit and dose. A lockout period between doses is set, as is a maximum dose. The patient-controlled analgesia pump minimizes the side effects of drug therapy by avoiding high blood levels that peak and drop with bolus therapy.

There are some limitations to PCA:

1. It is not applicable to most children under the age of 7 or to older children with cognitive deficits.
2. Many of the units are expensive.
3. Some of the units are inflexible with regard to agents used and dose ranges.
4. Often parents need to be reminded not to push the button for their child.
5. If the child fails to administer the medication, it is difficult to catch up, and a period of severe pain may ensue. Some units, however, circumvent this problem by including a low continuous infusion in addition to the self-administered boluses.

Standard of Care

1. Obtain physician's order to initiate PCA. This should occur after the physician has thoroughly examined the child.
2. Contraindications to PCA therapy include:
   a. Narcotic or drug abuse
   b. Psychiatric disorder
   c. Allergies to narcotics
   d. Chronic respiratory disease
   e. Lack of cooperation or understanding of PCA
   f. Altered respiratory or cardiac status without sufficient documentation
   g. Altered sensorium
   h. Patients under 7 years of age.
3. Narcan must be kept at the bedside or readily available; however, keeping it at the bedside may be hazardous, due to the child's ability to reach it.
4. Two nursing staff members must confirm PCA orders.
5. Follow pump instructions when entering PCA orders.
6. Use the 0–3 pain scale, color scale, or other rating systems, asking the patients to rate their pain (see Appendix 5).
7. Document the PCA dose on a flow sheet. Document the child's self-request for medicine and the child's rating of pain.
8. Monitor vital signs at least every 4 hours.

Assessment

1. Assess the child's ability to understand and utilize the PCA.

2. Assess the child's history of painful experiences through the use of a patient pain profile.
3. Assess the child for secondary health problems or other diseases.
4. Assess the child for history of respiratory difficulty.
5. Assess the child for emotional or psychological trauma.
6. Assess the child's ability to use the desired pain scale.
7. Assess the child's response to PCA management.

Nursing Diagnoses

The following is a list of possible diagnoses and could apply, depending on the child's age, clinical situation, and physical condition:

Anxiety

Pain

Planning

When planning to initiate pain control with a PCA, gather the following equipment:

PCA device

Medication to be infused

Flow sheet

Physician's order

Interventions

PROCEDURE	**RATIONALE/EXPECTED OUTCOME (EO)**
1. Assess the child's ability to understand and participate in pain management.	The PCA will work best with children who are able to self-administer pain relief. *EO: The child will willingly participate in his or her own pain management.*
2. Review PCA orders and compare to institutional policy and recommended doses of medication to be used.	To ensure accuracy and appropriateness. To identify changes that may result from analgesic use. *EO: The child's PCA orders will be within policy guidelines.*
3. Assess vital signs before placing the child on PCA and at least every 4 hours.	To identify changes that may result from analgesic use. *EO: The child's vital signs will be within normal limits. If vital signs are altered, appropriate action will be taken.*
4. Enter PCA orders in accordance with pump instructions (Fig. 28-1).	To ensure proper and effective pain management. *EO: The child will receive PCA therapy.*
5. Assess the child's pain, using pain scales, vital signs, and activity level (see Pain Assessment).	To effectively evaluate the child's response to PCA. *EO: Both the child and caregiver will agree on a decrease in the level of pain with the PCA.*
6. Document PCA dose, child's demanded dose, and activity on flow sheet (see Appendix 5).	To provide a comprehensive picture of child's pain experience and interventions, and to allow for evaluation. *EO: The child will have an objective summary of the pain management in the medical record.*
7. Chart summary of pain management by PCA and evaluate pain control.	The management is documented and can be reviewed for assessment and evaluation.

PROCEDURE   **RATIONALE/EXPECTED OUTCOME (EO)**

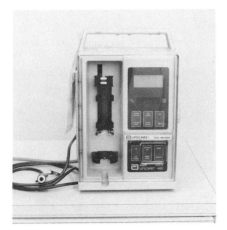

Figure 28-1.

8. Supplement pain control with factors that increase tolerance:

    a. Distraction (Fig. 28-2)

    b. Imagery

    c. Relaxation

    d. Cutaneous stimulation

EO: The child and parents will be taught techniques to supplement pain control via the PCA.

Distraction requires the child to focus attention on something other than the pain. The child may become involved in activities that are exciting, interesting, or absorbing.

The child concentrates on pleasurable activities or things and becomes less aware of the pain.

Relaxation reduces pain caused by muscle tension and anxiety. Fatigue tends to increase pain.

This technique stimulates the skin's surface to relieve pain. Techniques include massage, vibration, pressure, and application of heat or cold.

Patient/Family Education: Home Care Considerations

1. Give the child and parents a written list of medications used for pain control at home, dosages, schedule, and possible side effects.
2. Teach parents techniques that can be used to decrease pain (for example, distraction, imagery, relaxation, and cutaneous stimulation).

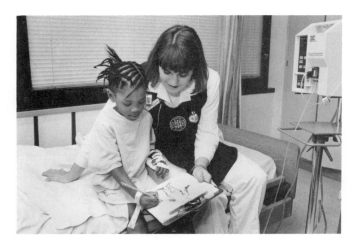

Figure 28-2.

References

Bender, L. H., Weaver, K., & Edwards, K. (1990). Postoperative patient-controlled analgesia in children. *Pediatric Nursing, 16*(6), 549–554.

Bucknell, S., & Sikorski, K. (1989). Putting patient-controlled analgesia to the test. *Maternal Child Nursing, 14*(1), 37–40.

Gregory, G.A. (1989). *Pediatric anesthesia*. Vol. 2. New York: Churchill Livingstone.

McIlvaine, W.B. (1989). Perioperative pain management in children: A review. *Journal of Pain and Symptom Management*, December, 215–229.

Rauen, K.K., Ho, M. (1989). Childrens' use of PCA after spinal surgery. *Pediatric Nursing, 15*(6), 589–637.

Schechter, N., Berrien, F., & Shoshana, K. (1988). The use of patient-controlled analgesia in adolescence with sickle cell pain crisis: A preliminary report. *Journal of Pain and Symptom Management, 2* (3), 109–113.

Scheidler, V. (1988). Patient-controlled analgesia. *Current Concepts in Nursing, 1,* 13–16.

Taylor, C., Lillis, C., & LeMure, P. (1989). *Fundamentals of nursing: The art and science of nursing care*. Philadelphia: J.B. Lippincott Company.

Vichinsky, E., Johnson, R., & Lubin, B. (1982). Multi-disciplinary approach to pain management in sickle cell disease. *American Journal of Pediatric Hematology/Oncology, 4* (3), 328–333.

Webb, C.J., Stergios, D. A., & Rodgers, B. M. (1989). PCA as post operative pain treatment for children. *Journal of Pediatric Nursing, 14*(3), 162–171.

Immunizations

29

Definition/Purpose

Immunity is resistance that an individual has against disease. Antigens, substances that induce the formation of antibodies in the body, react with antibodies, producing immunity. *Active immunity* is immunity produced by natural or artificial stimulation so that the body produces its own antibodies. It may be produced by an attack of a specific disease or by introduction of vaccines or toxoids by injection. Maternal antibodies affect the infant's susceptibility to disease. The half-life of immunoglobulin G antibodies is 3–4 weeks, with some effect up to 15–16 weeks. *Passive immunity* is acquired immunity produced by administration of preformed antibodies whose protection is of short duration. It is employed to protect children against a disease to which they have been exposed.

Active Immunity

Toxoid—A toxin treated by heat and a chemical agent to destroy its harmful properties without destroying its ability to stimulate antibody production

Vaccine—A suspension of attenuated or killed microorganisms administered for prevention, amelioration, or treatment of infectious diseases

Passive Immunity

Serums prepared in humans—found in a patient recently convalescent from disease or acquired from donors who have been recently vaccinated.

Serums prepared in animals—when a specific toxic effect of venom is best managed by antibody administration from the animal (Table 29-1).

Table 29-1. Vaccines and Their Route of Administration

Vaccine	Type	Route
BCG	Live bacteria	ID
Cholera	Inactivated bacteria	Subq, IM, ID
DPT	Toxoids or inactivated bacteria	IM
Hepatitis B	Inactivated viral antigen or yeast recombinant-derived antigen	IM
Haemophilus B	Polysaccharide	Subq, IM
Influenza	Inactivated virus	IM, Subq
Measles	Live virus	Subq
Meningococcal	Polysaccharide	Subq
MMR	Live virus	Subq
Mumps	Live virus	Subq
Pneumococcal	Polysaccharide	IM, Subq
Polio		
OPV	Live virus	Oral
IPV	Inactivated virus	Subq
Rabies	Inactivated virus	IM
Rubella	Live virus	Subq
Tetanus and Td, DT	Toxoids	IM
Typhoid	Inactivated bacteria	Subq

ID, intradermal; Subq, subcutaneous; IM, intramuscular.

Standard of Care

1. Vaccines work best when they are given at the recommended time and on a regular schedule.
2. Before any immunization is administered, the family should provide the following information:
   - Present status of immunization
   - Past response to immunizations
   - Past and current illnesses.

Assessment

1. Assess child for history of recent illness or exposure to infections, illness, or childhood diseases. Minor, nonfebrile illnesses should not contraindicate the use of vaccines, especially when a child continually has a minor upper respiratory infection or allergic rhinitis. For a child with an acute febrile illness, guidelines for immunization are based on the physician's assessment of the child's illness and the specific vaccine the child is scheduled to receive.
2. Assess the child for the following special clinical circumstances:
   a. Prematurity—Prematurely born infants should be immunized at the usual chronologic age. Eighty four percent of preterm infants show evidence of transplacental transfer of maternal antibodies to diphtheria and tetanus antigens compared with 100% of term babies. Only 16% of preterm infants show evidence of transplacental transfer of antibodies to pertussis versus 85% of term infants. If the infant is still in the hospital at the time the immunization is due, only DPT should be given. OPV can be initiated on discharge. Varicella-zoster immune globin should be given as soon as possible after delivery to infants whose mothers have had onset of varicella within 5 days before or 2 days after delivery.
   b. Pregnancy—In general, pregnant women should receive vaccines only when they are urgently needed. In the United States, the only vaccines recommended for administration during pregnancy are those for tetanus and diphtheria. Efforts should be made to immunize women against rubella, measles, and mumps before they become pregnant. Susceptible children living with a pregnant female should receive the rubella virus vaccine, since immunized children are less likely to acquire rubella and introduce it into the household.
   c. Immunodeficient or immunosuppressed children—Live virus vaccines of all types are contraindicated in patients with congenital disorders of immune function. Live vaccines should be administered no less than 3 months after all immunosuppressive therapy has been discontinued. A child recovering from a successful bone marrow transplant must be considered unimmunized and be reimmunized with inactivated vaccines. In immunocompromised children who develop chickenpox (varicella zoster), both vidarabine and acyclovir are effective in treating varicella or zoster. Those children exposed to the disease and younger than 15 years of age should receive varicella-zoster immune globulin (VZIG). Older children are likely to be immune but if susceptible, they also should receive VZIG. Children with malignancies receiving immunosuppressive therapy who have antibodies at the time of exposure and a negative history of past diseases may still be at risk if they recently received blood products.
   d. HIV infection—Live viral and bacterial vaccines are contraindicated in children with symptomatic HIV infection because of the risks of serious adverse effects. However, because of severe measles in symptomatic HIV-infected children, including fatalities, measles vaccinations are recommended regardless of symptoms. Asymptomatic HIV-seropositive children should be immunized according to schedule.

e. Asplenic children—Because of the high risk of fulminant bacteremia, polyvalent pneumococcal vaccine is recommended for children 2 years and older. Likewise, quadrivalent meningococcal polysaccharide and Haemophilus b conjugate should be administered to those 18 months and older.

f. Children with a history of seizures—Infants and children with neurologic disorders have an increased risk of adverse events following receipt of pertussis and measles vaccines. Children with a personal history of seizures are at increased risk of having a seizure following the measles and pertussis vaccine. A family history of seizures is no reason to defer immunizations.

g. Children with chronic diseases—Some chronic diseases render children more susceptible to the severe manifestations and complications of common infections. In general, immunizations recommended for healthy children should be given to children with chronic diseases (for example, cardiorespiratory, allergic, hematologic, metabolic, and renal disorders).

3. Assess for allergic reactions to previous immunizations or a sensitivity to eggs.

4. Assess the family's knowledge of the need for immunization and the potential side effects.

Nursing Diagnoses

The following is a list of possible diagnoses and could apply, depending on the child's age, clinical situation, and physical condition:

Anxiety

Pain

Impaired skin integrity

High risk for altered body temperature

High risk for injury

Planning

In planning to administer an immunization, the following equipment must be gathered:

Alcohol pads

Appropriate size syringe with needle ($\frac{5}{8}$-inch to 1-inch needle and 3 mL syringe)

Vaccine.

Interventions

PROCEDURE	RATIONALE/EXPECTED OUTCOME (EO)
1. Prepare the child appropriate to developmental level.	Prior knowledge will allay fears and encourage cooperation. *EO: The child will be prepared developmentally according to age for the injection.*
2. Parents should be informed about the benefits and risks of immunizations. Obtain signed consent for immunization.	The parent must be educated about the major benefits in preventing disease in the child as well as the community. Benefit and risk statements should be presented in lay terminology. *EO: Parent and child will exhibit decreased anxiety when they have their questions answered.*
3. Obtain equipment for the administration of the immunization.	

PROCEDURE	**RATIONALE/EXPECTED OUTCOME (EO)**
4. Have epinephrine (1 : 1000) available for immediate use should an anaphylactic or allergic reaction occur (0.01 mL/kg).	
5. Obtain the vaccine and draw up in syringe. Note the schedules of immunizations (Tables 29-2, 29-3, and 29-4).	Changing needles between drawing up the vaccine and injecting it into the child is not necessary.
6. Adequately restrain the child before the injection.	

Table 29-2. Recommended Schedule for Immunizations of Normal Infants and Children

Recommended age	Immunization	Comments
2 months	DPT-1, OPV-1, HbCV-1	Can be initiated as early as 4 weeks in areas of high epidemicity.
4 months	DPT-2, OPV-2, HbCV-2	2-month interval between initial and second OPV.
6 months	DPT-3, HbCV-3	
15 months	MMR, HbCV-4	TB test may be done at this time.
15–18 months	DPT-4, OPV-3	
4–6 years	DPT-5, OPV-4	
11–12 years	MMR	
14–16 years	Td	Repeat every 10 years.

(Provided by Illinois Department of Public Health, 1991).

Table 29-3. Recommended Schedule for Immunizations of Infants and Children Delayed in Beginning Immunizations up to Their 7th Birthday

Timing	Vaccines
Age at first visit	
a. 2–14 months	DPT-1, OPV-1
b. 15–24 months	DPT-1, OPV-1, MMR
c. 18 months or older	DPT-1, OPV-1, MMR, HbCV
2 months after DPT-1, OPV-1	DPT-2, OPV-2
2 months after DPT-2	DPT-3
10–16 months after DPT-3	DPT-4, OPV-3
4–6 yrs of age	DPT-5, OPV-4
11–12 years	MMR
10 years later	Td

(Provided by Illinois Department of Public Health, 1991.)

Table 29-4. Recommended Schedule for Immunizations for Children 7 Years of Age or Older Who Have Not Received Vaccines Previously

Timing	Vaccines
First visit	MMR, OPV-1, Td-1
2 months later	OPV-2, Td-2
8–14 months later	OPV-3, Td-3
11–12 years	MMR
10 years later	Td (Repeat every 10 years.)

(Provided by Illinois Department of Public Health, 1991.)

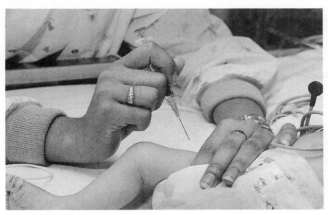

Figure 29-1.

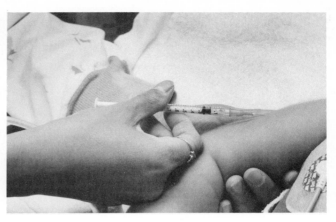

Figure 29-2.

PROCEDURE	**RATIONALE/EXPECTED OUTCOME (EO)**
7. Inject the vaccine in a site as free as possible from the opportunity for a local neural, vascular, or tissue injury.	In infants, the anterolateral aspect of the thigh provides the largest muscle and is preferred for IM injections. The upper, outer aspect of the buttocks should not be used because of the hazard of damaging the sciatic nerve. Subcutaneous injections can be given in the thigh or the upper arm (Fig. 29-1). Intradermal injections are given on the volar surface of the forearm (Fig. 29-2). *EO: The child will remain injury-free from the injection of the vaccine.*
8. Comfort the child after the immunization.	
9. Enter the following data into the child's medical record and the child's personal record: a. Month, day, and year of administration b. Vaccine administered c. Manufacturer d. Lot number e. Expiration date f. Site and route of administration g. Provider of administering vaccine.	*EO: The child will have his or her immunization history accurately recorded.*
10. Keep the child in the health facility for 20 minutes after the injection.	If the child is going to have a life-threatening reaction to the immunization, it will most likely occur within 20 minutes of administration.

Patient/Family Education: Home Care Considerations

1. Alert the family to the potential side effects of the immunization:
   a. Fever*
   b. Local irritation*
   c. Rash†
   d. Sterile abscesses at injection site†
   e. Seizures†
   f. Anaphylaxis—shock (24 hours after injection)†
   g. Encephalopathy (3–15 days after injection)†

---

* Common side effects that can be treated with an antipyretic medication such as acetaminophen 15 mg/kg given every 4 hours. (Aspirin is no longer recommended because of its potential to cause gastrointestinal bleeding and its recent link with Reye's syndrome.)
† Unusual side effects that warrant notification of a health care provider.

2. Emphasize to the parents the importance of keeping appointments for their child's immunizations.

3. Provide a written record of the immunization and have the family bring the record to future health visits so it can be updated.

References

American Academy of Pediatrics. (1991). *Report to the Committee on Infectious Diseases*. Elk Grove Village, I.L.: American Academy of Pediatrics.

Carroll, P., Maher, V. F. (1990). Legal aspects of vaccine administration. *Advancing Clinical Care*, *5*(1), 11–15.

Engel, N. (1990). Pertussis vaccine: Safety Update. *Maternal Child Nursing, 15*(5), 293.

Few, B. (1988). Hemophilus influenza type B vaccine. *Journal of Maternal Child Nursing, 13*(6), 407.

Hick, J.F. (1989). Optimum needle length for diphtheria-Tetanus-Pertussis Inoculation of Infants. *Pediatrics*, *84*(1), 136–137.

Illinois Department of Public Health. (1988). *Who needs them? Everyone*. Springfield, I.L.: Illinois Department of Public Health, Division of Infectious Disease Immunization Program.

Jurgrau, A. (1990). Why aren't we protecting our children? *RN,* 10(11), 30–34.

Mansell, K.A. (1985). New immunization against H. influenzae type b. *Pediatric Nursing, 11*(6), 433–435.

Messner, R.L., Mufson, M. A. (1990). Pneumococcal vaccine: A focus for nursing. *Advancing Clinical Care*, *5*(1), 11–15.

PARENT TEACHING GUIDE
Metered Dose Inhaler (MDI)

Introduction

Your doctor has prescribed an inhaler to help control respiratory symptoms not controlled by oral medications.

Medication to be administered: _____

Number of puffs: _____

Frequency of use: _____

Carefully follow your doctor's orders and these instructions.

To Prepare

1. If ordered, first inhale a bronchodilator to open your airways. Use your inhaler after the bronchodilator.

2. Shake medication before use. Hold canister upright.

3. Place medication cartridge in the plastic oral adapter and take the cap off the mouthpiece.

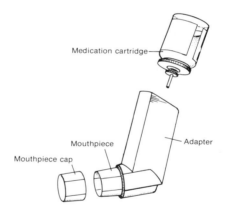

To Inhale

1. Breathe all your air out through pursed lips.

2. Place mouthpiece between lips or approximately $1\frac{1}{2}$ inches away from lips.

3. Keep your mouth wide open and take a slow deep breath. Do *not* seal your lips tightly around the mouthpiece.

4. While taking a deep breath, firmly press down on the metal medication vial to give one dose of the medication.

5. Keep your tongue down and out of the way.

6. Remove mouthpiece from mouth. Hold your breath for 10 seconds or as close to 10 seconds as you can, but no less than 1–3 seconds.

7. Breathe air out slowly. Wait 1 minute before taking a second puff, if prescribed.

Cleaning

1. Remove medication cartridge and wash plastic adapter once a day with soap and water.

2. Rinse and dry completely.

3. Store in a clean plastic bag in a cool place.

Precautions

1. Use MDI only as directed by your doctor. Do not use your inhaler for episodes of shortness of breath. The inhaler medication prevents breathing problems; it does not relieve shortness of breath once it happens.

2. Call your doctor if you find yourself using your inhaler frequently, or if you develop any of the following side effects:
Dizziness
Headache
Rapid heartbeat
Skipped heartbeats
Increased wheezing or shortness of breath.

References

Jenkins, S.C., Heaton, Fulton, & Moxham, J. (1987). Comparison of domiciliary nebulized salbutamol and salbutemol from a metered-dose inhaler in stable, chronic airflow limitation. *Chest, 91,* 804–807.

Levison, H., Reilly, P.A., & Worsley, G.H. (1985). Spacing devices and metered-dose inhalers in childhood asthma. *Journal of Pediatrics, 107,* 662.

Zahr, L.K., Connolly, M., & Page, D.R. (1988). Assessment and management of the child with asthma. *Pediatric Nursing, 15*(2), 109–114.

Introduction

Your doctor has prescribed a turboinhaler specifically designed for delivery of the powder in cromolyn capsules. Carefully follow your doctor's orders and these instructions.

To Prepare

1. The parts of the turboinhaler include:
   A. The body—A white tube with a gray sleeve that slides up and down.

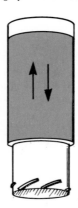

   B. The propeller—A piece that rests on the steel spindle and holds the capsule.

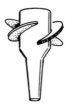

   C. The mouthpiece—A white tube with a flange and a stainless steel spindle.

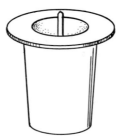

2. Wash and dry your hands.

3. Hold the turboinhaler vertically with mouthpiece held down. Unscrew body of inhaler counterclockwise.

4. Keep mouthpiece down and propeller on spindle. Insert colored end of capsule into propeller cup. Do not handle capsule excessively, because it will soften.

5. Screw body back into mouthpiece.

6. Keeping turboinhaler vertical and mouthpiece down, slide the gray sleeve down firmly until it stops. Then slide the gray sleeve up as far as it will go. Do this only once. This will pierce the capsule.

To Inhale

1. Hold turboinhaler well away from mouth and breathe out fully, emptying air from your lungs.

2. With head tilted back and teeth apart, close lips and teeth around mouthpiece. Inhale a deep and rapid breath. Do not exhale through the turboinhaler.

3. Remove turboinhaler from your mouth and hold your breath for a few seconds.

4. Exhale completely. Repeat steps 1, 2, and 3 until all the powder is inhaled. A light dusting of powder may remain in the capsule. This is normal.

Cleaning

1. Discard the empty capsule. Return the tuboinhaler to its container.

2. Once a week, take your turboinhaler apart and wash it in warm water. Pay particular attention to washing the inside of the propeller shaft. Shake off excess water and allow to air-dry. Reassemble parts.

Tips

1. The turboinhaler should be replaced every 6 months.

2. Because moisture from your hands will soften the capsules, do not handle them excessively and do not remove them from the foil wrapping until you are ready to use them.

3. Protect the capsules from extremes in temperature.

References

Baciewicz, A.M., & Kyllonen, K.S. (1989). Aerosol inhaler technique in children with asthma. *American Journal of Hospital Pharmacy, 46*(12), 2510–2511.

Brim, S. (1989). A quick guide for home use of inhalant medications. *Pediatric Nursing, 15*(1), 87–88, 94.

Definition/Purpose

Children ages three to ten often have great difficulty timing inhalations to match delivery of the mist from the metered dose device. The bad taste of the medication accentuates the problem. For these reasons we recommend a holding chamber to aid in the delivery of the drug prescribed.

All holding chambers catch the mist from the MDD and hold it until the child starts to breath in. This eliminates the need for good coordination between release of the mist and inspiration. In large volume holding chambers, air dilutes the unpleasant taste of the medication, making it easier to breath in. There are four basic chambers: Inspirease; Inhal-Aid; Aerochamber, and a paper tube.

Chamber Types

1. Inspirease (Key Pharmaceuticals) (Fig. 1)
   Requires replacement bags
   Requires a prescription

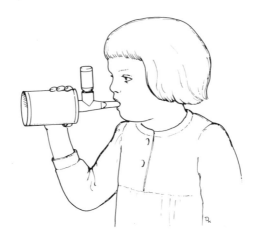

Figure 1. Inspirease holding chamber.

This is a collapsible, large-volume reservoir that is easy to carry. It is an excellent device for children 4 years and older, because it makes a musical sound if one breathes in too fast. Because slow inhalation leads to greater deposition of the medication mist, the sound is a helpful feedback feature.

Instructions

a. Extend bag. Attach medicine device.
b. Place the mouthpiece on the tongue and puff one whiff of medication into the chamber.

    c. Suck in slowly. Hold breath 5 seconds.

    d. Breathe out, keeping lips snugly around mouthpiece.

    e. Suck in again slowly and hold breath 5–10 seconds.

    f. Depending on the doctor's orders, repeat the above steps with a new puff.

2. Inhal-Aid (Key Pharmaceuticals) (Fig. 2)
   Requires a prescription

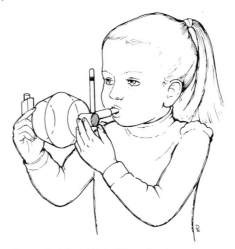

Figure 2. Inhal-Aid holding chamber.

This is a large-volume device that most 3-year-olds can learn to use. It can be used with good effect during a mild or moderate asthma attack, because the ability to hold one's breath is not required. A special feature is the incentive marker that indicates adequate depth of a breath.

Instructions:

    a. Attach medication device.

    b. Place mouthpiece on tongue.

    c. Puff one whiff of medication into the chamber.

    d. Suck in with lips snug around mouthpiece, and hold breath for 5 seconds. (If your child cannot hold his or her breath, encourage the child to inhale, raising the float to the top 10 times in a row.) The slower the rate and the higher the float, the better. Breathe out through the mouthpiece.

    e. Wait at least 1 minute and then repeat if more than one puff is ordered.

3. Aerochamber (Monaghan Medical Corporation) (Fig. 3)
   No prescription needed

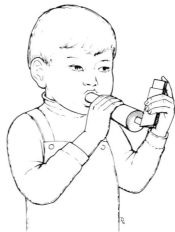

Figure 3. AeroChamber holding chamber.

This holding chamber has a valve that prevents accidental exhalation of the medication. It is recommended for children ages 3 years and older. It is the only device that has instructions for its use printed on the chamber.

Instructions:

    a. Attach medication device.
    b. Place the mouthpiece on the tongue and puff one whiff of medication into the chamber.
    c. Suck in slowly and hold breath for 10 seconds.
    d. Breathe out, keeping lips snug around mouthpiece.
    e. Wait at least 1 minute and then repeat routine.

4. Paper tube
   No prescription needed

Children 5 years and older who have difficulty coordinating the release of medication from a MDD with their inhalation will find a tube holding chamber helpful.

Instructions:

    a. Roll a piece of paper to form a tube 8 inches long and 2 inches in diameter.
    b. Puff one whiff of medication into the tube; then inhale with lips snug around the tube.
    c. Start to inhale slowly and hold your breath 5–10 seconds.
    d. Wait 1 minute and then repeat.

References

Levinson, H., Reilly, P.A., Worsely, G.H. (1985). Spacing devices and meter dose inhalers in childhood asthma. *Journal of Pediatrics, 107*(5), 662–668.

Plant, T.F. (1989). Holding chambers for aerosol drugs. *Pediatric Annals, 18*(12), 824–826.

Children under three years of age may have great difficulty timing their inhalations to match the delivery of mist from a metered dose inhaler (MDI). The bad taste of the medicine also inhibits smooth inhalation. For this reason, your child may use a compressor-driven nebulizer (CDN). The CDN produces a fine mist that your child inhales while breathing normally, even while sleeping.

As a parent of a child with asthma, you must know how to monitor the progress of an episode by observing the four signs of asthma trouble in children:

1. The child wheezes during inspiration and expiration.

2. Chest skin is sucked in (retractions) because the child cannot draw air into the lungs.

3. Breathing out takes longer than breathing in.

4. Breathing is rapid.

In general, if there is no significant improvement in these signs within 15 minutes of a treatment, or if the improvement does not hold for 4 hours, you need to contact your child's physician.

Using the CDN

Setting it up

1. Using the dropper that comes with the medication, draw up _____ mL of _____ and squirt it into the plastic cup.

2. Measure _____ mL of normal saline and put it into the cup. Tap water may be used in an emergency; however, constant use of tap water will cause minerals to build up and clog the nebulizer opening.

3. Replace the top of the chamber and tighten it.

4. Insert a "T" piece or mask on top of the cup.

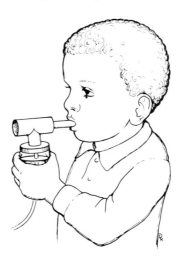

5. Attach the tubing to the machine and to the bottom of the nebulizer cup.

6. Treatment should take 5–12 minutes. If it takes longer, there is a crack in the cup and the cup needs to be replaced.

7. Treatment should be given every _____ hours.

Cleaning the machine

1. After each treatment, take the cup apart and clean it with hot tap water.

2. Once a day, clean the cup and mouthpiece with a weak solution of dishwashing detergent. Soak for a few minutes, rinse with water, and let air dry.

3. Once a week, clean the cup and tube with a solution of 1 cup of white vinegar to 3 cups of water. Let it soak for 10 minutes; then rinse under warm running water.

4. Wash equipment in a pan rather than the sink. (The sink may contain grease that will clog the nebulizer.)

5. Always keep 2–3 nebulizer cups on hand in case one breaks, or so that several doses can be set up for a babysitter or grandparent who is unfamiliar with asthma medicines.

References

Bacon, C. (1982). Nebulizer therapy for small asthmatic children. *Maternal and Child Health, 7*(6), 243–248.

Brim, S. (1989). A quick guide for home use of inhalant medication. *Pediatric Nursing, 15*(1), 87–94.

Lewis, M. (1984). The place of nebulizers in childhood asthma. *Maternal and Child Health, 9*(1), 36–41.

Plaut, T. (1989). Helping asthma patients breathe easier. *Contemporary Pediatrics, 89*(10), 59–76.

Robertson, C.F., Smith, F., & Beck, R. (1985). Response to frequent low doses of nebulized salbutamol in acute asthma. *Journal of Pediatrics, 106,* 672.

Respiratory System Procedures

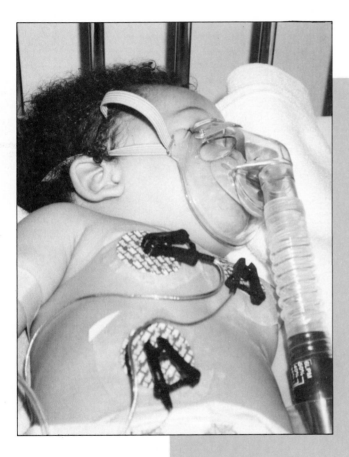

Unit V

Pleural Cavity Evacuation: Chest Tube

30

Definition/Purpose

To keep the lungs expanded, maintenance of a negative intrapleural pressure is essential. As the chest expands during inspiration, the pressure in the chest cavity falls, becoming less than atmospheric and allowing air to fill the lungs. Intrapleural pressure fluctuates from −5 cm of water during inspiration to +3 cm of water during expiration.

Thoracic surgery, a penetrating chest wound, or the rupture of a bulla allows air or fluid to enter the pleural space. When this occurs the pressure in the space remains near atmospheric pressure and does not allow for proper inflation and deflation of the lungs. The entry of air or fluid into the intrapleural space causes the lung on the affected side to recoil and collapse. If such collapse results from entry of air into the intrapleural space with little or no fluid, the condition is called *pneumothorax*. If it results from a large amount of serosanguineous fluid with a large amount of air, the condition is called *hemopneumothorax*.

With the setup of a chest tube system, one or more tubes are inserted through the chest wall to remove the air and fluid from the intrapleural space. If operating properly, a chest tube will permit the affected lung to reexpand. Because the insertion of a chest tube creates a new opening into the chest wall, the distal end of the chest tube is submerged underwater. This water permits the air to exist but not reenter; thus, it is called a "water seal." The chest tube and the water seal constitute the basic components of any chest tube system (Fig. 30-1).

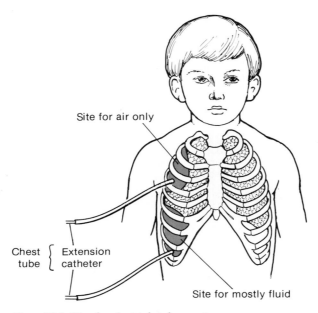

Figure 30-1. Sites for chest tube placement.

Types of Chest Tube Systems: Bottle (Gravity)

Two-bottle Gravity System

The child's air and fluid are drained into the collection bottle, which traps the fluid and passes the air onward through the water seal bottle and then allows it to exit the outlet tube. Air and fluid are forced through the bottles by gravity and positive expiratory pressure Fig. 30-2.

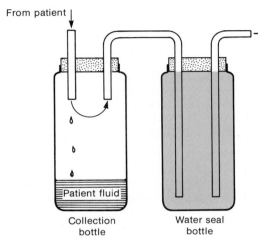

Figure 30-2. Two-bottle gravity system.

One-bottle Gravity System

This system is identical to the two-bottle system, except that the collection and water seal bottles are combined into a single unit (Fig. 30-3).

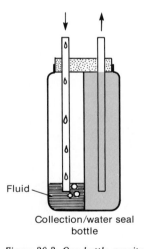

Figure 30-3. One-bottle gravity system.

Three-bottle System on Suction

The first two bottles are identical to the two bottles in the gravity system. However, instead of passing from the water seal into the atmosphere, the air is passed through a third bottle, the suction control bottle. The suction bottle contains water and an opening for the entry of the air from the atmosphere. Air from the child's lungs passes over the suction control water, while air from the atmosphere passes through it. It is the depth of the manometer

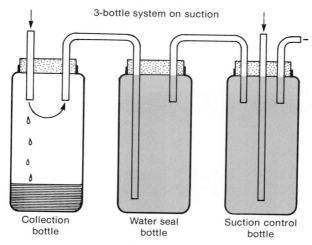

Figure 30-4. *Three-bottle system on suction.*

tube in the water that determines the amount of suction pressure applied to the intra-pleural contents (Fig. 30-4).

Two-bottle System on Suction

This system is identical to the three-bottle system on suction, except that the collection and water seal bottles are combined into a single bottle (Fig. 30-5).

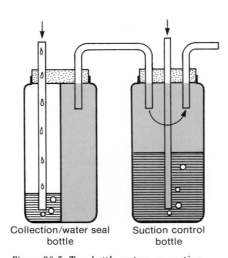

Figure 30-5. *Two-bottle system on suction.*

Disposable Unit

This system integrates the three compartments into one unit. The collection chamber for drainage is on the right. This chamber consists of calibrated columns that enable the user to measure the amount of drainage. Resealing diaphragms on the back of the collection chambers allow for withdrawal of drainage for analysis. The middle compartment is the water seal chamber. The standard water level (2 cm H_2O) is marked. At the top of the water seal chamber is a positive pressure relief value, which enables excess pressure to be vented into the atmosphere, preventing tension pneumothorax. The third chamber is the suction control chamber. The chamber may be filled to various suction levels. A rubber diaphragm on the back of the chamber allows the replacement of water that has been lost to evaporation (Fig. 30-6).

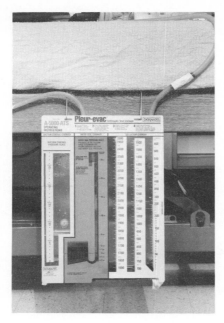

Figure 30-6.

Standard of Care

1. The drainage system must be kept at a level lower than the child's chest.
2. The drainage tubing should fall in direct line to the system to facilitate drainage.
3. Tape the connecting points to ensure that the system is airtight and will not pull apart.
4. The glass bottles or disposable unit will be taped to the floor to prevent accidental tipping.
5. A clamp should be taped to the child's bed for ready access.

Assessment

1. Assess the pertinent history and physical findings for precipitating events, prior experience with a chest tube, respiratory rate and effort, use of accessory muscles, shape of the chest, breath sounds, degree of restlessness, arterial blood gases, end tidal CO_2, and oxygen saturation.
2. Assess for allergies, especially iodine.
3. Assess psychosocial and developmental factors for age, usual comfort measures, habits, and previous experience with hospitalization.
4. Assess the child's and family's knowledge of the illness and their willingness and readiness to learn.

Nursing Diagnoses

The following is a list of possible diagnoses and could apply, depending on the child's age, clinical situation, and physical condition:

Anxiety

Fear

High risk for injury

Decreased cardiac output

Impaired skin integrity
Impaired gas exchange
High risk for infection
Pain

Planning

In planning to assist in the insertion of a chest tube, gather the following equipment:
Chest tube tray
1% lidocaine
Povidone-iodine
2-0 silk with a cutting needle
Sterile gloves and mask
Stethoscope
Drainage system
Sterile water (1000 mL bottle)
Adhesive tape
Clamp (padded)
5-mL syringe with needle
Alcohol swabs
Petrolatum gauze

Interventions

PROCEDURE	**RATIONALE/EXPECTED OUTCOME (EO)**
1. Explain to the child and parents the reason for the chest tube, how it will be inserted, and what it will look like.	The child and family will tend to cooperate with the procedure if they are well informed. *EO: The child and family will verbalize understanding of the procedure.* *EO: The child and family will have decreased anxiety about the procedure.*
2. Obtain a signed consent for the procedure from the guardian.	*EO: The guardian acknowledges through a signed consent that he or she has obtained information regarding the procedure and has agreed to the procedure.*
3. Assist the physician in preparing the child and the supplies necessary for the insertion. Prepare the drainage system according to the directions accompanying the system.	
4. Once the tube is in place and connected to the drainage system, obtain a chest x-ray.	The chest x-ray will confirm position of the tube and whether it has begun to evacuate fluid and/or air.
5. Make sure the water in the suction control chamber is bubbling gently. Also check the water seal for bubbles.	If bubbles are seen in the water seal chamber, it means air is entering the system from one or more of the following: a. a leak in the tubing b. a leak under the dressing c. a leak from the pleural cavity

PROCEDURE	**RATIONALE/EXPECTED OUTCOME (EO)**

PROCEDURE

RATIONALE/EXPECTED OUTCOME (EO)

d. the drainage of air from the pleural cavity (pneumothorax)

e. crack in the unit.

6. Make sure the connections between the chest tube and the drainage tubing and between the suction tubing and short latex tubing are tight and wrapped with adhesive tape (Fig. 30-7).

Loose connections will cause an air leak in the system and ineffective drainage of fluid and evacuation of air.

EO: The child's chest tube system will have tight connections that are reinforced with tape.

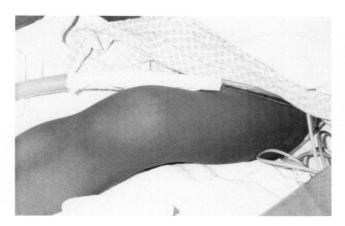

Figure 30-7.

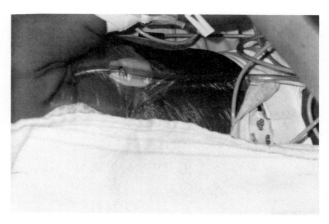

Figure 30-8.

7. Check the dressing to assure it is clean, dry, and intact (Fig. 30-8). The dressing should be covered with adhesive tape. Remove the dressing only if the chest tube has moved or if fluid is leaking around the insertion site and soiling the dressing. Inspect the entry site for drainage, inflammation, or subcutaneous emphysema.

EO: The child's skin will remain intact under the dressing.

EO: The child will be free from infection under the dressing.

8. Assess drainage through the chest tube. Mark the drainage level at the start of the collection and at the end of every shift (or more often if needed).

If the child is actively bleeding, assess the drainage frequently (every 10-15 minutes).

EO: The child will have the drainage measured and recorded.

9. Check the drainage tubing for kinks or obstructed flow. There should be no dependent loops of tubing or tubing laid horizontally on the bed. Do not strip or "milk" the tubing unless ordered by the physician.

Stripping or milking the tubing (manually compressing the drainage tubing between the chest tube and the unit) creates a hazardously high pressure in the pleural cavity. The high negative pressure (-350 cm H_2O) can suck lung tissue into the drainage holes, rupturing alveoli and causing a pleural air leak.

EO: The child will be free from injury caused by stripping or milking an occluded chest tube.

10. Assess the child's respiratory effort (rate, regularity, depth, ease, anxiety, and chest discomfort). Auscultate the lungs. Percuss the lung fields.

Decreased breath sounds could indicate the presence of air or fluid between the stethoscope and the lung.

A dull percussion note indicates fluid accumulation in the chest. A dull percussion may also mean that the fluid is walled off in a part of the lung that the tube can not reach (loculated). A distant hollow sound could mean air has accumulated in the pleural cavity.

EO: The child will demonstrate improved air exchange.

11. Assess the child for a tension pneumothorax (air

This can be a life-threatening complication that com-

PROCEDURE

under pressure within the pleural cavity). Signs of tension pneumothorax include:

    a. The high pressure alarm on the ventilator sounds continuously.

    b. The trachea is shifted away from the affected side.

    c. Breath sounds are absent on the affected side.

    d. The affected side of the chest does not move with respirations.

    e. The affected side is hyperresonant to percussion.

12. Have a clamp at the bedside for the following reasons:
    - To locate the source of an air leak if bubbling occurs in the water seal bottle while the system is on suction.
    - To replace the drainage system.

    Do not clamp the chest tube to get the child out of bed, to walk, or during transportation to another area in the hospital.

13. Assess the child's level of discomfort and medicate as ordered.

14. Record the insertion, the child's tolerance of it, and x-ray results, and make an ongoing assessment of respiratory status in the medical record.

RATIONALE/EXPECTED OUTCOME (EO)

presses the lung, heart and great vessels. The entire mediastinum is compressed and shifted decreasing cardiac output.

EO: The child will have a tension pneumothorax recognized and treated.

EO: The child will maintain normal cardiac output.

Clamp the tube momentarily at points along its length. Move from chest to drainage system. Once the clamp is placed between the air leak and the water seak, the bubbling will stop.

Whenever the chest tube is clamped no air or fluid can escape from the pleural space. This puts the child at risk for a tension pneumothorax.

The manipulation of the chest wall and the insertion of a tube is painful.

EO: The child will have a reduction in pain.

EO: The child's medical record will reflect the chest tube insertion and ongoing assessments.

Patient/Family Education: Home Care Considerations

1. Answer the child's and family's questions honestly and completely. Reinforce previous teaching.
2. Discuss signs and symptoms of improved respiratory status as well as complications.
3. Review follow-up care and complications.
4. Provide telephone numbers of persons to contact as questions arise.

References

Carroll, P.F. (1986). The ins and outs of chest drainage systems. *Nursing '86, 16*(12), 26–33.

Cohen, S. (1980). How to work with chest tubes. *American Journal of Nursing, 80*(4), 685–712.

Erickson, R. (1981). Chest tubes: They're really not that complicated. *Nursing '81, 11*(5), 34–43.

Gift, A.G., Bolgiano, C.S., & Cunningham, J. (1991). Sensations during chest tube removal. *Heart and Lung, 20*(2), 131–137.

Knauss, P.J. (1985). Chest tube stripping: Is it necessary? *Focus on Critical Care, 12*(6), 41–43.

Mim, B. (1985). You can manage chest tubes confidently. *RN, 48*(1), 39.

Oxygen Therapy

31

Definition/Purpose

Acute respiratory diseases are the most common causes of illness in infancy and childhood. Oxygen is administered to most critically ill children. Oxygen should be considered a medication; thus, the flow rate and concentration must be ordered by a physician and checked frequently.

Oxygen therapy can be considered either short- or long-term. Short-term oxygen therapy is administered for a duration of 30 days or less and generally is used for acute disorders. Long-term oxygen is administered for longer than 30 days and generally is used for chronic disorders.

Short-term oxygen therapy has two primary goals:

1. To relieve or prevent hypoxia

2. To reverse signs, symptoms, or physiologic abnormalities arising from tissue hypoxia.

Indications for short-term therapy include:

1. Documented PaO_2 less than 60 mm Hg or SaO_2 less than 90%

2. Postanesthesia

3. Postcardiopulmonary arrest

4. Reduced cardiac output

5. Hypotension, tachycardia, cyanosis, chest pain, dyspnea, or acute neurologic dysfunction

6. Endotracheal suctioning, bronchoscopy, or thoracentesis.

Continued needs for short-term oxygen need to be documented every 24 hours, depending on the condition of the child and the indication for its use.

Long-term oxygen therapy has three primary goals:

1. To relieve hypoxemia

2. To reverse signs, symptoms, and physiologic abnormalities arising from tissue hypoxia

3. To provide improved exercise tolerance, self-reliance, and cognitive ability.

Indications for long-term therapy include:

1. Failure of other therapy to optimize oxygenation

2. Significant hypoxia at rest or during sleep, documented by a pulse oximeter (PaO_2 of 55 mm Hg or less, or SaO_2 of 85% or less)

3. Significant hypoxia during exercise or feeding.

Continued need for long-term oxygen therapy is documented at 1 month, 6 months, 12 months, and yearly after that. Each child under consideration, however, has different pathology and considerations.

The most common method to deliver oxygen to infants is via a head hood or nasal cannula (Figs. 31-1 and 31-2). An air–oxygen humidified mixture at a flow rate of at least 7 L/min is administered to prevent carbon dioxide accumulation inside the hood. The nasal cannula, which is relatively comfortable and inexpensive, may be used for long- or short-

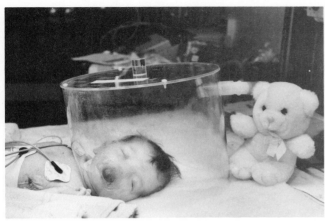

Figure 31-1.

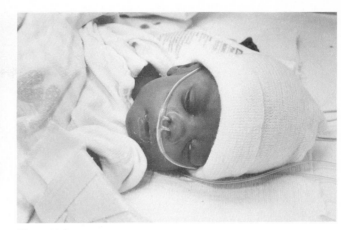

Figure 31-2.

term therapy and is routinely applied to infants for home care. Hoods have the disadvantage that the child must be removed from the oxygenated environment for feeding, weighing, etc.

An oxygen tent (mist tent) is used for children with croup, laryngotracheobronchitis, asthma, pneumonia, bronchiolitis, and bronchitis. The mist moistens airways, minimizes fluid loss from the lungs, provides a cool environment that aids in temperature reduction, liquifies secretions, reduces bronchial edema, and allows for small-to-moderate oxygen administration as indicated (up to 50% oxygen concentration). Tents, however, have several disadvantages that limit their usefulness. They make observation of the child difficult because of the high humidity. The oxygen concentration also falls quickly when the tent is opened for routine care and returns slowly to its previous level of oxygen after the tent is closed. (Fig. 31-3).

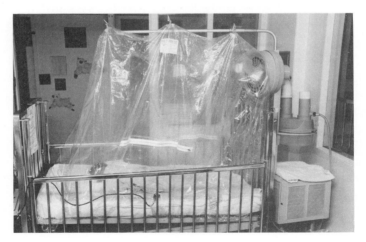

Figure 31-3.

Face tents and several kinds of oxygen masks are available for pediatric patients. Face tents are soft, plastic tent-shaped devices that fit around the child's chin and are held in place around the jaw by elastic straps. Gas flow should be a minimum of 7 L/min to ensure adequate carbon dioxide removal. Oxygen masks usually deliver inspired oxygen concentrations up to 55%; however, some are able to deliver concentrations up to 100% (Fig. 31-4).

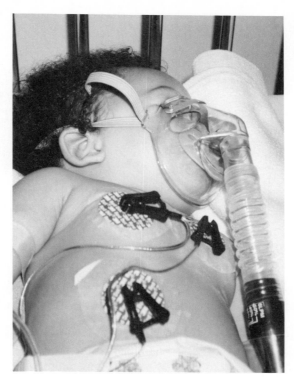

Figure 31-4.

Standard of Care

1. Oxygen therapy must be ordered by a physician.
2. In emergency situations, administer oxygen in generous amounts. Do not worry about alveolar hypoventilation; the need for immediate oxygenation takes precedence over the risk of hypoventilation.

Assessment

1. Assess the pertinent history and physical findings for events precipitating the need for oxygen, medications used, prior experiences with oxygen therapy, home treatment attempted, respiratory rate and effort, use of accessory muscles, shape of chest, breath sounds, restlessness, anxiety, heart rate, blood pressure, cyanosis, fatigue, diaphoresis, arterial blood gas results, and chest x-rays.
2. Assess the psychosocial and developmental factors such as age, ability to understand reasons for specific treatment, and previous coping mechanisms and habits.
3. Assess the child's and family's knowledge of the illness and interventions for respiratory compromise, and their willingness to learn.

Nursing Diagnoses

The following is a list of possible diagnoses and could apply, depending on the child's age, clinical situation, and physical condition:

Activity intolerance

High risk for altered body temperature

Impaired verbal communication

Fear

Anxiety

Impaired gas exchange
Hypothermia
Impaired physical mobility
High risk for injury
Pain

Planning

When planning to care for a child receiving oxygen therapy, the following equipment must be gathered:

Pulse oximeter
Thermometer
Stethoscope
Oxygen source, flow meter, and delivery device
Blood pressure monitoring device
Extra linen and towels.

Interventions

PROCEDURE	**RATIONALE/EXPECTED OUTCOME (EO)**
1. Monitor vital signs every 4 hours or more frequently as needed.	
2. Observe child for changes in respiratory rate, effort, or color. Notify physician of clinical changes.	
3. Auscultate breath sounds for symmetry and adventitious sounds.	
4. Review laboratory data: chest x-rays, arterial blood gases, and blood counts.	Blood gases are obtained 15–20 minutes after a change is made in the FIO$_2$ to document the effectiveness of the oxygen therapy.
5. Analyze inspired oxygen frequently (may be continuous or hourly, depending on the condition of the child and amount of oxygen being used).	Drifting of the oxygen concentration may be a problem; thus, continuous monitoring is necessary
6. Ensure that the inspired oxygen is humidified and warmed unless otherwise ordered by the physician.	Humidification prevents drying of the nasal mucosa. Warming prevents hypothermia and helps liquefy and mobilize secretions.
7. Position child appropriately: a. Semi-Fowler for a child in distress b. Prone for a child with copious mucus production.	*EO: The child will have the signs and symptoms of respiratory distress detected and controlled.*
8. Ensure that tubing associated with oxygen delivery is changed daily.	This will minimize the risk of micro-organisms multiplying in a warm moist environment and will decrease the risk of infection.
9. Keep infants and children dry. Change gowns and linens frequently to decrease dampness. Place additional clothing on children if they have difficulty maintaining a stable temperature (for example, socks, hat, and mittens). Wipe sides of the hood or tent to reduce moisture buildup.	The cool damp environment inside a tent or hood can decrease a child's body temperature.

PROCEDURE	**RATIONALE/EXPECTED OUTCOME (EO)**
10. Measure temperature in the hood or tent (usually 68°F–75°F).	*EO: The child's temperature will remain between 36°C and 37.2°C (97°F–99°F).*
11. Post *No Smoking—Oxygen in Use* signs on the patient's door.	
12. Do not allow friction, metal, electrical, or battery-operated toys in a tent.	*EO: Potentially combustible objects will be kept out of reach of the child undergoing oxygen therapy.* *EO: The child will not be injured while receiving oxygen therapy.*
13. Avoid oily, greasy, or alcohol-based substances.	
14. Place call light on the outside of the tent.	
15. Encourage parents to remain with the child whenever possible.	This will decrease the child's and parents' anxiety.
16. Allow a parent inside the tent with the child. Encourage the parent to hold, rock, and comfort the child.	*EO: The child will have anxiety related to parental separation decreased.*
17. Encourage parents to provide familiar toys and objects that are safe in an oxygen-rich environment.	
18. Consult the child-life specialist regarding play activities appropriate for growth, development, and health status.	The oxygen devices place physical limitations on the child; thus, creative activities need to be initiated.
19. Use medical play as an anxiety-reducing technique; for example, place the oxygen mask on a doll.	*EO: The child will engage in age-appropriate diversional activities.*
20. Assess for potential complications of oxygen therapy:	
a. Respiratory depression	May occur if the basic respiratory drive is hypoxia.
b. Retrolental fibroplasia	Occurs in newborns and premature infants in whom retinal vessels are not fully developed. The effect of high PaO_2 is retinal vasoconstriction, which causes hemorrhage in the vitreous, producing traction in the retina that may result in blindness.
c. Substernal pain occurs in children who receive 1.0 FIO_2 for 6 hours or 0.6 FIO_2 for 36 hours.	The pain may be related to pulmonary endothelial damage.
d. Atelectasis occurs when high concentrations of oxygen are used.	The alveoli are filled with oxygen and nitrogen is removed; thus, as oxygen is absorbed from the alveoli, atelectasis develops.
e. Pulmonary toxicity occurs in children who receive more than 0.5 FIO_2 for longer than several days, or who receive positive pressure ventilation.	Endothelial damage and alveolar damage lead to scarring and chronic lung disease, bronchopulmonary dysplasia, (BPD). *EO: The child will have complications recognized and treated.*

Patient/Family Education: Home Care Considerations

1. The child and family will be taught the purpose and operation of the oxygen equipment and the anticipated length of use.

2. If oxygen is to be used at home, the following issues need to be addressed in teaching sessions:
   a. Secure oxygen tanks in place, because they can be easily knocked over. A fall could knock the valve off and release an intense concentration of oxygen, increasing the risk of fire.
   b. Prohibit cigarette smoking in any room where oxygen is being used, and take precautions against lighted candles or a fireplace.

Table 31-1. Summary of Oxygen Delivery Systems

System	Description/Indications	Advantages	Disadvantages
Isolette	Oxygen piped into isolette. Useful for small infants who require temperature stabilization.	Environmental temperature can be controlled. Infant is visible.	Difficult to maintain uniform FIO_2. If humidity is added, microorganisms grow inside the water reservoir.
Hood	Lucite box placed over head. Has removable lid or ports for access to infant. Requires 7–12 L of gas flow. FIO_2 can be >90%. Useful for the infant or child who is too small for a mask.	Easy visibility and access to child. Can be used in cribs, in isolettes, and under warmers. Quick recovery time of FIO_2.	Moist environment may lead to skin irritation and prevent quick assessment of color or respiratory effort.
Cannula-Prongs	Two short vinyl prongs for each naris. Oxygen flow should not exceed 4–5 L/min. Useful for children who require oxygen concentrations up to 50%. FIO_2 / O_2 Flow 0.24 / 1 L 0.28 / 2 L 0.32 / 3 L 0.36 / 4 L 0.40 / 5 L 0.44 / 6 L	Child can eat and talk without altering FIO_2.	High flow rates may cause drying and bleeding of nasal mucosa.
Tents	Drape clear plastic over bed frame and tuck under the mattress. Useful for children who require high humidity and low concentration of oxygen.	Toddler can move around bed and play, yet still receive oxygen and humidity.	Child is difficult to see and assess. The cool mist will decrease body temperature, thus increasing oxygen requirements. Cannot provide reliable FIO_2 > 0.4–0.5. Difficult to maintain specific oxygen concentrations.
Aerosol mask	Mask fits over nose and mouth. Two ports on each side of mask provide CO_2 exhalation. Useful in children who require FIO_2 > 40%. FIO_2 / O_2 Flow 0.40 / 5–6 L 0.50 / 6–7 L 0.60 / 7–10 L	Comfortable for the older child, who is quiet and does not struggle.	Eating disrupts oxygen delivery. FIO_2 is limited by child's minute ventilation and tidal volume.
Partial rebreather mask	Mask as above plus a reservoir bag. The oxygen source is directed into the bag. Child inhales gas from the bag and room air through ports on the mask. On exhalation, a percentage of exhaled	Can deliver high FIO_2 concentrations.	Same as in the aerosol mask.

(continued)

Table 31-1. (*continued*)

System	Description/Indications	Advantages	Disadvantages
	gas returns to the reservoir bag. Gas flow must be adjusted so the bag does not collapse during inspiration by more than $\frac{1}{3}$ its volume. FIO_2 O_2 Flow 0.35–0.60 6–10 L		
Non-rebreather mask	Mask plus reservoir bag. Consists of two valves: a) The first, between mask and bag, allows one-way gas flow from bag to mask and prevents exhaled gas from returning to the bag. b) The second is at exhalation ports, so that as the child exhales, the valves close to prevent entrainment of room air. Useful in children who require high FIO_2 gas concentration if the flow is adjusted so the bag never collapses with inhalation. FIO_2 O_2 Flow 0.60–1.00 6–10 L	Can deliver FIO_2 of 0.9 or more.	Because the child inhales only from gases in bag, a kink in oxygen tubing will quickly cause hypoxia.
Venturi mask	Face mask with attached cone containing a "jet" orifice. Diameter of the inner orifice through which oxygen flows alters flow. Air entrainment on either side of "jet" blends oxygen with air. Useful when precise oxygen concentration must be delivered. FIO_2 O_2 Flow 0.28 4–5 L 0.31 6 L 0.35 8 L 0.40 8 L 0.60 10 L	Delivers precise oxygen concentration.	Air entrainment ports can become occluded. Child cannot eat or talk while wearing the mask.

c. The oxygen system should be at least 10 feet away from any open fires, including pilot lights in stoves, furnaces, and water heaters.

d. The oxygen system should be at least 10 feet away from electric equipment that may spark. Keep heating pads and electric blankets off the bed.

e. Avoid using petroleum jelly, face creams, lip balms, alcohol, or oils, since all are flammable and have the potential to explode in oxygen-rich environments.

   f. Have child wear 100% cotton garments. Silk, wool, and synthetic fabrics are subject to static electricity, which could ignite materials in the presence of oxygen.
   g. Have an all-purpose fire extinguisher available and visible.
3. Emphasize to the family that oxygen is considered a drug. It should be used only as prescribed. Too much or too little may cause medical complications. If the child seems to be in respiratory distress, the family should notify their physician and follow the advice given. Do not change the flow rate unless ordered by the physician.

References

Clarke, P., & Deeds, N. C. (1988). The child in a mist tent. *Pediatric Nursing*, *14*(6), 446–450.

Ellmyer, P., & Thomas, N. J. (1982). A guide to your patient's safe home use of oxygen. *Nursing '82*, *12*(1), 56–57.

Postural Drainage: Chest Physical Therapy

32

Definition/Purpose

An integral part of treatment of both acute and chronic respiratory disorders is administration of chest physical therapy to improve pulmonary hygiene and to maintain normal airway function. These techniques promote effective coughing, removal of secretions, and deep breathing.

Chest physical therapy requires the use of four techniques:

1. *Positioning of the child.* Postural drainage requires gravity to promote drainage of the tracheobronchial tree. If the child is positioned so that each bronchus drains downward, mucus collected in the bronchus is forced toward the trachea, where it can be expelled by a cough or through suctioning. Drainage of the bases of the lungs is facilitated by placement of the child in a Trendelenburg position, while drainage of the apical segment of the upper lobe of the lung is facilitated with the child in a sitting position. These positions may need to be modified in unstable children. (The head-down position would be inappropriate for a child with increased intracranial pressure or abdominal distention.) Infants can be positioned while in an incubator or crib, or on the lap of the therapist. Children may be positioned in bed with the use of pillows.

2. *Percussion, clapping, or pummelling.* During postural drainage, percussion is performed over the drainage bronchopulmonary segment for 1–2 minutes. Percussion is thought to hasten drainage by shaking secretions free from the walls of the airways. A cupped hand or soft mask is used to create an air pocket that cushions the blow of the percussion and transmits an energy wave into the lung. Percussion is not performed over bony prominences or the abdomen.

3. *Vibration.* Vibration is a fine, shaking motion applied during exhalation after postural drainage and percussion to help move secretions from peripheral airways toward the trachea. Vibration is achieved by applying a shaking motion to the drainage bronchopulmonary segment immediately after percussion as the child exhales. In the case of the neonate, this may be accomplished with the hand or a padded electric toothbrush.

4. *Coughing.* Coughing should follow percussion and vibration and is most effective if the child is sitting up so that diaphragmatic excursion is maximal. Ideally, the child should take several deep breaths and then follow the last breath with a deep cough. A tracheal tickle may be effective in producing a cough. This is accomplished by applying gentle pressure below the thyroid cartilage. A check of breath sounds will determine if the cough was effective. Children with suppressed or ineffective coughs should be suctioned.

Standard of Care

1. Contraindications to chest physiotherapy include the presence of displaced or fractured ribs, hemoptysis, or pulmonary hemorrhage.

2. Percussion is not performed directly over a recent incision, an open wound, drainage tubes, or an implantable venous port.

3. Chest physiotherapy should not be scheduled any sooner than 1 hour before feedings and should never be performed immediately after meals, since loss of appetite or emesis may occur. Children receiving continuous nasogastric feedings should have their feedings discontinued 30 minutes before the treatment and during therapy. Children with a history of gastric reflux will require close monitoring throughout the therapy and may require more time between feedings and treatments.

4. If the child is in pain, analgesics should be administered 1 hour before the treatment to reduce pain and increase cooperation.

Assessment

1. Assess the pertinent history and physical findings for precipitating events (for example, upper respiratory infections, allergens, stress); duration of respiratory difficulty; radiologic findings; medications taken; respiratory rate and effort; use of accessory muscles; shape of chest; breath sounds; degree of restlessness; heart rate; blood pressure; signs of respiratory failure; and arterial blood gases.

2. Assess psychosocial and developmental concerns in relation to age, degree to which this illness has interfered with normal lifestyle, and the child's and family's coping mechanisms.

3. Assess the child's and family's knowledge of the disease process and how chest physiotherapy aids in resolution. Also assess the family's willingness to learn the techniques for home care.

Nursing Diagnoses

The following is a list of possible diagnoses and could apply, depending on the child's age, clinical situation, and physical condition:

Altered nutrition, less than body requirements

High risk for aspiration

High risk for altered body temperature

Ineffective breathing pattern

High risk for injury

Pain

Planning

The following equipment must be gathered before beginning treatment:

Stethoscope

Vibrating padded toothbrush, cup or mask for percussion

Suction equipment (depending on the condition of the child)

Pillows.

Interventions

PROCEDURE	**RATIONALE/EXPECTED OUTCOME (EO)**
1. Explain the procedure to the child and family. It should be emphasized to both the child and parent that the nurse/therapist is not "hitting" the child.	Since constriction of the smooth muscles of the tracheobronchial tree may develop because of fear, tension, or discomfort, a happy cooperative child will have a more

PROCEDURE

2. Record vital signs and breath sounds before beginning the therapy.
3. Take the necessary measures as outlined in "Standard of Care" to prevent pain and aspiration.
4. Keep the infant or child covered with a gown or blanket.

5. Make yourself aware of chest x-ray results and the goal of the therapy. (Check physician's order.)

Infant

6. Bronchial drainage positions for the main segments of all lobes. The hand indicates the area to be vibrated.
   a. Apical segment of the left lower lobe (Fig. 32-1A).
   b. Posterior segment of the left lower lobe (Fig. 32-1B).
   c. Anterior segment of the left upper lobe (Fig. 32-1C).

RATIONALE/EXPECTED OUTCOME (EO)

effective therapy session. The therapy session should be fun and provide positive reinforcement.

EO: The child and family will express concerns about the therapy and have their questions answered. The child will cooperate with the treatment and not view it as a punishment.

This will allow for the collection of baseline data for evaluation of therapy.

EO: The child will have minimal discomfort. Measures will be taken to prevent the child from aspirating gastric contents.

Infants in temperature-regulated environments require special attention to prevent heat loss during the treatment.

EO: The child will maintain a normal body temperature throughout the treatment.

Often there is an order for drainage of a particular section of the lung that is affected.

The procedure is most easily performed on the therapist's lap.

EO: The child will obtain chest physiotherapy appropriate to the physical diagnosis and findings.

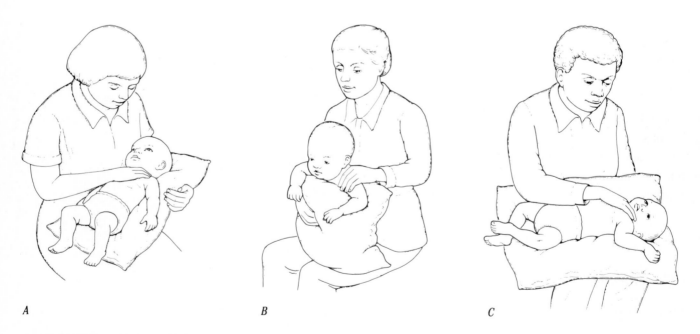

A   *B*   *C*

Figure 32-1. Bronchial drainage positions for the main segments of all lobes in infants.

PROCEDURE

    d. Superior segment of the right lower lobe (Fig. 32-1D).

    e. Posterior segment of the right lower lobe (Fig. 32-1E).

    f. Lateral segment of the right lower lobe (Fig. 32-1F).

    g. Anterior basal segment of the lower lobe (Fig. 32-1G).

    h. Right middle lobe (Fig. 32-1H).

    i. Lingular segments of left upper lobe (Fig. 32-1I).

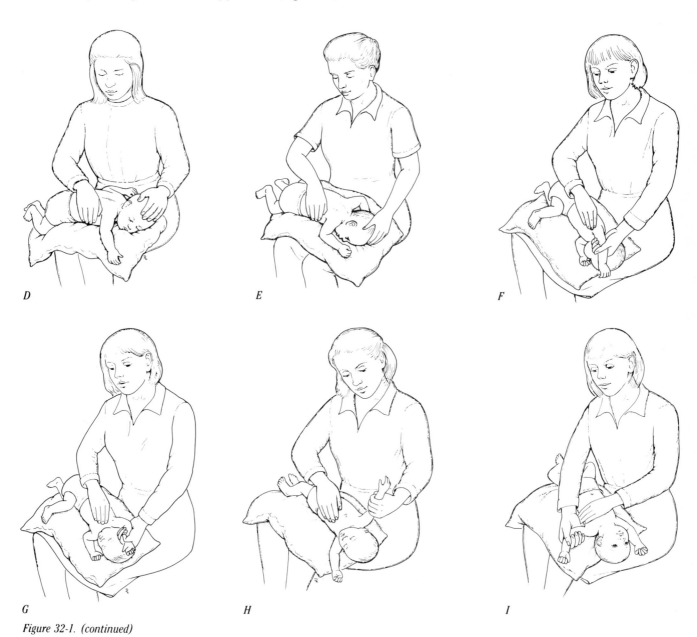

D   *E*   *F*

G   *H*   *I*

Figure 32-1. (continued)

PROCEDURE

Child

7. Bronchial drainage positions for major segments of all lobes.
   a. Apical segment of the right upper lobe and apical subsegment of apical-posterior segment of the left upper lobe (Fig. 32-2A).
   b. Posterior segment of right upper lobe and posterior subsegment of apical-posterior segment of left upper lobe (Fig. 32-2B).
   c. Anterior segments of both upper lobes (Fig. 32-2C).
   d. Superior segments of both lower lobes (Fig. 32-2D).

RATIONALE/EXPECTED OUTCOME (EO)

The drainage platform is padded but firm, and pillows are used to maintain each position with comfort.

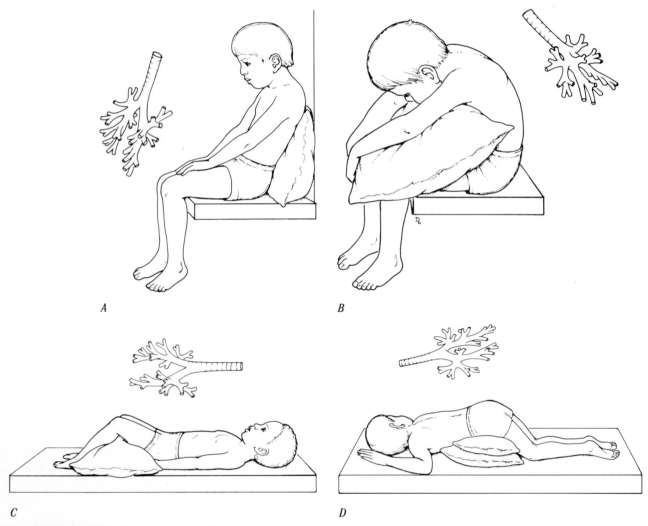

A

B

C

D

Figure 32-2. Bronchial drainage positions for the main segments of all lobes in children.

PROCEDURE

   e. Posterior basal segments of both lower lobes (Fig. 32-2E).

   f. Lateral basal segment of the right lower lobe (Fig. 32-2F).

   g. Anterior basal segment of the left lower lobe (Fig. 32-2G).

   h. Right middle lobe (Fig. 32-2H).

   i. Lingular segments of left upper lobe (Fig. 32-2I).

RATIONALE/EXPECTED OUTCOME (EO)

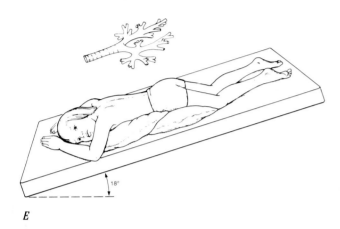

E

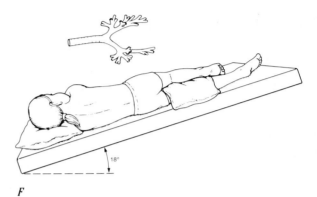

F

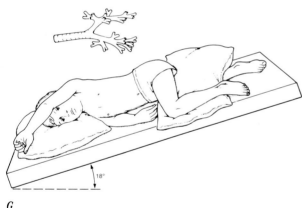

G

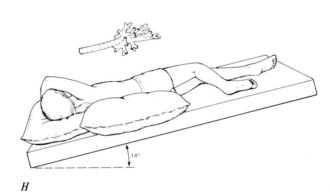

H

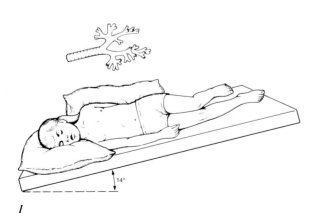

I

Figure 32-2. (continued)

PROCEDURE	**RATIONALE/EXPECTED OUTCOME (EO)**
8. Record vital signs and breath sounds after ending therapy and suctioning (if necessary).	*EO: The child's breathing pattern before and after the therapy will be compared and documented.*
9. Assess the child's tolerance of the therapy and how often the therapy needs to be performed. The procedure should be stopped if the child is fatigued.	Excessive fatigue is the most common problem seen in seriously ill children.

Patient/Family Education: Home Care Considerations

1. Teach child and family the use of positioning and breathing exercises to improve respiratory status.

2. Teach child and family the importance of coughing or percussion to clear the airway.

3. Provide an opportunity for the child and extended family and friends to observe a demonstration of and practice the skills essential for chest physiotherapy.

References

Fedorovich, C., & Littleton, M. T. (1990). Chest physiotherapy: Evaluating the effectiveness. *Dimensions of Critical Care Nursing, 9*(2), 68–74.

Rosdahl, C. (1991). *Textbook of basic nursing* (5th ed.). Philadelphia: J. B. Lippincott Company.

Suddarth, D. S. (1991). *The Lippincott manual of nursing practice.* (5th ed.). Philadelphia: J. B. Lippincott Company.

Tracheostomy

33

Definition/Purpose

A tracheostomy is the surgical creation of a stoma into the trachea. The reasons for tracheostomies vary:

1. Airway obstruction at or above the larynx
2. Inability to remove secretions from the tracheobronchial tree
3. The need for long-term positive pressure ventilation.

Airway obstruction may be caused by central nervous system vocal cord paralysis, subglottic web, cystic hygroma, subglottic stenosis, or epiglottitis. Also, children with Treacher Collins and Pierre Robin syndromes may experience airway obstruction due to enlarged tongues. Children who require tracheostomies for inability to remove secretions may include those with bronchopulmonary dysplasia, pneumonia, hyaline membrane disease, or diaphragm dysfunction.

The length of time a child has a tracheostomy depends on his or her progress, related conditions, and diagnoses.

Standard of Care

1. Because the tracheostomy is an open surgical wound, strict asepsis is mandatory.
2. Tracheostomy tubes are changed weekly.
3. An extra tracheostomy tube of the same size the child has inserted is to be kept at the bedside.
4. An ambu bag and adaptor (if necessary) are also to be kept at the bedside.
5. The tracheostomy ties are changed daily or when wet or dirty.

Assessment

1. Assess the pertinent history and physical findings for the date of placement of the tracheostomy; the reason for placement; the type and size of the tube; the condition of the skin around the stoma; the child's color, vital signs, and breath sounds; the consistency and amount of secretions; and the presence or absence of a cuff.
2. Assess the psychosocial and developmental factors of age, change in body image, fear of shortness of breath, and fear of the inability to communicate.
3. Assess the family's knowledge of the purpose of the tracheostomy, their understanding of the anatomy, the routine care necessary, the indications for contacting a physician, and their readiness and willingness to learn.

Nursing Diagnoses

The following is a list of possible diagnoses and could apply, depending on the child's age, clinical situation, and physical condition:

Ineffective airway clearance

High risk for infection

Impaired verbal communication

Impaired skin integrity

Anxiety

Fear

Body image disturbance

Altered growth and development

Ineffective family coping

Planning

When planning to care for a child with a tracheostomy, the following equipment must be gathered:

Slate, pen, paper, and picture board

Stethoscope

Tracheostomy collar with humidification source

Suction catheter

Sterile gloves

Sterile water

Rolled-up towel

Sterile saline drops

Aspirator

Ambu bag

Hydrogen peroxide

Cotton-tipped applicators or pipe cleaners

Tracheostomy ties (twill ties)

Tracheostomy tube

Scissors

Interventions

PROCEDURE

Preoperative

1. Describe and illustrate with diagrams the altered physiology that requires the tracheostomy.

2. Explain what the tracheostomy will look like and what care will be required postoperatively.

3. Reinforce and clarify what the physician has told the family and child.

4. Explain that the child will not be able to speak or cry after the tracheostomy is placed. Reassure the child and family that the child will learn how to cover the opening of the tracheostomy to vocalize, or that he or she will be taught to use sign language or a vocalization device that fits over the tracheostomy.

RATIONALE/EXPECTED OUTCOME (EO)

A well-informed family will experience less anxiety and will be more receptive to teaching.

EO: The family will express their fears and anxieties in caring for a child with a tracheostomy.

Placement of the tracheostomy cannula renders the child aphonic due to the interrupted passage of air from the lungs to the oral and nasal cavities that modifies the air for speech purposes.

PROCEDURE

5. Provide slate, pen and paper, or a picture board for communication.

6. Stress to the family that they will need to talk to the child frequently and provide tactile stimuli.

7. Encourage parents to let the child explore the environment; remind the parents to set limits on the child as they would if the child did not have a tracheostomy.

Postoperative—General Considerations

8. Auscultate chest every 2–4 hours, noting symmetry of breath sounds, respiratory rate and depth, presence of wheezing, congestion, etc.

9. Observe child for restlessness, anxiety, stridor, cyanosis, tachypnea, tachycardia, nasal flaring, and difficulty eating.

10. Monitor blood gases as ordered.

11. Ensure at least maintenance fluid intake unless contraindicated.

12. Provide humidification using a tracheostomy collar (Fig. 33-1).

RATIONALE/EXPECTED OUTCOME (EO)

EO: The child will establish an effective method of communication.

Children with tracheostomies are at risk for delays in receptive and expressive language development, as well as deficits in oral, speech, and voice production.

Developing and maintaining abilities to cope with illness along with the child's normal developmental tasks are important for the child's welfare.

EO: The child will attain developmental milestones.

EO: The child has clear breath sounds on auscultation.

EO: The child's respiratory rate and heart rate are within normal limits for age.

Maintenance fluid and humidification of inspired air keep secretions thin and moist and prevent mucus plugs from forming.

EO: The child will maintain a patent airway.

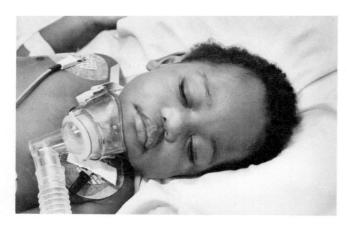

Figure 33-1.

13. Perform postural drainage and percussion if ordered.

This will maximize airway clearance.

Postoperative Suctioning

14. Suction every 2–4 hours or as needed.

15. Wash hands.

16. Open suction catheter package so that the catheter can be attached to the suction tubing, but remain sterile in the package (Fig. 33-2).

The suctioning procedure is carried out in a sterile manner.

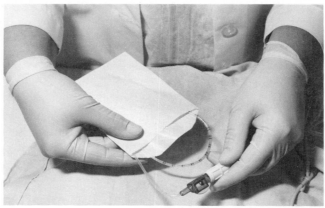

Figure 33-2.

PROCEDURE

17. Open cup of sterile water.
18. Open saline drops.
19. Put on sterile gloves. (The dominant hand is sterile; the nondominant hand is not sterile.)
20. Insert 2–3 drops of saline into the tracheostomy tube, using the nonsterile hand (Fig. 33-3). Hyperventilate child with ambu bag connected to oxygen (Fig. 33-4). If child has a metal tracheostomy tube in place, remove the inner cannula before instilling the saline.

RATIONALE/EXPECTED OUTCOME (EO)

A two-gloved technique is used under universal precaution guidelines.

This will help liquefy the secretions, making it easier to suction them out. Hyperventilation before suctioning prevents hypoxia during suctioning.

EO: The child will not become hypoxic during the procedure and will maintain presuctioning vital signs and pulse oximeter readings.

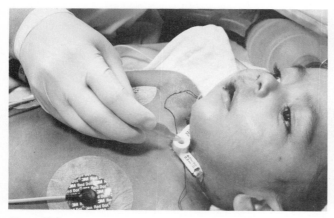

Figure 33-3.

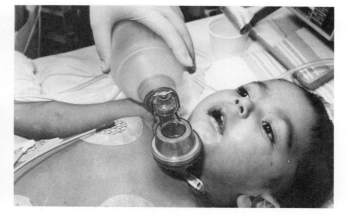

Figure 33-4.

21. Pick up the suction catheter with the sterile hand and pass the catheter gently into the trachea until resistance is met (Fig. 33-5). Do not apply suction when inserting the catheter.
22. Apply suction (80–100 mm Hg) and withdraw catheter using twisting motion. Limit suctioning to 5–15 seconds.

Gentle suctioning removes secretions, but does not damage the tracheal mucosa, causing bleeding.

EO: Suctioning will not cause mucosal trauma.

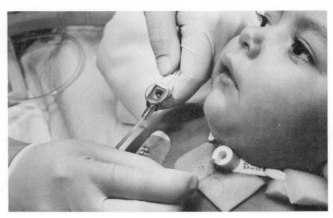

Figure 33-5.

PROCEDURE	**RATIONALE/EXPECTED OUTCOME (EO)**
23. If child desaturates during suctioning, hyperventilate child with 5–10 breaths, using the ambu bag connected to oxygen. Allow 30 seconds for recovery between suction attempts.	
24. Repeat steps 20–23 as needed. Rinse catheter with sterile water.	
25. Discard catheter, gloves, saline, and water. If the child has a metal tracheostomy tube, clean the inner cannula with ½ strength peroxide and pipe cleaners before reinserting it after suctioning.	
26. Record the color, amount, and consistency of the secretions and how the child tolerated the procedure.	*EO: The child's medical record will reflect the suctioning procedure and the results.*

Postoperative—Stoma Skin Care

27. Assess for signs of infection (for example, change in color or smell of mucus; fever; redness, swelling, tenderness, or warmth around the stoma).	When the skin is not intact (because of the stoma) and the upper airway is bypassed by the tracheostomy tube, there is an access route for infection to enter the respiratory tract. Secretions also tend to pool at or around the stoma, which provides a medium for growth of organisms and breakdown of the skin.
28. Clean around the stoma every 8–12 hours (or more often if necessary) to prevent skin irritation.	
29. Wash hands.	
30. Mix one part hydrogen peroxide with one part sterile water in a sterile cup.	
31. Open sterile applicator sticks.	
32. Put on sterile gloves.	
33. Soak applicator stick in peroxide solution and then roll stick over the skin beneath the tracheostomy tube to remove crusted secretions (Fig. 33-6). Repeat as needed to remove all secretions.	*EO: The child will remain free from inflection.*

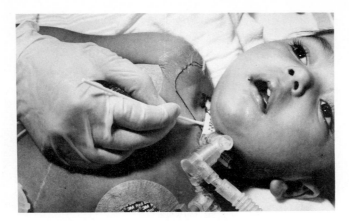

Figure 33-6.

PROCEDURE

34. Change external dressing (if present) and ties when wet or soiled with secretions or food.

35. Discard used supplies.

36. Record the cleaning process, condition of the skin and tracheostomy stoma, and how the child tolerated the procedure.

Postoperative—Tube Change

37. Schedule tube changes 2–3 hours after meals.

38. Attach ties to the clean tracheostomy tube.

39. Insert obturator into tube (Fig. 33-7).

RATIONALE/EXPECTED OUTCOME (EO)

EO: The child will maintain intact skin around the stoma and under the ties.

EO: The child's medical record will reflect the cleaning procedure and the condition of the skin.

This will prevent vomiting and the possibility of aspiration.

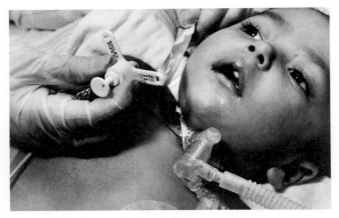

Figure 33-7.

40. Set tube back on a sterile field (such as the package).

PROCEDURE	**RATIONALE/EXPECTED OUTCOME (EO)**
41. Position the child supine with a small roll under shoulders.	This will help expose the area.
42. Suction the child.	
43. Cut old tracheostomy ties and remove old tube.	
44. Gently and quickly insert the new tube with obturator. Hold tube in place at flange with one hand and remove obturator.	
45. Observe for correct placement of the tube: • Chest movement • Color • Vital signs	*EO: The child's tracheostomy tube will be changed with minimal discomfort and anxiety on a weekly basis or if occlusion occurs.*
46. Secure tracheostomy ties around neck snugly enough to fit one finger under the ties.	
47. Record the child's tolerance to the procedure in the medical record.	*EO: The child's tolerance to the procedure will be recorded in the medical record.*

Postoperative—Tie Change

48. Place a roll under the child's shoulders.	This will expose the area for visualization.
49. Slide the old ties from the center of the hole to the top on both sides of the tracheostomy tube.	
50. Insert the new ties under the old ones using a Lark's knot.	A Lark's knot is used because with a slip knot, the material used may fray and come undone if the hole is placed too close to the edge.
51. Secure tie at back of the neck so that one finger can be placed under the tie.	This will prevent the ties from being placed too tightly or loosely.
52. Cut and remove old ties.	
53. Examine the neck for sores or erythremia. Document the condition of the skin in the medical record.	*EO: The child's ties are changed daily (or as needed) when wet or dirty.*

Patient/Family Education: Home Care Considerations

1. Instruct the child and family on the basic anatomy and function of the respiratory system, with emphasis on the trachea.
2. Demonstrate to the family skin care, suctioning, and changing the ties and tube. Have at least two members of the family return the demonstrations.
3. Teach the family safety precautions to take with a child who has a tracheostomy:
   a. Keep obstructive materials such as sheets, pillows, stuffed animals, and blankets away from the stoma.
   b. Check toys for small parts that could be inserted into the tracheostomy tube.
   c. Use nonplastic bibs to keep food and fluids out of the tracheostomy.
   d. Avoid powders or aerosols that act as irritants to the respiratory tract.
   e. Position the child on his or her side after eating or in an infant seat with the head supported and neck slightly hyperextended to prevent aspiration.
   f. Carry a travel kit when leaving home. It should include everything needed to care for the child with a tracheostomy (for example, suction catheter, battery-operated aspirator, extra tracheostomy tube, scissors, and twill ties).
   g. Keep the child away from swimming pools, tubs, or basins, where large amounts of water could enter the trachea.

4. Teach the family CPR.
5. Teach the family what to do should the tracheostomy become displaced.
6. Encourage the child to wear a Medic-Alert bracelet.
7. Have parents post a list of emergency numbers near the telephone.
8. Notify the telephone and electric companies that a child with a tracheostomy is present in the home and needs uninterrupted service for safe medical care.

References

Hall, S. S., & Weatherly, K. S. (1989). Using sign language with tracheotomized infants and children. *Pediatric Nursing, 15*(4), 362–367.

Kaufman, J., & Hardy-Ribakow, D. (1988). *What parents need to know about trache care. RN, 51*(10), 99–100; 103–104.

Kennedy, A. H., Johnson, W., & Sturdevant, E. W. (1982). An educational program for families of children with tracheostomies. *Maternal/Child Nursing, 7*(1), 42–49.

Sherman, L., & Rosen, C. (1990). Development of a preschool program for tracheostomy-dependent children. *Pediatric Nursing, 16*(4), 357–361.

Simon, B. M., & McGowan, J. S. (1989). Tracheostomies in young children: Implications for assessment and treatment of communication and feeding disorders. *Infants and Young Children, 1*(3), 1–9.

Endotracheal Tube Care

34

Definition/Purpose

Endotracheal intubation involves passing an endotracheal tube (ETT) through either the nares or the mouth to the midtrachea (approximately at the T2 level). It is indicated during cardiopulmonary resuscitation, respiratory failure with hypoxemia or hypercarbia, absent pharyngeal reflexes, coma, brain stem dysfunction, and if the airway is unstable from facial trauma or airway abnormality. Endotracheal intubation may also be used to provide mechanical ventilation or higher concentrations of the oxygen, and to facilitate bronchial hygiene.

A few anatomic considerations are important to the procedure for infants and children when compared with the adult:

1. The larynx is located more anterior and cephalad than in adults.
2. The infant's gums are soft, vascular, and easily indented.
3. The larynx and trachea are small; in the neonate the tracheal diameter is about 5 mm.
4. Deciduous teeth are poorly anchored and easily dislodged.
5. The epiglottis is shorter in the infant than in the adult. It is U-shaped in the infant, whereas it is flat in the adult.
6. The angle formed by the epiglottis and vocal cords is more acute in the infant.
7. The larynx is funnel-shaped in the infant and cylindrical in the adult.
8. The narrowest part of the trachea in infants and children is the subglottic area (the cricoid ring).

Endotracheal suctioning involves the passing of a catheter through the endotracheal tube for the mechanical removal of secretions from the tube and the tracheobronchial areas. A buildup of secretions in the ETT can result in hypoxia or hypercapnia. Care must be taken when suctioning a child with suspected or documented increased intracranial pressure.

Standard of Care

1. A child must be connected to a cardiorespiratory monitor with limits set and alarms on during and after intubation.
2. Obtain vital signs of the intubated child every 1–2 hours.
3. Auscultate breath sounds every 1–2 hours.
4. Measure the length of the ETT (from the child's lips to the tip of the tube) every 2 hours. To prevent accidental extubation, assess the security of the tube every 1–2 hours as well.
5. Administer mouth care every 4 hours. Apply lotion or mouth moisturizer to prevent cracking and splitting of lips.
6. Restrain the child if he or she is capable of dislodging the tube.
7. Place a bite block or oral airway for children with teeth, who may chew the endotracheal tube.

8. Aseptic technique must be used when suctioning an endotracheal tube.

9. Sterile gloves must be worn on both hands while suctioning.

10. A new setup of gloves, catheter, and irrigation containers is required for each suctioning procedure.

11. Hyperoxygenate the child with an ambu bag and 100% oxygen before suctioning.

12. Obtain actual endotracheal tube cuff pressure every 4 hours.

Assessment

1. Assess the child's medical history, with emphasis on respiratory disorders, congenital defects, and conditions affecting the tracheobronchial passages.

2. Assess physical findings such as general appearance, pallor, cyanosis, and decreased systemic perfusion.

3. Assess behavior for anxiety, lethargy, or restlessness. Monitor the child for a change in vital signs such as tachycardia, bradycardia, tachypnea, hypotension, or hypertension.

4. Assess for signs and symptoms of respiratory distress, such as retractions, nasal flaring, wheezing, cyanosis, and restlessness.

5. Assess the endotracheal tube for excessive movement (shown by change in length measurement) and the need to resecure the tube.

6. Assess the child's and family's coping mechanisms and previous experience with intubation and the ICU environment.

Nursing Diagnoses

The following is a list of possible diagnoses and could apply, depending on the child's age, clinical situation, and physical condition:

Ineffective airway clearance

Ineffective breathing pattern

Impaired verbal communication

Fear

Impaired gas exchange

High risk for infection

Sleep pattern disturbance

Altered tissue perfusion

Impaired physical mobility

Oral mucous membrane, altered

Impaired swallowing

Planning

To assist in the preparation of endotracheal intubation, the following equipment must be gathered:

Laryngoscope handle

Laryngoscope blades (Table 34-1)

Endotracheal tube (Table 34-2)

Stylet

Magill forceps

Lubricant

Table 34-1. Laryngoscope Blade Size

Age	Blade
Premature	Miller 0
Term–1 year	Wis-Hipple 1 or Miller 1
1–1.5 years	Wis-Hipple 1½
1.5–12 years	Miller or Flagg, 2–4
13 years or older	MacIntosh 3

Table 34-2. Endotracheal Tube Size

Age	Tube Size
Premature	2.5
Term–3 months	3.0
3–7 months	3.5
7–15 months	4.0
15–24 months	4.5
2–15 years	Internal diameter = (16 + age in years) − 4 (Round to nearest 0.5)

Table 34-3. ETT Size versus Suction Catheter Size

Size of ETT	Size of Suction Catheter
2.5–3.0	5½–6 F
3.5–4.5	8 F
5.0–6.7	10 F
7.0–9.0	14 F

Ambu bag with appropriate size mask and manometer

Oxygen source

Suction source

Yankeur suction or closed-port suction

Sterile suction kit (appropriate size for ETT) (Table 34-3)

Sterile single-use water container

Sterile single unit of 0.9% sodium chloride

Benzoin

Tape

2 × 2 gauze

Hypoactive dressing

Tape remover

3-way stopcock

Pressure manometer

5-mL syringe

Stethoscope

Interventions

PROCEDURE

RATIONALE/EXPECTED OUTCOME (EO)

Preparation of the child

1. If the child is unconscious or an infant, no preparation is needed other than positioning. If the child is conscious, explain in simple terms that you are go-

EO: The child or parent will demonstrate knowledge of the intubation procedure, duration of the tube placement, and prognosis.

PROCEDURE	**RATIONALE/EXPECTED OUTCOME (EO)**

ing to make it easier for him or her to breathe and that he or she will soon feel sleepy from the medication given (sedative and neuromuscular block).

Intubation is uncomfortable, terrifying, and a prolonged procedure if the child is not totally cooperative; thus sedation and a neuromuscular block are necessary.

EO: The child will have periods of restful sleep.

2. Notify the family of the intended procedure, the reasons for the intubation, the expected duration, and the risks of the intubation.

Although stressed, the family will cooperate with the plan of care if they understand the reasons for intubation.

EO: The family will verbalize the relationship between the intubation and the child's condition.

Positioning the Child

3. Position the child supine, with the face forward, the neck slightly flexed, and the head extended. A firm pad may be placed under the shoulders. (This is Sniffing position.)

Excessive extension should be avoided, especially if the child has increased intracranial pressure. Excessive extension decreases cerebral bloodflow.

Intubation

4. Assemble and check equipment. Check laryngoscope batteries and bulb.

5. Put on gloves and suction the child's mouth of secretions using a Yankeur suction or closed-port suction catheter.

This will assist in visualization of the trachea.

6. Ventilate the patient with 100% oxygen using a mask and ambu bag for 2–3 minutes.

Ventilating preintubation minimizes hypoxia during intubation and decreases intracranial pressure.

7. The physician will now intubate the child (Fig. 34-1). Assist with suctioning and ventilation. Also check vital signs during intubation.

Bradycardia may be due to vagal stimuli and hypoxia; hypotension may be due to sedation.

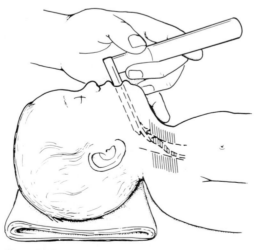

Figure 34-1.

8. Once the tube is in place, remove the mask from the ambu bag and attach bag to ETT. Ventilate with 100% oxygen.

9. Watch for bilateral movement of the chest wall; auscultate lungs for equal breath sounds.

If the ETT is placed properly, both sides of the child's chest should expand. If the chest expands on one side only, the tube is in the corresponding mainstem bronchus and should be withdrawn 0.5–1.0 cm until both

PROCEDURE

RATIONALE/EXPECTED OUTCOME (EO)

sides move. If the chest does not expand, but the abdomen distends, the tube is in the esophagus rather than the trachea. If this happens, the ETT is removed, the child hyperventilated with bag and mask, and intubation attempted again.

EO: The child will have an endotracheal tube inserted without complications.

Securing the Endotracheal Tube

10. Obtain assistance of another staff member.

EO: The child will maintain a patent airway and adequate oxygenation.

11. Cut two squares of hypoactive dressings large enough to fit over cheeks.

12. Tear two pieces of tape long enough to reach from one cheek to the other. Split each piece of tape for two thirds of its length.

13. Paint tincture of benzoin onto each cheek and above the mouth over the nasal philtrum.

14. After the benzoin is dry (tacky), fix the hypoactive squares on each cheek.

This will protect the child's delicate facial skin from a tape burn.

15. Next, fix the unsplit end of one of the tapes to the square on one cheek. The upper split tail is carried over the nasal philtrum onto the opposite cheek. (Make sure it adheres well.) The lower split tail is brought under the tube and then is wrapped around it in a spiral fashion. The last 5 mm of the tail is folded over on itself to make a tab to grasp when the tape is removed. The second split tape is applied in a similar fashion using the other cheek (Fig. 34-2).

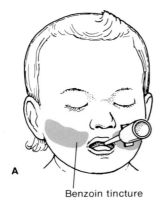 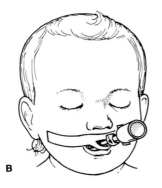 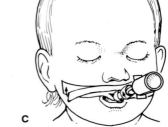

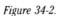
Benzoin tincture

Figure 34-2.

16. Record length of ETT.
17. Auscultate breath sounds.

The ETT should be 1–2 cm above the carina or at the level of the third rib.

EO: The child has no aventitious breath sounds.

18. Obtain a chest x-ray to check the tube placement.
19. Insert nasogastric tube.

This will prevent aspiration of stomach contents and

PROCEDURE

RATIONALE/EXPECTED OUTCOME (EO)

prevent air trapping and abdominal distention due to positive pressure ventilation.

Suctioning the Endotracheal Tube

20. Assemble equipment:
    ambu bag
    suction source
    sterile suction kit with gloves
    catheter of .9% sodium chloride.

EO: The child will maintain pulmonary function.

21. Adjust amount of suction:
    • 50–80 mm Hg for infants
    • 80–110 mm Hg for children.

This provides adequate vacuum to remove secretions without causing trauma to tracheal tissues.

22. Explain the procedure to the child (if appropriate) and the family.

EO: The child and family will experience a decreased feeling of anxiety and will cooperate with interventions designed to alleviate dyspnea.

23. Open suction kit near the head of the bed, maintaining a sterile field. If a kit is not available, use inner surface of sterile glove wrapper for a sterile field.

24. Using a sterile technique, glove both hands.

25. Wrap catheter around the dominant "sterile" hand, leaving suction port exposed.

EO: The child is protected from nosocomial infections.

26. With nondominant "clean" hand, grasp suction tubing and attach to suction port. Thumb of "clean" hand will control suction port.

The "clean" hand manipulates the non-sterile equipment.

27. Using the "clean" hand, disconnect ventilator or other oxygen source and place on sterile field.

28. Using the "clean" hand, hyperventilate the child with ambu bag for 8–10 breaths with 100% oxygen (Fig. 34-3).

Hyperventilation reexpands sections of the lungs and minimizes hypoxia due to suctioning.

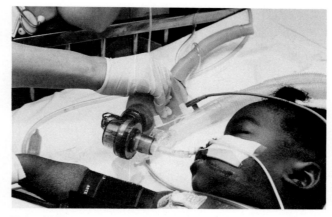

Figure 34-3.

29. Instill into the endotracheal tube 0.5–1.0 mL of normal saline for infants or 1–5 mL for children.

30. Using sterile hand, gently and quickly introduce the catheter without suction through the ETT until the child coughs or resistance is felt.

Never push catheter against resistance because of the possibility of tracheal injury.

PROCEDURE	**RATIONALE/EXPECTED OUTCOME (EO)**

31. Pull catheter back 0.5 cm, then apply intermittent suction with the thumb of the "clean" hand, while pulling out the catheter and rotating it with the "sterile" hand (Fig. 34-4).

Suctioning should not exceed 5 seconds. Prolonged suctioning may cause hypoxia.

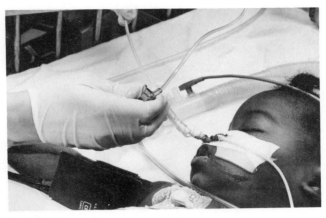

Figure 34-4.

32. Monitor heart rate and color throughout procedure. If bradycardia, cyanosis, or mottling occurs, stop suctioning and hyperventilate with 100% oxygen until stable.

Vagal nerve stimulation may cause bradycardia.

EO: The child will inspire and exhale without wheezing or use of accessory muscles.

EO: The child will regain and maintain normal color, vital signs, and cardiac function.

33. Repeat suctioning as many times as needed using the above technique.

The child's status (oxygen saturation) and type of secretions will dictate both the number of times that the catheter is passed and the frequency with which the suction procedure is performed.

34. Reconnect oxygen source of ventilator.

35. Flush catheter with sterile water.

36. Assess need for further suctioning:
    a. Coughing
    b. Secretions in ETT
    c. Noisy breath sounds.

37. If consistency of secretions is thick, instill 0.9% sodium chloride into the ETT as before. Repeat steps 25–32. Reposition the child's head when suctioning.

Turning the head to the left should help direct the catheter into the right mainstem bronchus; and to the right into the left bronchus.

38. Using the same catheter, suction the oropharynx and nose. Do not reintroduce this catheter into trachea.

Once the catheter is introduced into the nose and mouth, it is no longer sterile.

39. Discard all contaminated equipment. Wash hands.

40. Record color, amount, consistency, and odor of secretions. Record change in lung sounds before and after suctioning. Also record any adverse reactions to suctioning (for example, apnea, bradycardia, or decreased heart and respiratory rates).

| **PROCEDURE** | **RATIONALE/EXPECTED OUTCOME (EO)** |

PROCEDURE

Testing Cuff Pressure

41. Measure and record cuff pressure every 4 hours using one of these methods:
    • Minimal leak volume (MLV)
    • Actual leak volume (ALV).

RATIONALE/EXPECTED OUTCOME (EO)

If a cuffed ETT is inserted, the pressure of the inflatable balloon at the distal end must be measured to prevent necrosis and stenosis of the trachea. The optimum cuff pressure is <15 mm Hg. The cuff should be deflated every 2 hours to prevent necrosis of the trachea.

EO: The child will have the cuff pressure of the ETT tested.

42. ***MLV:***
    • Positive pressure inflation needs to be delivered by a ventilator or an ambu bag (Fig. 34-5).

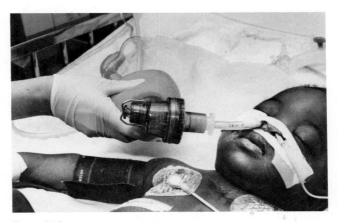

Figure 34-5.

• Insert the tip of a 5-mL syringe filled with air into the cuff, filling valve.
• Place stethoscope on neck over larynx.
• Slowly inflate the cuff while auscultating the neck.
• Inflate only until an air rush is not heard during a positive pressure inflation.
• Slowly withdraw air from the cuff until a small leak is heard.
• Remove syringe.

This is the minimal occlusive volume needed to prevent an air leak and aspiration.
A small air leak avoids undue pressure on the trachea.

ALV:

• Connect syringe and monometer to a 3-way stopcock. Connect the other stopcock port to the cuff, filling valve.
• With the ETT's cuff inflated, use aseptic technique to suction oronasal pharyngeal secretions from above the cuff.
• With the stopcock in the Off position to the monometer, withdraw air from the filling valve to deflate the cuff.
• Place stethoscope to neck.
• Slowly inject air from the syringe into the cuff until no rush of air is heard during a pressurized breath.
• Turn stopcock off to the syringe and record the cuff pressure from the monometer.

Prevents aspiration of secretions that may have pooled above the cuff.

Optimum cuff pressure < 15 mm Hg.

PROCEDURE	**RATIONALE/EXPECTED OUTCOME (EO)**
43. Be aware of complications associated with tracheal intubation: • Trauma from instrumentation • Expulsion or obstruction of the tube • Infection from contaminated equipment • Edema of larynx or trachea • Laryngospasm • Ulceration of tracheal mucosa • Granuloma of vocal cords • Nasal septum necrosis • Sinusitis • Eustachian tube dysfunction.	*EO: The child is free from preventable injury due to the tracheal intubation.*

Patient/Family Education: Home Care Considerations

1. Explain to the child and family the importance of the tube and measures that must be taken to secure it in place (for example, restraints, or sedation).

2. Explain to the child and family that the child will be unable to talk or vocally cry until the ETT is removed.

3. Instruct the child and family on alternative measures of communication (for example, hand signals, or pen and pad for writing or drawing).

4. Instruct family on comfort measures (for example, lotion for lips, glycerin swabs to cleanse mouth, and back rubs).

5. If neuromuscular blocking agents are used, explain to the family the reason for their use and that the effects are temporary. Explain that the child may be able to hear discussions in the room; therefore, the family will want to discuss concerns and prognosis out of the child's hearing range. Also, encourage them to talk to the child, play records or tapes, and orient the child to the day and time.

6. Explain any procedures (for example, suctioning, or retaping) to the family and reasons for a certain technique.

References

Czarnik, R.E., Stone, K.S., Everhart, C.C., et al. (1991). Differential effects of continuous versus intermittent suction on tracheal tissue. *Heart and Lung, 20*(2), 144–151.

Engler, A.J. (1989). Verifying endotracheal tube placement with the Trache Mate intubation system. *Pediatric Nursing, 15*(4), 390–392.

Eubanks, D.H., & Bone, R.C. (1985). *Comprehensive respiratory care.* St. Louis: C.V. Mosby Co.

Howard-Glenn, L., & Koniak-Griffin, D. (1990). Evaluation of monometer use in manual ventilation of infants in neonatal intensive care units. *Heart and Lung, 19*(6), 620–626.

Johanson, B.C., Dungca, C.U., Hoffmeister, D., & Wells, S.J. (1981). *Standards for critical care.* St. Louis: C.V. Mosby Co.

Kleiber, C. (1986). Clinical implications of deep and shallow suctioning in neonatal patients. *Focus on Critical Care, 13*(4), 36–39.

Turner, B.S. (1990). Maintaining the artificial airway: Current concepts. *Pediatric Nursing, 16*(5), 487–493.

Transcutaneous Oxygen Tension

35

Definition/Purpose

Critically ill infants and children require frequent blood gas determination. One noninvasive method to determine oxygen saturation is the use of a *transcutaneous oxygen tension monitor*. TcPO$_2$ monitoring is theoretically based on the physiology of oxygen supply to the skin. The amount of oxygen delivered to the skin depends on three factors: the thickness of the skin, blood flow to the skin, and arteriovenous oxygen difference.

TcPO$_2$ monitoring has three influences on the skin. First, it changes the diffusion barrier. A local hyperemia is produced by an electrode, which dilates underlying capillaries, increasing blood flow and shifting the oxygen dissociation curve to the right, thus displacing oxygen from hemoglobin. Second, by using a small amount of solution over the area being measured, the conductivity of the oxygen through the epidermis is increased. Third, because local hyperemia is used, maximum vasodilation occurs.

The electrodes are more accurate in infants less than 1 year old because they have a greater capillary density per cubic millimeter of skin than older children. The more capillaries, the more oxygen there is to be released. The TcPO$_2$ electrodes are also more accurate when the PaO$_2$ is 30–150 mm Hg. Accuracy can be improved outside this range by calibrating the electrode.

If the child's body temperature is less than 35.5°C (96.0°F) or the mean arterial pressure more than two standard deviations below the average for a child of that age, the electrode will not accurately reflect PaO$_2$. Both of these conditions constrict large proximal arteries, which local heating of the electrode cannot overcome.

Standard of Care

1. Reposition the sensor every 3–4 hours to prevent skin irritation or burning.
2. Check the monitor's sensitivity daily by putting the sensor in the calibration chamber and depressing the power button for 5 seconds.
3. Zeroing solution expires in 1 month. Do not use it if it is over 1 month old.

Assessment

1. Assess the pertinent history for the need for oxygen monitoring, and frequent blood samples where repeated blood gas determination presents a risk.
2. Assess the physical findings for respiratory rate, use of accessory muscles, breath sounds, degrees of restlessness and anxiety, heart rate, blood pressure, diaphoresis, cyanosis, and arterial blood gases. Assess the skin for potential areas of electrode placement.
3. Assess the family's understanding of the disease process and the support and information that the transcutaneous oxygen monitor will yield.

Nursing Diagnoses

The following is a list of possible diagnoses and could apply, depending on the child's age, clinical situation, and physical condition:

Anxiety

Fear

Impaired skin integrity

Planning

When planning to measure TcPO$_2$, the following equipment must be gathered:

TcPO$_2$ monitor

Sensor and cable

Zeroing solution

Distilled water and 3-mL syringe

Contact jelly

Adhesive ring

Gauze pad

Alcohol swab

Preparation block

Interventions

PROCEDURE

1. Explain the purpose of the transcutaneous oxygen tension monitor to the parent. Include the fact that blood samples will still need to be obtained, but not as frequently as if the monitor were not available. Also, certain conditions may necessitate drawing of blood.

2. Zeroing and calibration of the monitor must be done in accordance with the operator's manual. Each machine is different.

3. Apply the TcPO$_2$ probe:
   a. Abrade the skin with an alcohol swab.
   b. Apply the two-way, self-adhesive ring to the probe.
   c. Apply a tiny drop of contact gel to the center of the probe membrane.
   d. Secure the probe to the selected site with gentle pressure. Run finger around ring to seal it to the skin.

4. Record the TcPO$_2$ reading:
   a. Immediately on application of the sensor, the pO$_2$ mm Hg display will show a sharp drop.
   b. In 3–10 minutes the value will increase.

RATIONALE/EXPECTED OUTCOME (EO)

EO: The family will have their questions answered, thus decreasing their fear and anxiety.

The TcPO$_2$ no longer has a linear correlation with the TcPO$_2$ when the cardiac output falls to 65% of the control value.

EO: The monitor will be calibrated and zeroed according to the manufacturer's recommendations.

This will remove salt deposits that would alter skin conductivity.
This will help position the probe on the child's skin.

This increases the conductivity of the oxygen through the epidermis to the probe.
The site selected for placing the probe is in an area with a high density of capillaries and with little or no subcutaneous fat layers. The thorax and abdomen are recommended sites because of increased capillary density. Avoid sites where postural pressure would be evident. Also avoid areas of poor perfusion and those sites where edema is present.

EO: The child will have the probe applied in an area of high capillary density with no fat layers and in an area away from postural pressure on the probe and child.

Unit calibration and skin warming varies from 5 to 30 minutes for each position of the electrode.

The value will increase as hyperemia develops.

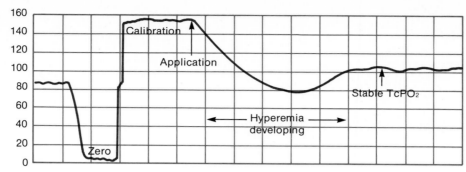

Figure 35-1.

PROCEDURE

c. After 10 minutes (total of 20 minutes from probe application), the true $TcPO_2$ will be reflected (Fig. 35-1).

d. Document the value in the medical record and notify the physician of significant changes in monitor reading or the child's clinical condition (Table 35-1).

RATIONALE/EXPECTED OUTCOME (EO)

EO: The child will have the $TcPO_2$ reading correlated with the clinical condition.

Table 35-1. Blood Gases and pH in Pediatric Patients

Age	PaO_2 (mm Hg)	$PaCO_2$ (mm Hg)	pH (mm Hg)
Preterm	60 ± 8	37 ± 6	7.37 ± .03
Term	70 ± 11	39 ± 7	7.40 ± .02
1 Month	95 ± 8	40 ± 6	7.41 ± .04
1 Year	93 ± 10	41 ± 7	7.39 ± .02

5. Reposition the probe every 3–4 hours. Document the condition of the skin under the probe.

The probe warms the child's skin to a temperature above normal (44°C or 111.2°F). Irritation or burning of sensitive skin may occur if the probe is left in the same position for long periods of time.

EO: The child's skin under the probe will remain intact.

Patient/Family Education: Home Care Considerations

1. Explain to the family that erythematous marks may occur at the electrode site, resulting from the heat produced by the electrodes. The erythematous sites will disappear in several days to several weeks.

2. Explain to the family that if the $TcPO_2$ readings do not correspond to the child's general condition, arterial or venous blood gases will need to be drawn to clarify the child's respiratory status.

References

Gregory, G.A. (1989). *Pediatric Anesthesia.* New York: Churchill Livingstone.

Hader, C.F., & Sorensen, E.R. (1988). The Effects of body position on transcutaneous oxygen tension. *Pediatric Nursing, 14*(6), 469–473.

Marsden, D., Chiu, M.C., Paky, F., et al (1985). Transcutaneous oxygen and carbon dioxide monitoring in intensive care. *Archives of Diseases in Childhood, 60,* 1158–1161.

Pewey, K.J., & Hall, M.W. (1985). Transcutaneous oxygen monitoring: Economic impact on neonatal care. *Pediatrics, 75*(6), 1065–1067.

Yip, W.C.L., Tay, J.S.H., Wong, H.B., et al (1983). Reliability of transcutaneous oxygen monitoring of critically ill children in a general pediatric unit. *Clinical Pediatrics 22*(6), 431–35.

End-Tidal CO_2

36

Definition/Purpose

Accurate assessment of ventilation is fundamental to the care of critically ill infants and children. The *end-tidal carbon dioxide* ($ETCO_2$) monitor is a noninvasive technique that provides continuous data regarding the adequacy of ventilation. Until recently, the only method to adequately assess ventilation was an arterial blood gas (ABG) measurement. ABGs are painful, time-consuming, and costly. Moreover, ABGs provide only intermittent data, which limits their usefulness in documenting transient events. End-tidal CO_2 monitoring, however, provides a noninvasive, continuous, real-time measurement of exhaled carbon dioxide gas and should be equal to an arterial CO_2 measurement.

The most common devices used to measure CO_2 concentration in exhaled gases are the infrared analyzer and the capnometer. Both function on the principle that CO_2 absorbs infrared light within a wavelength. The greater the concentration of CO_2, the greater the absorption and the less infrared detection by the analyzer.

Standard of Care

1. Effective clinical use of an $ETCO_2$ monitor requires an understanding of what is measured, how it is measured, and the patient care required when using this type of monitoring.

Assessment

1. Assess the history and physical findings for: events precipitating the current crisis (for example, respiratory infection, stress, or allergens); prior experiences with similar episodes; respiratory rate and effort; breath sounds; arterial blood gas values; chest x-ray, and other laboratory values (for example, CBC and theophylline level).
2. Assess psychosocial and developmental factors for previous experience with hospitalization, coping mechanisms, normal lifestyle, and usual comfort measures.
3. Assess the child's and family's knowledge of the prescribed treatment and support services, and their willingness and readiness to learn.

Nursing Diagnoses

The following is a list of possible diagnoses and could apply, depending on the child's age, clinical situation, and physical condition:

Impaired gas exchange

Ineffective airway clearance

Anxiety

Fear

Planning

When planning to measure $ETCO_2$, the following equipment must be gathered:

Sensor

Capnometer

Flow sheet

Interventions

PROCEDURE	**RATIONALE/EXPECTED OUTCOME (EO)**
1. Explain the nature of the monitoring devices. Teach the child and parent how to control anxiety by breathing slowly and deeply.	Children in severe respiratory distress experience a feeling of suffocation; once the distress is reduced, their anxiety will decrease. (Unfamiliar surroundings and devices will likewise produce anxiety.) *EO: The child and parent will experience decreased anxiety.*
2. Encourage the child and parents to express their feelings about the illness.	
3. Allow parents to remain with the child as much as possible.	*EO: The child and parents will cooperate with interventions designed to monitor and alleviate distress.*
4. Monitor respiratory rate, blood pressure, and heart rate every 15–30 minutes.	Pulse and blood pressure will increase to compensate for hypoxia.
5. Auscultate breath sounds and observe color every 15–30 minutes.	Mucous plugs and inflammation of the airways interfere with normal airflow and gas exchange.
6. Observe and record respiratory effort every 15–30 minutes.	
7. Position the child in whatever position is most comfortable.	*EO: The child maintains a patent airway.*
8. Monitor the child for the response and side effects of medications administered.	
9. Administer oxygen as ordered.	
10. Maintain patent IV.	
11. Use a cardiopulmonary monitor to observe for apnea and dysrhythmias.	*EO: The child will maintain a normal respiratory rate, color, and cardiac function.*
12. Have emergency equipment available (for example, endotracheal tube if not already in place, ambu bag, and intubation equipment).	*EO: The child's deterioration in respiratory status will be recognized and treated.*
13. Monitor the ETCO$_2$ (according to two types of gas sampling):	
a. Sidestream—Aspirates the gas sample from the respiratory circuit through a small-bore tubing to a sensing chamber in the monitor (Fig. 36-1).	**Advantages:** Can be used in the intubated and nonintubated child.

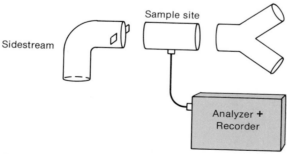

Figure 36-1. Sidestream capnometer.

PROCEDURE

b. Mainstream—Incorporates the sensor between the ventilator circuit and the artificial airway (Fig. 36-2).

RATIONALE/EXPECTED OUTCOME (EO)

Disadvantages: a. Falsely low ETCO₂ if high flow rates are used in children with small tidal volumes.
b. Contamination of analyzer from water and mucous.
c. Delay between sampling and measurement.

Advantages: a. No delay between sampling and measurement.
b. A decreased effect of moisture on the sensor.

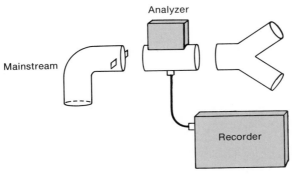

Figure 36-2. Mainstream capnometer.

c. More accurate ETCO₂ measurements when the child has rapid respiratory rates.

Disadvantages: a. Requires intubation.
Sensors are heavy and require support to avoid tension on the endotracheal tube.

EO: The child's ETCO₂ will be monitored, taking into account the advantages and disadvantages of the two types of gas sampling.

14. Support the sensor on the end of the endotracheal tube.

15. Analyze the capnogram waveform if available:
   a. Normal waveform (Figs. 36-3 and 36-4).

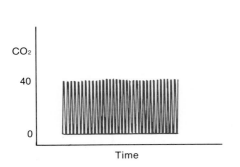

Slow Speed Capnogram

Figure 36-3. Slow speed capnogram.

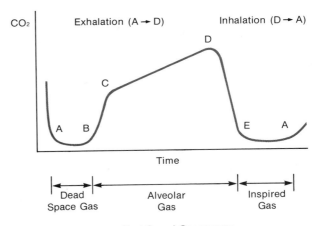

Fast Speed Capnogram

Figure 36-4. Fast speed capnogram.

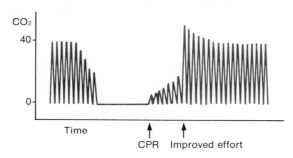

Figure 36-5.

PROCEDURE

b. Cardiac arrest waveform (Fig. 36-5).

c. Ventilator weaning waveform (Fig. 36-6).

d. Apnea waveform (Fig. 36-7).

RATIONALE/EXPECTED OUTCOME (EO)

During a cardiac arrest circulation ceases and $ETCO_2$ disappears, reappearing when circulation is restored.

During the weaning process, the $ETCO_2$ may be higher with the ventilator breath and lower with the child's breath. Stability between the two types of breaths indicates the child's readiness to be weaned.

During apnea the $ETCO_2$ wave disappears because CO_2 is no longer transported from the lungs to the sensor.

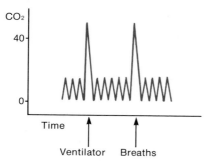

Figure 36-6. Ventilator weaning waveform.

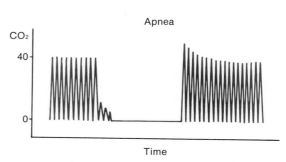

Figure 36-7. Apnea waveform.

e. Displacement of the endotracheal tube waveform (Fig. 36-8).

f. Pneumothorax waveform (Fig. 36-9).

When the endotracheal tube is displaced, the $ETCO_2$ disappears since little or no CO_2 can be detected in the esophagus.

A "staircase effect" on the descending limb of the curve is seen in pneumothorax or when chest tubes are in position but occluded.

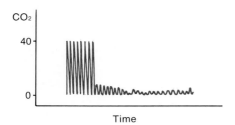

Figure 36-8. Displacement of the endotracheal tube waveform.

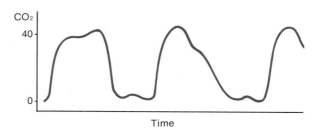

Figure 36-9. Pneumothorax waveform.

PROCEDURE	RATIONALE/EXPECTED OUTCOME (EO)
g. Asthma waveform (Fig. 36-10).	Here the plateau disappears, caused by a kinked endotracheal tube or prolonged exhalation secondary to small airway obstruction.
h. Bronchial waveform (Fig. 36-11).	An increase in plateauing correlates with a positive response to bronchodilator treatments.

EO: The child's waveform will be analyzed to provide a means of early detection of dangerous trends and as a means of assessing the effectiveness of treatments.

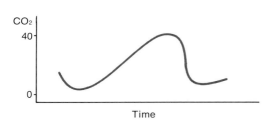

Figure 36-10. Asthma waveform.

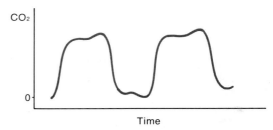

Figure 36-11. Bronchial waveform.

Patient/Family Education: Home Care Considerations

1. Instruct parents regarding the signs and symptoms of recurrent illness and actions to be taken.
2. Provide written material to enhance verbal instructions.
3. Provide parents with telephone numbers and names of contact persons if they have questions or concerns.
4. Stress the importance of follow-up appointments.

References

Curley, M.A.Q., & Thompson, J.E. (1990). End-tidal CO₂ monitoring in critically ill infants and children. *Pediatric Nursing, 16*(4), 397–403.

Hayward, C.A. (1988). *Advanced concepts in capnography.* Nellcor, Inc.

Nuzzo, P.F. (1986) Practical applications of capnography. *Respiratory Therapy,* November/December, 12–17.

Pascucci, R.C., Schena, J.A., & Thompson, J.E. (1989). Comparison of a sidestream and mainstream capnometer in infants. *Critical Care Medicine, 17*(6), 560–562.

Pulse Oximetry

37

Definition/Purpose

Pulse oximetry is a reliable and noninvasive method used to measure arterial hemoglobin oxygen saturation (SaO_2). The SaO_2 is expressed either as a percentage or as the ratio of saturated hemoglobin to the total hemoglobin. A pulse oximeter measures the absorption, or amplitude, of two wavelengths of light (red and infrared) passing through body parts with a high perfusion of arterial blood. The measurement of oxygen saturation is based on the differences between the absorption of light in reduced and saturated hemoglobin.

A lightweight probe is clipped onto the child's earlobe, finger, or toe. The probe is connected by a cable to the oximeter unit. One surface of the probe contains two light-emitting diodes; the opposite surface contains a light-sensitive photodetector. A modulated or pulsating signal is then emitted. Other tissues and fluids present at the probe site also absorb light, but they do not pulsate; thus, they do not modulate the light. The pulsatile signal from the arterial blood flow is isolated for SaO_2 calculations.

Some environmental and physiologic variables produce discrepancies between oximeter readings and blood sample analysis:

- Dyes used in cardiac output studies will cause transiently high readings.
- Elevated levels of carboxyhemoglobin, methemoglobin, and sulfhemoglobin may alter oximeter accuracy by producing an overestimation of blood SaO_2 levels. The degree of error increases in proportion to the amount of dyshemoglobin.
- Children with elevated bilirubin concentrations (>20 mg percent) may have falsely lower oximeter readings. It has also been noted that while infants are undergoing phototherapy, the oximeter probe should be covered with an opaque material.
- Another limitation is signal failure caused by poor tissue perfusion. Poor perfusion may be caused by hypothermia, hypotension, vasopressor drugs, hypovolemia, decreased cardiac output, or peripheral vascular disease.
- Children in mist or croup tents may have difficulty keeping the probe in place because of the moisture in the environment.

Standard of Care

1. When weaning a child from oxygen, note and record the oxygen saturations continuously. The major goal of continuous oxygen monitoring is to limit the number of episodes of hypoxemia.
2. To obtain an accurate reading, the apical heart rate and the heart rate indicator on the machine must correlate.

Assessment

1. Assess the pertinent history and physical findings, with emphasis on precipitating events of the respiratory distress.
2. Assess the child's respiratory rate and effort, use of accessory muscles, shape of chest, breath sounds, degree of restlessness, anxiety, perfusion, and vital signs.

3. Assess the child's developmental level, coping mechanisms, and previous experience in the medical environment and with supplemental oxygen.

Nursing Diagnoses

The following is a list of possible diagnoses and could apply, depending on the child's age, clinical situation, and physical condition:

Impaired gas exchange

High risk for injury

Altered tissue perfusion

Impaired skin integrity

Planning

To monitor a child's oxygen saturation, the following equipment must be obtained:
Oximeter

Probe

Interventions

PROCEDURE	**RATIONALE/EXPECTED OUTCOMES (EO)**
1. Gather equipment.	
2. Wash hands.	
3. Turn power switch on and allow for a 2-minute warm-up.	This warm-up stabilizes the probe light source.
4. Position the sensor on the appropriate body part (Figs. 37–1 and 37–2): Big toe or foot for infant, finger for toddler through adolescent.	Light source and detector must face each other with a tissue pad in between.

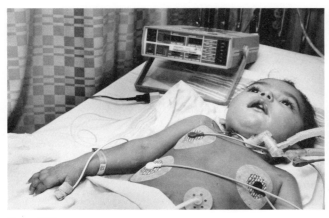

Figure 37-1.

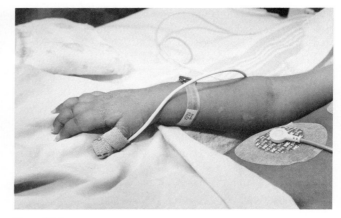

Figure 37-2.

5. Set the pushwheel switch or other alarm limits determined by physician order.	If the child's SaO_2 falls below that prescribed limit, an audible and visual alarm is activated.
6. Obtain SaO_2 and pulse rate values from the oximeter unit after stabilization for 10 seconds.	

PROCEDURE	**RATIONALE/EXPECTED OUTCOME (EO)**
7. Obtain an ABG and check for correlation with oximeter.	If oximeter readings and ABG correlate, the oximeter can then be used confidently as a continuous monitor of SaO_2 levels and provide early warnings of potential hypoxic episodes. *EO: The oximeter unit reading will correlate accurately when compared to an initial ABG.*
8. Auscultate breath sounds every 2 hours and prn.	
9. Monitor vital signs every one to two hours and prn.	
10. Administer oxygen and monitor mechanical ventilator changes as needed when oximeter readings change.	*EO: The child will have adequate gas exchange as demonstrated by:* *a. ABG within normal limits for that child* *b. Normal breath sounds* *c. Oximeter readings within normal limits for the child (normal range is 94–97% SaO_2.)*
11. Assess probe site for adequate tissue perfusion every 2 or 4 hours.	*EO: The child's skin integrity will be maintained as demonstrated by:* *a. Good skin turgor at probe site* *b. Warm, pink probe site with rapid capillary refill.*
12. Rotate probe site every 4 hours.	

Patient/Family Education: Home Care Considerations

1. Provide simply stated information to the child and family on the function of the oximeter.

2. Inform the family of the events that may affect the accuracy of the readings (for example, movement of the child, hypotension, hypothermia, and dislodged probe).

3. Review the signs and symptoms of respiratory distress with the family and how the oximeter readings are altered.

References

Bakow, E. (1988). Respiratory care update. *Critical Care Nursing, 11* (3), 39–40.

Bucher, H.U., Fanconi, S., & Baeckert, P. (1989). Hyperoxemia in newborn infants: Detection by pulse oximetry. *Pediatrics, 84*(2), 226–230.

Dziedzc, K. et al (1989). Pulse oximetry in neonatal intensive care. *Clinical Perinatology,* March, 177–1977.

Harbold, L.A. (1989). A Protocol for neonatal use of pulse oximetry. *Neonatal Network, 8*(1), 41–42; 55–7.

Jennis, M. & Peabody, J. (1987). Pulse oximetry: An alternative method for the assessment of oxygenation in newborn infants. *Pediatrics, 79* (4), 524–527.

Rutherford, K.A. (1989). Principles and applications of oximeter. *Critical Care Nursing Clinics of North America, 1*(4), 649–57.

Schroeder, C. (1988). Pulse oximetry: A nursing care plan. *Critical Care Nurse, 8* (8) 50–68.

Waxman, K. (1983). Transcutaneous oxygen monitoring of emergency department patients. *The American Journal of Surgery, 146*(7), 35–38.

Aspiration of Secretions from Nose and Mouth

38

Definition/Purpose

Sick children cannot move secretions effectively; therefore, these secretions must often be removed by suction. Gentle stimulation of the upper airway surface will elicit spontaneous coughs that are effective in moving secretions toward the large airways. If such cough stimulation is not effective, suctioning will be required. The purpose of suctioning is to maintain a patent airway and promote adequate ventilation. It is indicated for secretions audible in the airway, signs of airway obstruction, or signs of an oxygen deficit.

Standard of Care

1. Suction containers and connecting tubing are changed every 24 hours.
2. A new sterile suction catheter will be used each time suctioning is anticipated.
3. Two people are required to suction an active, alert child.

Assessment

1. Assess the history and physical findings for color and vital signs with emphasis on respirations and breath sounds; color, consistency, and amount of secretions; tolerance to suctioning; fever, cough, nasal discharge, anorexia or feeding difficulty; and prior respiratory illness.
2. Assess the psychosocial concerns and developmental factors relevant to the child's age, ability to understand the rationale for suctioning, coping mechanisms, and habits.
3. Assess the child's and family's knowledge of prior experiences with respiratory illnesses and their understanding of the need for intervention in respiratory distress.

Nursing Diagnoses

The following is a list of possible diagnoses and could apply, depending on the child's age, clinical situation, and physical condition:

Anxiety

Fear

Ineffective airway clearance

High risk for injury

High risk for infection

Planning

When planning to suction a child, the following equipment must be gathered:

Wall suction unit with container and connecting tubing (Fig. 38–1)

Sterile tracheobronchial suction catheters

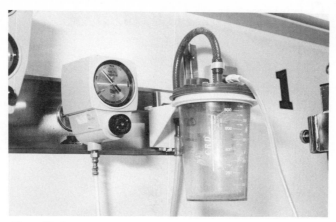

Figure 38–1.

Sterile gloves
Cup filled with normal saline (sterile)
Goggles
Water soluble lubricant

Interventions

PROCEDURE	**RATIONALE/EXPECTED OUTCOME (EO)**
1. If applicable, explain the procedure briefly to the child and the family.	Both child and family will tend to cooperate with the suctioning if they understand the purpose. *EO: The child and family will express their fears and concerns.*
2. Turn on suction. Nasopharyngeal and oropharyngeal: 75 mm Hg for neonates to 100–125 mm Hg for older children.	Excessive suction will damage delicate mucous membranes, causing bleeding. *EO: The child's mucous membranes will be protected from excessive suction.*
3. Open saline cup.	
4. Leaving the wrapper on, attach a sterile suction catheter to the connecting tubing of the suction bottle without contaminating the catheter.	
5. Auscultate breath sounds.	*EO: The child's breath sounds will be assessed prior to suctioning.*
6. Put on goggles.	Goggles protect the suctioner's eyes from airborne particles coughed out during the procedure.
7. Put gloves on both hands.	
8. Remove the sterile catheter from the wrapper, grasping the catheter with dominant hand. Use only dominant hand for manipulation of the catheter. To determine how far to insert the catheter, measure the distance between the tip of the nose and the external opening of the ear.	Insertion of the catheter further than this measurement may cause vomiting and aspiration.
9. Suction the nasopharynx first, then the oropharynx: a. Hold the catheter so that its natural curve is aligned with the child's trachea. Lubricate the end of the catheter.	Lubricant decreases the trauma of the catheter on the nasal mucosa.

PROCEDURE

    b. Gently insert the lubricated catheter into the external nares, using an upward motion until the nasal septum is passed; then use a downward motion.

    c. Tracheal tickle may be applied to stimulate a cough.

10. Place thumb on suction port. Suction should be applied upon withdrawal of the catheter only. Use a rotating movement of the catheter, not an up-and-down movement, while removing the catheter.

11. Each suctioning attempt should last only 5–15 seconds: 5 seconds in infants, and 15 seconds for the older child. Allow at least 30 seconds for reoxygenation and recovery between suction passes.

12. Repeat steps 9–11 in the other nostril.

13. Last, suction secretions from the mouth.

14. After suctioning, remove and discard the gloves and suction catheter.

15. Flush connecting tubing with saline solution until clear. Discard the cup after a single use. Wash hands.

16. Turn suction off.

17. Auscultate breath sounds.

18. Comfort the child after the procedure (hold an infant, and praise a child for cooperation).

19. Document in the medical record the child's tolerance to the suctioning and the amount and characteristics of the sputum removed.

RATIONALE/EXPECTED OUTCOME (EO)

Mucosal hemorrhage and erosion can occur if mucosa is elevated into the suction catheter holes. This also becomes a focus for infection. Turning the catheter as it is withdrawn helps clean all surfaces of the respiratory passages.

EO: The child will be free from infection due to mucosal injury.

EO: The child will be free from hypoxia and dysrhythmia associated with suctioning.

This prevents transmission of microorganisms.

EO: The child will demonstrate clear breath sounds upon auscultation.

EO: The child's medical record will indicate the suctioning procedure, tolerance to the procedures, and results.

Patient/Family Education: Home Care Considerations

1. Instruct the family in the technical skills to be carried out at home. Help the parents decide what aspects of management of the illness should be the child's responsibility.

2. Teach the signs and symptoms of illness complications, including crisis situations and how to obtain emergency care.

3. Reinforce the importance of regular medical follow-up.

4. Refer to community health agency to provide reinforcement of health teaching at home.

References

Taylor, C., Lillis, C., & LeMone, P. (1989). *Fundamentals of nursing—The art and science of nursing care.* Philadelphia: J.B. Lippincott Company.

Young, C.S. (1988). Airway suctioning: A study of paediatric physiotherapy practice. *Physiotherapy, 74*(1), 13–15.

You have recently learned that your baby will require a special kind of home monitoring device. The apnea/monitor is easy to operate and is a adapted for home use. This home care aid will review the basics of apnea monitoring.

What is Apnea?

Apnea is a common phenomenon in premature infants, who have periods of rapid breathing separated by periods of slow breathing or periods during which there is no visible breathing. *Apnea* is defined as a lapse of spontaneous breathing for 20 seconds or more followed by a decreased heart rate and color change. It reflects immature neurologic and respiratory control mechanisms.

Purpose of the Monitor

The most common conditions requiring home apnea monitoring include abnormal pauses in breathing or abnormal slowing of the heart rate. Other infants require monitoring because they have artificial airways (tracheostomy).

It is important to understand that monitoring is not a cure for any symptom or disease. It is, however, a means of helping your infant through a part of the development process by detecting abnormal episodes of breathing or heart rate and instructing you to take corrective action.

Initial Anxieties

Anxiety is normal when you arrive home with your infant and monitoring equipment. It is the first time that you are on your own. Each family's ability to adjust to the monitoring will hinge on the support of other family members, the number and ages of other children in the home, other medical problems experienced by your family, and the services offered in the community and by the hospital and medical instrument company that manufactures the monitor.

The strain you are likely to experience will surface as a lack of sleep, a tendency to hover over the baby, a reluctance to disconnect the monitor at any time, and a growing feeling of "cabin fever." These reactions are normal and will pass.

Going out, even for short periods, is important to the health of the entire family. It is difficult, however, to find a babysitter who is competent and willing to watch a child on a monitor. Babysitting responsibilities should not be forced on reluctant relatives or friends. It is suggested that the sitter be trained in infant cardiopulmonary resuscitation (CPR). The following community organizations may provide assistance in locating a babysitter:

American Heart Association

American Red Cross

Visiting Nurses' Association

Local nursing schools

Local parents' monitoring programs.

Operating the Infant Monitor

The figure illustrates the apnea monitor you will be taking home. Your monitor may also show a digital display of the heart rate. Always refer to the manufacturer's manual for specific setup instructions.

Refer to the manufacturer's instruction manual and follow these steps to set up your child's monitor.

Step 1

Plug monitor into wall outlet. Turn it on by pressing the power button. When you do this, the alarm will sound because nothing is hooked up to the monitor.

Step 2

Turn the monitor off. Set the alarm delay to _____ seconds. This setting determines the number of seconds allowed to pass from the time an infant stops breathing until the apnea alarm sounds. Because normal pauses in breathing vary between infants, your doctor should determine which setting should be used.

Step 3

Plug the electrode cable into the monitor.

Step 4

Attach the lead wires or belt to the cable.

Step 5

Apply electrodes on the infant's body where the greatest amount of respiratory movement occurs. When using disposable electrodes, placement is most commonly around the lower rib cage. With electrode belts, contact to the side, halfway between the armpit and the bottom of the rib cage. The points on the infant's skin where the electrodes will be placed must be clean, dry, and free of powder or oils. Areas with rashes or chafing should be avoided.

Step 6

Attach the lead wires to the electrodes. If you use snap leads, snap the leads onto the electrodes and then position the electrodes on the child.

Step 7

Turn on the monitor and watch the respiration indicator. (Your monitor may also have a heart rate indicator.) It should light up each time your child breathes. If it does not, try adjusting the sensitivity control, or move the electrodes until the lights respond.

Responding to an Alarm

Each alarm should be treated as though a real episode has occurred.

1. Observe the condition of your infant:
   When you arrive at your infant's side, you may observe any of the following:
   a. The baby is breathing and color is normal. If you find this, observe the infant for a few more seconds, reset the alarm, and resume your normal activity.
   b. The baby is not breathing or heart rate is low, but color is normal. If you find this, observe the infant for 10 seconds. If the situation corrects itself, reset the alarm and document the event on a flow sheet. If the problem persists, begin stimulation.
   c. The baby is not breathing or heart rate is low, and color is abnormal. If you find this, begin stimulation immediately.

2. Stimulation:
   Proper stimulation should progress from gentle to moderate to vigorous, as needed.
   a. Gentle stimulation
      This involves lightly touching your baby's back, cheeks, feet, or trunk. Removing the baby's blanket may also work.
   b. Moderate stimulation
      If light stimulation does not return the baby to normal, gently squeeze the baby's feet or the skin on the chest, or give the baby a gentle shake.
   c. Vigorous stimulation
      If stronger stimulation is necessary, slap the baby's feet.

If all above fails begin CPR.

General Care of the Infant Monitor

1. Do not immerse the infant monitor or any of its cords or wires in water.

2. The monitor should never be used while your infant is being bathed.

3. Do not attempt to repair or modify your monitor. Only an authorized dealer should perform such work.

4. Do not place your monitor near or on top of other electrical devices such a radio or television, because this may interfere with the unit's sensitive monitoring features.

5. The monitor should not be exposed to high temperatures, and therefore should not be set on or near a radiator or heater or placed in direct sunlight.

6. Keep the monitor out of reach of young children and pets.

7. Place the monitor on a sturdy level surface and 4–6 inches away from the wall or curtains that may muffle the sound of the alarm. Do not place it on a mattress, because this will also muffle the alarm. Arrange the baby's room for convenience and safety (Fig. 1).

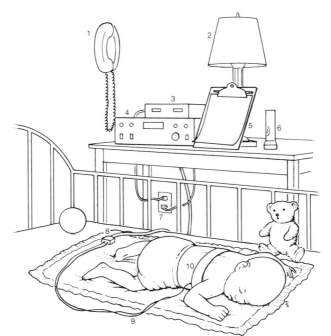

1. Telephone
2. Working light
3. Portable intercom
4. Infant monitor
5. Clipboard and pencil
6. Flashlight
7. Grounded outlet
8. Patient cable (to rear of monitor)
9. Lead wires
10. Electrode belt (electrodes underneath)

Figure 1.

8. Check the battery each day.

9. Be aware that strong radio signals from nearby TV or radio stations, airports, ham radios, or police stations could interfere with the monitor.

Conclusion of Home Monitoring

As your baby grows older, his or her respiratory pattern becomes more predictable and alarm conditions become less frequent. Most referral centers now use the following standard criteria to conclude home monitoring:

- The baby has been free of events requiring vigorous stimulation for at least 3 months.
- The baby has not experienced a real monitor alarm for at least 2 months.
- During the "normal" period, the baby has experienced the stress of a cold or DPT vaccination.
- The initial reason behind the decision to monitor has been resolved.

**Important Telephone Numbers
(Place near each telephone.)**

Police (Emergency Medical Services)
Pediatrician
Hospital Nursing Contact
Hospital Social Work Contact
Electric Company
Visiting Nurses' Agency
Pharmacy
Monitor Dealer Representative
Other Contacts:

_____ _____
_____ _____

PATIENT TEACHING CHECKLIST: HOME APNEA MONITORING

Child and Parent Should Be Able To:	Nurse Demonstration (Date and initial.)	Parent Return-Demonstration (Date and initial.)
1. Verbalize an understanding of apnea and the purpose of the apnea monitor.		
2. Know how to operate the monitor (set up on infant).		
3. Respond to an alarm situation and provide the necessary stimulation.		
4. Describe proper skin care.		
5. Perform general maintenance of the monitor.		
6. Perform infant CPR.		

References

Ad Hoc Committee of the National Sudden Infant Death Syndrome Foundation. (1982). *A Handbook for infant monitoring.* Marietta, GA: Healthdyne, Inc.

Berkemeyer, S.N., & Hutchins, K.H. (1986). Home apnea monitoring. *Pediatric Nursing, 12*(4), 259–304.

Davis, N. et al (1989). Infantile apnea monitoring and SIDS. *Journal of Pediatric Health Care,* March/April, 67–75.

Department of Health and Human Services. (1990). Cautions in infant apnea monitors. *FDA Drug Bulletin, 20*(1), 3.

Duncan, J.A., & Webb, L.Z. (1983). Teaching families home apnea monitoring. *Pediatric Nursing, 3,* 171–175.

Graber, H.S., & Stevens, S.B. (1984). A discharge tool for teaching parents to monitor infant apnea at home. *Journal of Maternal Child Nursing, 9*(3), 178–180.

Grisemer, A.N. (1990). Apnea of prematurity: Current management and nursing implications. *Pediatric Nursing, 16*(6), 606–611.

Lang, A. (1987). Nursing of families with an infant who requires home apnea monitoring. *Issues in Comprehensive Pediatric Nursing, 10*(2), 123–133.

Nulhall, P. (1988). Maternal responses to home apnea monitoring of infants. *Nursing Research, 37*(6), 354–357.

Saylor, C.F., et al (1989). Anxiety in mothers of infants on apnea monitors. *Childrens' Health Care,* Spring, 117–120.

Saylor, C.F., et al (1980). *Using monitors.* Horsham, PA: Intermed Communications, Inc.

Weese–Mayer, D.E., Browletter, R.T., Morrow, A.S., et al (1989). Assessing validity of infant monitor alarms with event recording. *Journal of Pediatrics, 115*(5), 702–708.

What is a Tracheostomy?

A tracheostomy is the surgical creation of an opening into the trachea (windpipe) (Fig. 1).

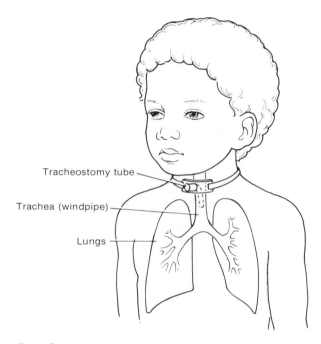

Tracheostomy tube

Trachea (windpipe)

Lungs

Figure 1.

Tracheostomy tubes, which fit into this opening, vary in size and type. The two types most often used are the metal Holinger and the plastic Shiley tracheostomy tubes.

The metal Holinger tube is made of silver and has three parts: the outer cannula (which holds the hole open), the inner cannula (which is a hollow tube that locks in place to the outer cannula) and the obturator (which guides the tube into place when it is being changed).

The plastic Shiley tube (Fig. 2) is soft and flexible and consists of two pieces: the outer cannula (which stays in the neck to hold the hole open) and the obturator (which guides the tube into place).

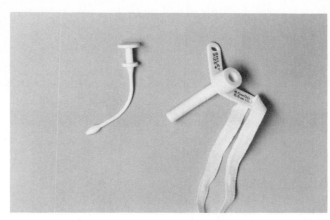

Figure 2.

Why Does My Child Need a Tracheostomy?

There are two reasons for tracheostomies: airway obstructions and the inability to cough out secretions that may lead to pneumonia. The length of time your child has the tracheostomy depends on the reason for the tube insertion and your child's progress.

What Are the Implications of the Tracheostomy?

Your child is different from other children only in breathing and vocalization. Your child will breath air directly into the windpipe rather than through the nose and mouth. As a result of this, he or she will not be able to talk as before because the air does not pass over the vocal cords. It is important that you:

Watch your child carefully because verbalizing pain, injury, or difficulty in breathing may be impossible.

Watch for the following signs of obstruction of the airway and report them to the doctor immediately if they do not improve with suctioning or changing of the tracheostomy tube:

- Restlessness, labored breathing, or increased respiratory rate
- Noisy respirations
- Retractions (drawing in of the chest or rib cage)
- Blue or ashen color of lips or nailbeds
- Mouth breathing with no air passage through the tracheostomy tube.

Always keep an extra tracheostomy tube available in case the one your child has in place becomes plugged and requires changing.

Report to the doctor if there is any food or water leakage through the tracheostomy tube or if there is bleeding around the tube.

Have your child wear a Medic Alert symbol.

You must also learn the following procedures to adequately take care of your child:

- Suctioning
- Changing the tracheostomy tube
- Cleaning the tracheostomy tube
- Skin care around the stoma
- Daily care
- Emergency care.

We realize that having to care for a child with a tracheostomy is anxiety-producing. Your child's doctors and nurses are here to help you and your family feel more comfortable about bringing your child home. *Do not hesitate to ask questions.*

Suctioning

Why Suction Your Child?

Suctioning clears the tracheostomy tube of mucus. It helps clear the tube of secretions and makes it easier for your child to breathe. The suction machine acts like a vacuum cleaner, pulling mucus out of the tracheostomy tube, through the suction catheter, and into a collection bottle.

When Should You Suction Your Child?

Suction your child on an average of every 4–6 hours, or more often if necessary. When your child has a cold or is sick, suctioning more frequently than usual may be required.

The following signs indicate the need to suction:
- Noisy respirations
- Pulling inward of the chest walls or ribs
- Pulling inward of the hollow in the neck
- Fast breathing
- Frightened look
- Difficulty eating or sucking
- Mucus bubbling around the tracheal opening
- Flaring of nostrils
- Change in color of the mouth and lips (pale, blue, or dusky)

How Should You Suction Your Child?

Gather the following equipment:

Suction machine

Connecting tubing for suction machine

Suction catheters (6F for infants; 8F–10F for toddlers and school-age; 12F–16F for adolescents)

Gloves (sterile)

Normal saline packets (3 mL each)

Pipe cleaners

2 Jars (sterile) containing normal saline

Hydrogen peroxide

Ambu bag with appropriate adaptor.

Follow these steps when suctioning a metal tube with inner cannula:

1. Wash your hands to minimize the chance of infection.
2. Assemble the necessary equipment (above).
3. Connect the suction catheter to the connecting tubing of the suction machine, being careful to keep the catheter inside the sterile wrapper.
4. Unlock the inner cannula from the outer cannula of the tracheostomy by twisting the knob upward (toward the chin). Remove the inner cannula with one hand while holding the outer tube in place with the other hand.
5. Place the inner cannula to soak in the sterile jar with saline while you suction your child.
6. Put on sterile gloves.
7. Check that the suction is working by placing one finger over the suction vent. Place the catheter end in a jar of sterile saline, suctioning a small amount of saline into the catheter.
8. With finger off the suction vent, insert the catheter into the trachea as far as it will go. This will cause your child to cough.
9. Apply suction as you gently pull the catheter out, rotating it between your thumb and forefinger. Do not leave the catheter in the tube for more than 5 seconds in infants and 15 seconds in older children, as you are blocking your child's airway. To avoid prolonged

suctioning, hold your own breath while suctioning to give you an idea of the feeling of breathlessness experienced by your child.

10. Rise the suction catheter in sterile saline solution between suctionings.

11. If your child is on an oxygen supplement or needs Ambu bagging, offer these between suction attempts. Allow 30 seconds for recovery between suctioning attempts.

12. If secretions are thick, instill 2–3 drops of normal saline into the tracheostomy tube and suction again.

13. When suctioning is finished, replace the inner cannula into the outer cannula. Twist the knob back in a downward position to lock it in place.

Follow these steps when suctioning a plastic tube without inner cannula:

1. Wash hour hands to minimize the chance of infection.

2. Assembly the necessary equipment.

3. Connect the suction catheter to the connecting tubing of the suction machine, being careful to keep the catheter inside the sterile wrapper.

4. Put on sterile gloves.

5. Check that the suction is working by placing one finger over the suction vent. Place the catheter end in a jar of sterile saline, suctioning a small amount of saline into the catheter.

6. With finger off the suction vent, insert the catheter into the trachea as far as it will go. This will cause your child to cough.

7. Apply suction as you gently pull the catheter out, rotating it between your thumb and forefinger. Do not leave the catheter in the tube for more than 5 seconds in infants and 15 seconds in older children, as you are blocking your child's airway. To avoid prolonged suctioning, hold your own breath while suctioning to give you an idea of the feeling of breathlessness experienced by your child.

8. Rinse the suction catheter between suctionings in sterile saline.

9. If your child is on an oxygen supplement or needs Ambu bagging, offer these between suction attempts. Allow 30 seconds for recovery between each suctioning attempt.

10. If secretions are thick, instill 2–3 drops of normal saline into the tracheostomy tube and suction again.

Changing the Tracheostomy Tube

Why is it Necessary to Change Your Child's Tracheostomy Tube?

The complete tracheostomy tube needs to be changed to prevent a buildup of secretions within the tube that cannot be suctioned out, and to prevent infections of the trachea and stoma.

When Should You Change the Tube?

The tracheostomy tube needs to be changed once a week, or more frequently, depending on the amount of secretions.

How Should You Change the Tracheostomy Tube?

Gather the following equipment:

Twill tape

Scissors

Roll to place under shoulders

Mummy restraint

Clean tracheostomy tube.

To change the tracheostomy tube, follow these steps:

1. Wash hands well.

2. "Mummy" young children and infants, or have an assistant restrain the child.

3. Remove the inner cannula (if there is one) of the tube to be inserted, and insert the obturator.

4. Attach the ties to the clean tracheostomy tube.

5. Lubricate the outer tube and obturator tip with sterile solution.

6. Place a small folded towel under your child's shoulder to extend the head and neck.

7. Cut the twill tape on the tube that is in your child.

8. Remove the old tube and gently insert the new tube. The tube should be directed back and then down (Fig. 3).

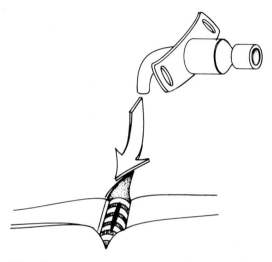

Figure 3.

9. Once the new tube is in place, hold the outer cannula with one hand and remove the obturator.

10. With your child's neck flexed, securely tie the twill tapes around the neck using a square knot. An index finger should fit snugly under the tape while the neck is flexed.

11. If your child's tube has an inner cannula, insert and lock it into place.

Cleaning and Sterilizing the Tracheostomy Tube

How Should You Clean a Plastic Tracheostomy Tube?

Once the tube is removed from your child, rinse it under cool tap water. Next, wash the tube with a mild soap, using pipe cleaners and a toothbrush to remove any dried secretions. Rinse tube thoroughly. Soak the tube and obturator in hydrogen peroxide for 8 hours. Rinse the tube with water, dry with a paper towel, and store the clean tube in an unused plastic sandwich bag.

How Should You Clean a Metal Tracheostomy Tube?

Once the tube is removed from your child, rinse it under cool tap water to remove most of the mucus. Next, wash the tube with a mild soap, using pipe cleaners and a toothbrush to remove any dried secretions. Rinse soap off tube. Last, boil the inner cannula, the outer cannula, and the obturator for 15 minutes in a pan of water. Remove the three parts of the tube from the water, let cool, and store in a plastic sandwich bag or a clean jar with a lid.

Tracheostomy Stoma Skin Care

What Equipment is Needed to Care for the Area Around the Stoma?

Water

Cotton-tipped swabs

Hydrogen peroxide

Clean jar

How Often Should You Clean Around the Stoma?

The area around the stoma must be cleaned once a day, usually at the same time that the twill ties are changed. If an odor is present, or if there is an increase in the amount of secretions pooling around the stoma, clean the area more frequently.

How Should You Clean the Skin Around the Stoma?

1. In a clean jar, mix equal parts of hydrogen peroxide and water, to make a solution of $\frac{1}{2}$ strength hydrogen peroxide.
2. Wet the cotton-tipped applicator with the solution and roll the applicator over the skin under the tracheostomy tube where secretions have crusted.
3. When through, rinse the area with an applicator dipped in clear water and let dry.
4. Never use powders or lotions on the area around the stoma. If an ointment is ordered by your physician, apply a thin layer as directed.

General Care Instructions: Daily Care of Tracheostomy

What Equipment Must You Take With You When You and Your Child Leave Home?

Battery-operated suction machine

Suction catheters

Extra tracheostomy tube

Scissors

Box of tissues

Ambu bag

All these items will fit into an accessory bag that can be used as a travel kit for trips away from home.

What Precautions Must You Take on Cold or Windy Days When You Take Your Child Out?

If it is cold, avoid having your child breath the cold air directly into the tracheostomy. This can cause tracheal spasm and form small ice particles in the mucus if exposed for extended periods of time. A scarf or turtleneck around the tracheostomy tube or a blanket over an infant's head and neck will prevent aspiration of cold air. The same technique should be used on dusty, windy days when dust particles may enter the trachea and cause dry crusty mucus.

What Can Your Child Eat, Now That Your Child Has a Tracheostomy?

Your child may eat the same food that he or she ate before the tube was inserted. Always burp your baby, and never prop the child's bottle. If your child chokes on a piece of food, suction the tracheostomy tube immediately.

How Should You Bathe Your Child?

You may bathe your child in the bathtub as long as you keep water from entering the tracheostomy tube. If water enters the tracheostomy, suction your child immediately. Never leave your child alone in the bathtub. Don not let your child take showers.

How Can You Provide Extra Humidity for Your Child?

Because the mouth and nose, which provide natural humidification, are bypassed by the tracheostomy, it is necessary to provide an alternative source of moisture to avoid crusting of secretions. There should be at least 50% humidity in the home of a child with a tracheostomy. This can be accomplished by using a humidifier or vaporizer. If your child's mucus remains thin, he or she is receiving enough humidity. If the mucus becomes thick, you will need to provide more humidity.

What Environmental Irritants Should Your Child Avoid?

- Pets with fine hair

- Lint, dust, or sand
- Aerosol sprays
- Powders
- Smoke or fumes

Can Your Child Have Immunizations?

It is important that your child's immunizations are kept up-to-date.

Emergency Care

What Should You Do if Your Child Stops Breathing?

1. Suction the tracheostomy tube immediately.
2. If the tracheostomy tube is plugged with mucus and you cannot suction it out, change the tube.
3. If your child still does not breathe when the new tube is inserted, begin CPR.
4. Call for help. Continue CPR until help arrives or your child responds by breathing on his own.
5. Pinch your child's nose shut and cover his or her mouth.
6. Seal your lips around the tracheostomy tube and breathe in twice.
7. Check your child's pulse at the inner aspect of the arm. If a strong pulse is present but your child is still not breathing, continue mouth-to-tube breathing: 20 breaths/minute for an infant; 16 breaths/minute for a child; and 12 breaths/minute for an adolescent. If no pulse is felt, compress the chest using routine CPR techniques.

PATIENT TEACHING CHECKLIST: TRACHEOSTOMY CARE

Child and Parent Should Be Able To:	Nurse Demonstration (Date and initial.)	Parent Return–Demonstration (Date and initial.)
1. Verbalize an understanding of what a tracheostomy is and why the child needs an artificial airway.		
2. a. Verbalize how and when to suction.		
b. Perform suctioning.		
3. a. Verbalize how to change tracheostomy tube.		
b. Perform tube change.		
4. Perform cleaning and sterilizing the tracheostomy tube.		
5. Perform skin care around the stoma.		
6. a. Verbalize specific daily care instructions.		
b. Perform daily care.		
7. a. Verbalize emergency care.		
b. Perform CPR on mannequin.		

References

Children's Memorial Hospital. (1985). *Pediatric home tracheostomy care: A parents' guide.* Chicago: Children's Memorial Hospital.

Jennings, P. (1988). Nursing and home aspects of the care of a child with tracheostomy. *Journal of Laryngology and Otology* (Suppl.), 25–29.

Kaufman, J., & Hardy-Ribakow, D. (1988). What parents need to know about trache care. *RN, 51*(10), 99–100; 103–104.

Kennedy, A. H., & Johnson, W. (1982). An educational program for families of children with tracheostomies. *MCN, 7*(1), 42–49.

Longo, A. (1983). Teaching Parents CPR. *Pediatric Nursing, 6,* 445–447.

Michael Reese Hospital and Medical Center. (1982). *Instructions in tracheostomy care at home.* Chicago: Michael Reese Hospital and Medical Center.

Simon B. M., et al (1989). Tracheostomy in young children: Implications for asessment and treatment of communication and feeding disorders. *Infants Young Children,* January, 1–9.

PARENT TEACHING GUIDE
Peak Flow Meter

Introduction

Early changes in the airway cannot be felt by your child. By the time the child feels tightness in the chest or starts to wheeze, he or she are already far into an asthma episode. The most reliable early sign of an asthma episode is a drop in the child's peak expiratory flow rate, or the ability to breathe out quickly, which can be measured by a peak flow meter. Almost every asthmatic child over the age of 4 years can and should learn to use a peak flow meter (Figs. 1 and 2).

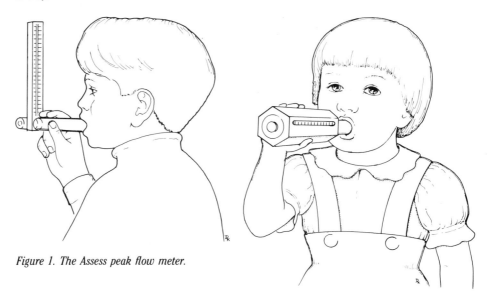

Figure 1. The Assess peak flow meter.

Figure 2. The Mini-Wright peak flow meter.

Steps to Accurate Measurements:

1. Remove gum or food from the mouth.
2. Move the pointer on the meter to zero.
3. Stand up and hold the meter horizontally, with fingers away from the vent holes and marker.
4. With mouth wide open, slowly breathe in as much air as possible.
5. Put the mouthpiece on the tongue and place lips around it.
6. Blow out as hard and fast as you can. Give a short, sharp blast, not a slow blow. The meter measures the fastest puff, not the longest.
7. Repeat steps 1–6 three times. Wait at least 10 seconds between puffs. Move the pointer to zero after each puff.
8. Record the best reading.

Guidelines for Treatment:

Each child has a unique pattern of asthma episodes. Most episodes begin gradually, and a drop in peak flow can alert you to start medications before the actual symptoms appear. This early treatment can prevent a flare from getting out of hand. One way to look at peak flow scores is to match the scores with three colors:

Green	*Yellow*	*Red*
80–100% personal best No symptoms Full breathing reserve	50–80% personal best Mild-to-moderate symptoms Diminished reserve	Below 50% personal best Serious distress Pulmonary function is significantly impaired.
Mild trigger may not cause symptoms. Continue current management.	A minor trigger produces noticeable symptoms. Augment present treatment regimen.	Any trigger may lead to severe distress. Contact physician.

Remember, treatment should be adjusted to fit the individual's needs. Your physician will develop a home management plan with you. When in doubt, consult your physician.

References

Mendoza, G. (1988). *Peak performance: A strategy for asthma self assessment.* Fairfax, VA: Mothers of Asthmatics.

Plaut, T. (1988). What a peak flow meter can do for children with asthma. *Contemporary Pediatrics, 10*(89), 33–52.

Cardiovascular System Procedures

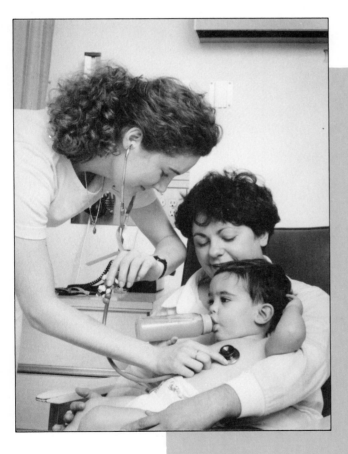

Unit VI

Cardiopulmonary Resuscitation and Airway Obstruction

39

Definition/Purpose

CPR (cardiopulmonary resuscitation) is a series of basic lifesaving techniques that support the respiratory and circulatory systems. Rescue breaths and external chest compressions provide adequate oxygenation of the tissues to maintain life. CPR is performed as an initial response to respiratory or cardiac arrest and is continued during advanced life support efforts.

There are no data for pediatric resuscitations performed annually in the United States. An estimate of incidence of potential resuscitations can be determined by examining the data on infant and childhood mortality. The majority of children who require resuscitations are at the younger end of the age range, with a mean age of 1.98 years. The most common primary diagnosis of hospitalized pediatric patients requiring resuscitation involves the respiratory system. There are no demographic studies to identify the socioeconomic, racial, familial, or community characteristics of the pediatric patient requiring life support interventions.

Standard of Care

1. All health care professionals should be certified in Basic Life Support (BLS) as defined by the American Heart Association or Red Cross.
2. Emergency Medical Services (EMS) system phone numbers should be known and displayed.
3. Safety and injury prevention education should be included in all child and parent health care.

Assessment

1. Assess baseline vital signs, including level of consciousness, of all patients.
2. Assess history for episodes of apnea, respiratory distress, cardiac anomalies, and infection. Assess family history for siblings with sudden infant death syndrome (SIDS).
3. Assess ABCs (airway, breathing, circulation) before proceeding with resuscitative actions.
4. Assess parent knowledge concerning child development, safety, accident prevention, and basic life support.

Nursing Diagnoses

The following is a list of possible diagnoses and could apply, depending on the child's age, clinical situation, and physical condition:

Decreased cardiac output

Gas exchange, impaired

Breathing pattern, ineffective

Body temperature, high risk for altered

High risk for injury

Planning

No equipment is needed to provide CPR.

Interventions

PROCEDURE

1. Identify children at risk and place them near the nurses' station, on a monitor, or have an arrest cart nearby. Monitors must have alarms turned on at all times.

RATIONALE/EXPECTED OUTCOME (EO)

Diagnosis of children potentially requiring life support

Respiratory:
- Pneumonia
- Asthma
- Epiglottitis
- Bronchopulmonary dysplasia
- Primary apnea
- Bronchiolitis

Cardiovascular:
- Congenital heart disease
- Septic shock
- Dehydration
- Myocarditis and pericarditis
- Congestive heart failure

Central Nervous System:
- Hydrocephalus
- Head trauma
- Seizure
- Tumor
- Meningitis
- Drug ingestion

Gastrointestinal:
- Trauma
- Enterocolitis
- Bowel perforation and obstruction
- TE fistula

EO: The child's risk of injury will be reduced.

2. Monitor vital signs, including temperature and level of consciousness at least every 4 hours if not more frequently.

Hypothermia and anxiety can be signs of impending arrest.

EO: The child will have a normal body temperature.

3. If arrest is suspected, gently shake and call by name.

This will help to determine unresponsiveness. Stimulating the infant may produce spontaneous respirations.

4. Call out for help.

Others can activate EMS and help with CPR.

5. Position child on his back.

6. Open airway with head tilt/chin life or jaw-thrust maneuvers.
   a. *Head tilt/chin left:*
      Standing next to the child, tilt the child's head back by placing one hand on the forehead and pushing down. At the same time, lift the chin with the fingers of the other hand. Do not overextend (Fig. 39-1).

Overextension of the infant's head past the "sniffing" position or neutral position may collapse the airway on itself, causing an obstruction.

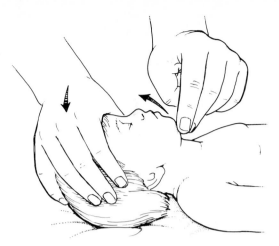

Figure 39-1. Head-tilt/chin-lift.

b. *Jaw-thrust maneuver:*
From behind the head, place 2–3 fingers of each hand under both angles of the lower jaw and lift upward. Because the jaw thrust can be done with or without a head tilt, this is the safest technique for opening the airway if a neck injury is suspected (Fig. 39-2).

7. While maintaining the open airway, look, listen, and feel for breathing.

8. Place cheek and ear close to child's mouth and nose. Listen and feel for airflow.

9. Look at chest and abdomen. Observe for movement (Fig. 39-3).

EO: The child will experience no further neck or spinal injury.

The infant displays abdominal movement during normal respiration.

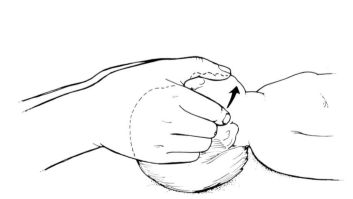

Figure 39-2. Jaw-thrust.

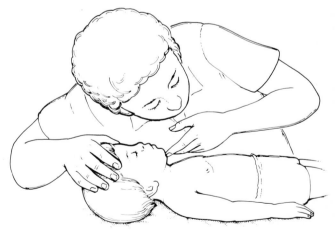

Figure 39-3. Determining breathlessness while maintaining head-tilt/chin-lift.

10. If there is no breathing, provide two initial breaths.
    a. For the infant (1 year old or younger) cover both the nose and mouth with rescuer's mouth (Fig. 39-4).

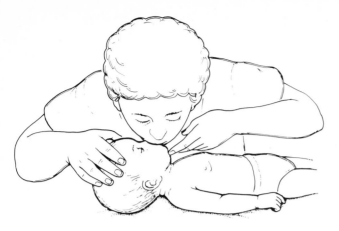

Figure 39-4. Rescue breathing with an airtight seal around the mouth and nose.

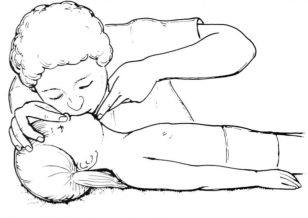

Figure 39-5. Mouth-to-mouth seal.

PROCEDURE

b. For the child between 1 and 8 years of age, the rescuer covers the child's mouth, creating a mouth-to-mouth seal, while pinching the child's nostrils shut (Fig. 39-5).

11. Evaluate breaths by watching for the chest to rise and fall.

12. Reposition head and airway if air does not enter freely. Treat for airway obstruction if continued rescue breaths are thwarted. (See Step 21.)

13. Locate and palpate the brachial pulse in the infant (Fig. 39-6).

14. Locate and palpate the carotid pulse of the child (Fig. 39-7).

RATIONALE/EXPECTED OUTCOME (EO)

EO: The child will have an artificial breathing pattern established.

The brachial and carotid pulses are the most central and accessible arteries for determining cardiac activity.

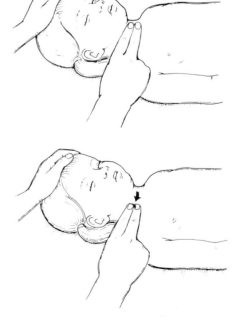

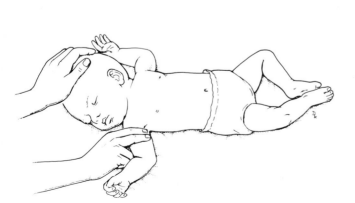

Figure 39-6. Locating the brachial pulse in an infant.

Figure 39-7. Locating and palpating the carotid artery pulse.

PROCEDURE	**RATIONALE/EXPECTED OUTCOME (EO)**

PROCEDURE

15. If there *is* a pulse, proceed with rescue breaths only. Provide one breath every 3 seconds for the infant. Provide one breath every 4 seconds for the child.

16. If there is *no* pulse, locate finger and hand position for chest compressions:
    a. For the infant, place two fingers' breadth below the nipple line (Fig. 39-8).
    b. For the child, place the heel of one hand one finger's breadth above the xyphoid notch (Fig. 39-9).

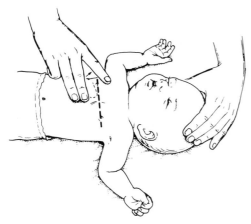

Figure 39-8. Locating finger position for chest compression in an infant.

17. Compress the *infant's* chest to a depth of ½–1 inch at a rate of 100 compressions per minute. Provide a rescue breath every fifth compression.

18. Compress the *child's* chest to a depth of 1–1½ inches at a rate of 80–100 compressions per minute. Provide a rescue breath after every fifth compression.

19. Reassess for spontaneous respirations and pulse after 1 minute (10 cycles of five compressions to one breath).

20. If no help is immediately available, stop CPR and telephone for help.

21. Reestablish CPR once help has been called. Continue until trained in advanced life support respond.

Obstructed Airway Management

Infant

22. If airway obstruction is suspected in the *infant,* hold the infant on his or her abdomen with the legs straddling the rescuer's arm. With the infant's head held downward, apply four back blows between the shoulder blades (Fig. 39-10).

RATIONALE/EXPECTED OUTCOME (EO)

Most pediatric arrests are respiratory in origin. Prompt management will usually prevent cardiac arrest.

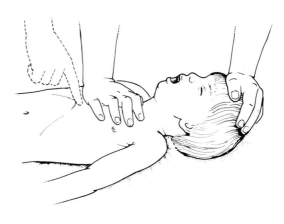

Figure 39-9. Locating hand position for chest compression in a child.

Infant CPR is best achieved by one rescuer, whereas child CPR can be equally effective with either one or two rescuers.

EO: The infant or child will have an artificial circulation established.

EO: The infant or child will have adequate gas exchange to maintain life.

EO: The child will have heart rate and breathing pattern reestablished.

When rescue breathing in the *unconscious* victim is unsuccessful despite repositioning of the airway, actions to relieve foreign body obstruction should be implemented.

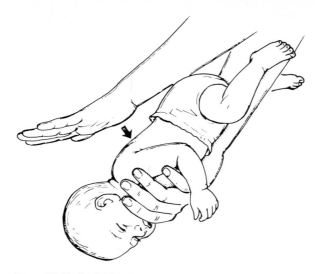

Figure 39-10. Back blow in an infant.

PROCEDURE	**RATIONALE/EXPECTED OUTCOME (EO)**
23. Turn the infant to his or her back and with the infant's head downward, apply four chest thrusts in the same location for CPR compressions (Fig. 39-11).	Intra-abdominal injuries to infants are prevented by avoiding the use of Heimlich maneuver.

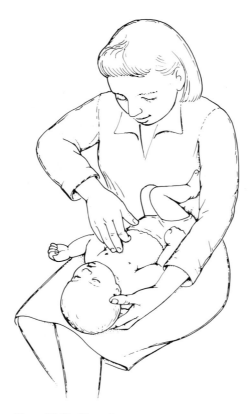

Figure 39-11. Chest thrust in an infant.

PROCEDURE

RATIONALE/EXPECTED OUTCOME (EO)

24. Open the airway and remove only visible particles.

The infant's airway can become further obstructed in the attempt to digitally remove a foreign body.

25. Reposition airway and provide two strong rescue breaths.

Some air may be forced past the obstruction.

26. Continue alternating back blows, chest thrusts, and rescue breaths.

27. Call for help.

28. Begin CPR if no pulse is palpable.

   Child (over 1 year of age)

29. If airway obstruction is suspected in the *child*, place the child on his or her back on the floor.

EO: The infant's or child's obstruction will be relieved.

30. Place the heel of one hand on the child's abdomen at the midline, above the navel and below the rib cage. (The rescuer may straddle or sit astride the child.)

31. Provide several upward thrusts (toward the rib cage) (Fig. 39-12).

The amount of force and whether to use one or two hands depends on the size of the child.

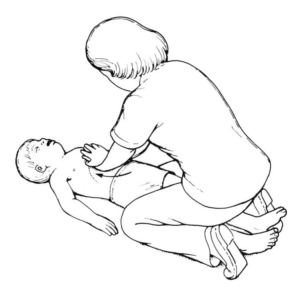

Figure 39-12. Chest thrust in a child.

32. Open the child's airway. Turn head to the side and sweep out visible objects.

33. Reposition airway and provide two strong rescue breaths.

34. Call for help.

35. Continue by alternating abdominal thrusts with rescue breaths until obstruction is relieved.

36. Begin CPR if pulse is not palpable.

Patient/Family Education: Home Care Considerations

1. Instruct parents of high-risk infants and children in CPR and obstructed airway management.

2. Refer to the American Heart Association or Red Cross for Basic Life Support certification classes.

3. Provide emergency phone numbers, especially for EMS access and the poison control center.

4. Instruct parents in home safety measures and car seat safety as related to the ongoing development of the child.

References

American Academy of Pediatrics. (1988). *Textbook of Pediatric Advanced Life Support.* Dallas: American Heart Association.

American Heart Association. 1987. *Instructor's manual for basic life support.* Dallas: American Heart Association.

American Heart Association. 1986. Standards and guidelines for cardiopulmonary resuscitation and emergency cardiac care. *JAMA, 255* (21), 2954.

Fleischer, G. & Ludwig, S. (1988) *Textbook of pediatric emergency medicine.* Baltimore: Williams & Wilkins.

Gillis, J., Dickson, D., Rieder, M., et al. (1986). Results of inpatient pediatric resuscitation. *Critical Care Medicine, 14,* 469.

Pacemakers

40

Definition/Purpose

A pacemaker may be used in children who have developed or who have the potential to develop atrioventricular (AV) conduction block that may cause low cardiac output. The function of the pacemaker is to provide an external electrical stimulus to generate intracardiac electrical activity when the heart's own electrical system fails.

The external pacemaker unit consists of an energy source and two terminals—one grounded terminal and one output terminal (Fig. 40–1). There are two modes of pacemakers that are commonly used:

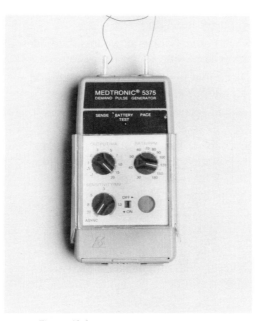

Figure 40-1.

1. *Fixed Rate* (asynchronous). These pace the heart at a set rate without regard for the child's rate.
2. *Demand.* These allow the child's cardiac rhythm to continue, provided that the ventricular rate equals or exceeds the rate at which the pacemaker is set. AV sequential pacemakers are either demand or control pacemakers that can provide both atrial and ventricular impulses in sequence.

The components of the demand pacemaker (the one most used in children) are:

1. *Output control*—Adjusts the amount of current delivered to the myocardium. The amount of current is measured in millamperes (mA). The correct setting is the one that maintains consistent capture of the heart impulse at the lowest possible output. This is set by the physician.

2. *Rate control*—Adjusts the pacing rate up to 800 pulses/minute, depending on the model. If the fixed rate model is used, the physician may set the rate above the child's own rate, overriding the child's rhythm. If demand pacing is desired as a backup, the rate will be set at the lowest possible rate that will provide adequate cardiac output.

3. *Sensitivity control*—Defines the minimum ECG signal that will inhibit a pacemaker impulse or initiate pacer firing.

4. *Sense-pace indicator*—Is a light that will indicate whether the pacemaker is sensing the child's R wave or generating an electrical impulse.

Standard of Care

1. Monitor the child's ECG rhythm at all times.

2. If an external pacemaker is in place, the following information should be recorded every 8 hours:
   a. Pacemaker mode
   b. Demand rate
   c. Sensitivity
   d. Electrical output
   e. On/off position
   f. ECG strip to verify proper pacemaker function

3. Monitor vital signs every 4 hours with apical pulse as well as cardiovascular function through perfusion, color, temperature, and blood pressure.

4. If the pacemaker is temporary, check that the wires are grounded and secured to the chest. Cover generator with a childproof cover.

5. Place ECG rhythm strip in the medical record at least every 8 hours to verify proper pacemaker function.

6. Obtain an informed consent (see Chap. 4) from the guardian for an elective insertion of a pacemaker. Many times, however, a pacemaker is inserted as part of another cardiovascular procedure or during resuscitation attempts.

7. Provide emotional and physical support to the child and family.

Assessment

1. Assess the medical history of the child, with emphasis on the cardiovascular system in regard to congenital anomalies and conditions affecting the heart's conduction system.

2. Assess physical status such as height, weight, peripheral perfusion, apical rate and rhythm, skin color, temperature, and level of consciousness.

3. Assess the developmental level of the child as well coping mechanisms and support systems.

Nursing Diagnoses

The following is a list of possible diagnoses and could apply, depending on the child's age, clinical situation, and physical condition:

Anxiety

Decreased cardiac output

High risk for injury

High risk for infection

Planning

In planning to care for a child with a pacemaker, the following equipment must be gathered:

For temporary pacemaker care:

Rubber glove

Fresh battery

Replacement generator

Tape

Alligator clips

20-gauge needle

Cardiac monitor

For permanent pacemaker care:

Cardiac monitor

Interventions

PROCEDURE	**RATIONALE/EXPECTED OUTCOME (EO)**
1. Prepare the child for the insertion of the pacemaker in a developmentally appropriate manner.	The child and family will cooperate if they understand the need for the pacemaker and the care required. *EO: The child and family will express their anxieties and fears in regard to the pacemaker.*

2. **External Pacemaker:**
 a. Connect epicardial wire to the negative (−) pole and ground wire to the positive (+) pole.
 b. Secure all connections.
 c. Check generator for fresh battery, which should be dated less than 30 days from the current date.
 d. Initiate proper setting on the generator as ordered by the physician:
   • Rate—If child's rate is adequate, set rate 10 lower
   • mA—Set just above child's threshold
   • Sensitivity—Set at a point where for each QRS complex, the red sense light flashes.
 e. Cover generator dials with a childproof cover.
 f. Slip generator and wires into a rubber glove.
	EO: The child will have the external pacemaker set up and initiated in a safe manner.
	
	This will prevent accidental movement of the dials. Exposed metal wire tips can provide low resistance pathways for electrical current to travel to the heart. The glove will also protect the generator unit and wires from moisture.

3. **Internal Pacemaker** a. Check incision site for signs and symptoms of infection (for example, redness, tenderness, drainage, and fever). b. Check the generator pocket for signs of trauma (bruising of the skin over the generator).	*EO: The child will have the internal pacemakers monitored for signs of infection or trauma to the generator.*
4. Attach a cardiac monitor to the child using at least three leads (Fig. 40-2). Place ECG strip in medical record.	*EO: The child will have cardiac rhythm assessed while in the hospital.*

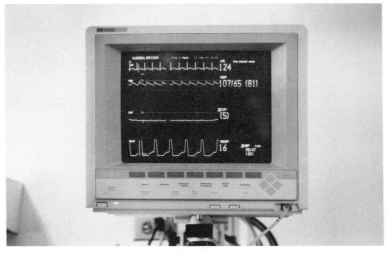

Figure 40-2.

PROCEDURE	**RATIONALE/EXPECTED OUTCOME (EO)**
5. Assess vital signs and cardiac function through capillary refill, skin color, and temperature every 4–8 hours. If the child is pacer-dependent, the function should be checked hourly.	The presence of a satisfactory heart rate on a monitor does not ensure effective cardiac contraction and cardiac output. *EO: The child will have cardiac output assessed.*
6. Observe the child and monitor for complications that may occur:	
a. Arrhythmias	May result from myocardial injury caused by the wires.
b. Pulmonary emboli	May be caused by dislodged thrombi at the tip of the wires.
c. Perforation	May result when a transvenous wire is used in the right ventricle.
d. Infection	May be from the invasive procedure.
e. Shocks	May occur at the skin near the wire insertion site if the mA output is too high.
f. Hiccups	May result if the pacer output is too high or if the wires stimulate the phrenic nerve.
g. Wire fracture	Wires may break. *EO: The child will be free from injury and complications of the pacemaker.*

Patient/Family Education: Home Care Considerations

Instruct child and parents of the need for the pacemaker, whether permanent or temporary. If temporary, explain when generator and wires will be removed. If pacemaker is permanent:

1. Review conduction system of the heart as well as "an EKG rhythm."

2. Explain parts of a pacemaker, including circuitry, battery, connector, insulated wire, and electrode tip. Inform the family of the preset rate of the pacemaker.

3. Discuss generator "pocket" and function in relation to body image.

4. Instruct family to maintain normal healthy lifestyle without limitations, unless restricted by physician.

5. Explain importance of follow-up appointments to check pacemaker function.

6. Instruct family to inform other doctors, dentists, and their school that they have a pacemaker.

7. Instruct child and family to carry a pacemaker identification card with them at all times. (It should include settings, date and location where implanted, the doctor responsible, and the model of pacemaker.)

8. Identify signs and symptoms of possible pacemaker problems:
   a. Recurrence of symptoms that were present prior to pacemaker implantation
   b. Swollen ankles
   c. Redness and drainage at incision site
   d. Prolonged fever
   e. Fainting or dizziness
   f. Excessive hiccupping
   g. Chest pain
   h. Muscle twitching
   i. Shortness of breath
   j. Any unusual sensations.

   If these occur, the doctor should be notified.

9. Distribute pamphlets on pacemakers (if available).

10. Identify any other special instructions regarding individual pacemaker care, such as taking an apical pulse daily and recording result. Also identify when to call the physician if apical rate is below the pacemaker setting.

Table 40-1. Troubleshooting Pacemaker Problems

Pacemaker Problem	EKG	Implications	Interventions
Failure to sense (competition)	Random spikes at fixed rate which may or may not capture— some paced beats, some fusions, and some spikes noncaptured	Potential for spike falling on a T wave to induce V tach— dangerous situation	• Check connection (especially + pole). • Turn sensitivity dial away from asynch until light flashes once for each QRS. • Decrease pacer rate or turn it off if patient rate is adequate. • Use a sub-Q ground to improve sensitivity.
Failure to capture	Spikes + on EKG not followed by a QRS.	If no escape, rhythm + cardiac output will equal zero!	• Check connections. • Increase mA (epicardial wires frequently need more voltage over time). • Switch poles if two RV wires are present. • Replace battery. • Consider atropine or Isuprel if unable to pace. • Consider pace port, Swan or transvenous wire via the cordis.
Failure to pace	No spikes on EKG	If patient rhythm is inadequate, there will be marked hypotension.	• Check connections (especially the negative pole). • If pace light is flashing, increase mA. • If pace light does not flash, make sure it is not oversensing—decrease the sensitivity. • Change pacer boxes. • Switch wires if 2 RVs are present. • Consider atropine or Isuprel. • Consider pace port or transvenous pacer.

References

Alpern, D. (1989). Psychosocial responses of children to cardiac pacemakers. *Journal of Pediatrics, 114*(3), 494–501

Besley, D., McWilliams G., Moody, D., & Castle, L., (1982). Long-term follow-up of young adults following permanent pacemaker placement for complete heart block. *American Heart Journal, 103*(3), 332–337.

Eiken, F. (1989). How to care for patients with temporary cardiac pacemakers. *Advancing Clinical Care,* November/December, 18–22.

Freeman, S., Young, D. (1981). Cardiac pacing in children and adolescents: Pediatric cardiology. *Pace, 4,* 550–558.

Hartler, C.O., Maloney, J.D., Curtis, J.J., & Barnhorst, D.A. (1977). Hemodynamic benefits of atrioventricular sequential pacing after open heart surgery. *American Journal of Cardiology, 40,* 232–236.

Porterfield, L. (1987). What do you need to know about today's pacemakers: *RN,* March, 44–49.

Young, D. (1981). Permanent pacemaker implantation in children: Current status and future considerations. *PACE, 4,* 61–67.

Cardiac Catheterization

41

Definition/Purpose

Cardiac catheterization is the passage of a catheter through a major blood vessel under direct visualization with a fluoroscope into the chambers of the heart. With it, the following information can be obtained:

1. Determination of intracardiac and intravascular pressure
2. Determination of pulmonary blood flow and cardiac output
3. Determination of oxygen content, saturation and tension
4. Detection of shunts
5. Visualization of the coronary artery by injection of contrast material
6. Visualization of the anatomy of the cardiac chambers and identification of congenital and acquired lesions.

Standards of Care

1. The cardiac catheterization procedure will be carried out under sterile conditions.

Assessment

1. Assess the pertinent medical history in relation to the anticipated cardiac lesion, the child's physiologic response to the lesion (such as activity limitations and cyanosis), current medications, and any previous surgical procedures.
2. Assess physical findings, including vital signs, pulses, presence of murmur, thrill, clubbing, level of hydration, height, weight, respiratory status, and complete blood count.
3. Assess the child's developmental level, coping mechanisms, and previous experience with hospitalization.
4. Assess the child's and family's knowledge of the planned procedure, potential complications, and the convalescent period.

Nursing Diagnoses

The following is a list of possible diagnoses and could apply, depending on the child's age, clinical situation, and physical condition:

High risk for infection

Fluid volume deficit

High risk for injury

Decreased cardiac output

Anxiety

Altered urinary elimination

Ineffective breathing pattern

Pain

Planning

To assess a child before and after catheterization, the following equipment is needed:

Thermometer

Stethoscope

Scale

Blood pressure cuff of appropriate size

Tape measure.

Interventions

PROCEDURE	**RATIONALE/EXPECTED OUTCOME (EO)**

Precatheterization:

1. Wash hands.

2. Gather equipment.

3. Take the child's apical pulse, respiration, temperature, and blood pressure on all four extremities.

   These vital signs serve as a baseline during and after the procedure.

4. Mark the pedal pulses with a pen, using an "X" where the pulsation is felt (Fig. 41-1).

   This serves as a landmark for pulses after the procedure.

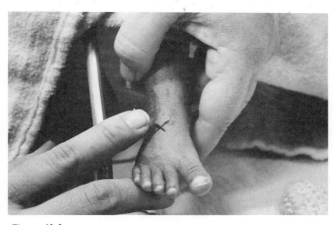

Figure 41-1

5. Measure the child's length (height) and weight. Explain that the child will have a blood test, chest x-ray, and echocardiogram prior to the catheterization.

   These measurements help determine the size of the catheter to be used, as well as the amount of the contrast medium.

6. Instruct the child and parent about what they may experience before and during the catheterization:
    a. Palpitations or missed beats secondary to the stimulation of the heart by the catheter
    b. Generalized warmth or a surge of heat secondary to the dye
    c. Nausea, dizziness, or headache due to the dye
    d. Discomfort from lying flat for several hours.

   EO: The child and parent verbalize an understanding of the environment and the catheterization procedure.

7. Take the child and parent on a tour of the cardiac catheterization laboratory.

PROCEDURE

8. Explain the meaning and reason for NPO.
9. Explain that the child will be transported on a stretcher for the test.
10. Explain to the child that parents will be waiting in the lounge or waiting room while the test is in progress.
11. Notify the physician of any allergy to iodine products or seafood.
12. Sedate the patient according to the physician's order.
13. Withhold anticoagulants and Lanoxin, as ordered by the physician.

Postcatheterization:

1. Observe operative site every half hour for bleeding, swelling, and hematoma formation.

2. If frank bleeding is present, apply direct pressure to insertion site immediately and notify physician. A sandbag may be used for extra pressure.
3. Monitor vital signs and extremity pulses, warmth, sensation, capillary refill and movement every 15 minutes for 1 hour; every 30 minutes for 1 hour; and then every hour for 2 hours. If stable, then every 4 hours.
4. Keep child in bed for 6 hours and discourage flexion at the hip. Provide quiet bed activities.

5. Encourage fluid intake.

6. Maintain strict intake and output.

7. Advance diet as tolerated.
8. Assess hydrational status every 4 hours.
9. Take temperature every 4 hours and notify physician for temperature over 38.5°C (101.4°F).
10. Assess the operative site every hour for redness, swelling, or drainage. If edema is present, elevate the extremity to facilitate venous return.
11. Give analgesics as ordered.

12. Auscultate breath sounds and heart tones every hour.

RATIONALE/EXPECTED OUTCOME (EO)

The contrast medium is an iodine preparation and can cause an allergic reaction.

Sedation will help immobilize the child during the test.

The pressure dressing will be removed in 24 hours by the physician.

EO: The child will suffer no adverse reactions from the catheterization.

The pulse distal to the puncture site may weaken, then gradually increase in strength.

The most common insertion site is the femoral area. Keeping the child quiet will prevent bleeding at the test site and disruption of the dressing.

The contrast medium can cause decreased renal perfusion.

EO: The child will have adequate urinary output (0.5–1.0 mL/kg/hr).

The child will show no clinical signs of dehydration, as evidenced by moist mucous membranes and good skin turgor.

EO: The child will be free of infection.

EO: The child will demonstrate adequate pain control by participation in play activities.

EO: The child will have baseline sinus rhythm and breath sounds.

PROCEDURE	**RATIONALE/EXPECTED OUTCOME (EO)**
13. Discuss the implications of the test results with the child and family and clarify any misconceptions.	Obtain the family's perceptions of the physician's recommendation. *EO: The child and family will understand the implications of the cardiac catheterization.*

Patient/Family Education: Home Care Considerations

1. Support the parents after they receive the results of the catheterization.
2. Discuss with the child and family the care of the wound (how to keep it dry) and the signs and symptoms of a wound infection (for example, fever, redness, and drainage).
3. Review dosage and administration of medications (if any).
4. Arrange for follow-up appointments.
5. Provide child and family with appropriate telephone numbers (such as the primary nurse and the cardiologist).

References

Perdue, B. (1990). Cardiac catheterization—before and after: What the patient should understand! What the nurse needs to know! *Advanced Clinical Care, 5*(2), 16–18.

Roberts, P.J. (1989). Caring for patients undergoing therapeutic cardiac catheterization. *Critical Care Nursing of North America, 1*(2), 275–288.

CVP Determination

42

Definition/Purpose

Indications for venous pressure monitoring in children include:

1. Infusions of large volumes of fluid or blood via a secure route
2. Infusions of hypertonic solutions
3. Infusion of vasoactive drugs
4. Monitoring of right heart pressures for the purpose of assessing venous return, blood volume, and right ventricular function, or obtaining indirect information about the pulmonary vascular system.

CVP catheters may be inserted percutaneously or by cutdown through several sites. The preferred sites are the external jugular and the subclavian veins. The CVP may be measured either by a transducer and monitor or by use of a water manometer (Fig. 42–1).

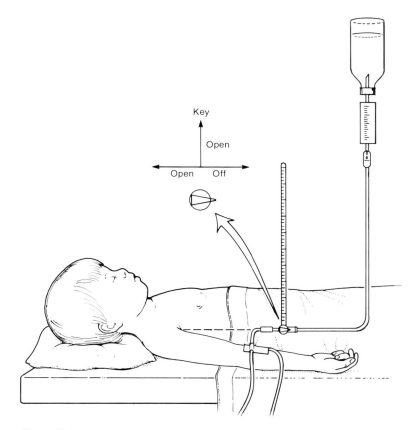

Figure 42-1.

The conversion factor from the mercury (mm Hg) reading to milliliters of water is:

$$1 \text{ mm Hg} = 1.36 \text{ mL water}$$

Normal CVP values are:

$$4.0\text{–}8.0 \text{ mm Hg or } 6.0\text{–}11.0 \text{ mL water.}$$

Standard of Care

1. Ensure that IV solution is infusing continuously.
2. Perform dressing change daily using aseptic technique.
3. Change all tubing and solution every 24 hours.
4. Secure catheter with tape/benzoin/transparent dressing to prevent dislodgement.
5. If drawing blood through the catheter, lower stopcock below atrium to prevent air from entering line.
6. Clear the IV line of fluid before sampling blood so that erroneous laboratory results are avoided.

Assessment

1. Assess the pertinent history and physical findings for the need for a CVP catheter (see Indications), the child's age, weight, and condition requiring a catheter insertion.
2. Assess the psychosocial and developmental factors, such as body image, fear, anxiety, and effect of the disease on self-concept and family interaction.
3. Assess the child's and family's knowledge of the rationale for function and care of the catheter and their expectations of therapy.

Nursing Diagnoses

The following is a list of possible diagnoses and could apply, depending on the child's age, clinical situation, and physical condition:

High risk for injury

Impaired skin integrity

High risk for infection

Planning

In planning to determine a child's CVP measurement; the following equipment must be gathered:

Infusion solution

Manometer

Pen and paper.

Interventions

PROCEDURE

1. Determine a single position of the child to be used for all measurements and post it on a sign above the bed.

RATIONALE/EXPECTED OUTCOME (EO)

It was first thought that the child had to be flat to obtain an accurate measurement. However, it is now agreed that the child may be elevated up to 45° as long as the *same* position is used for each measurement.

EO: The child will have the CVP measurement determined in a uniform position.

PROCEDURE

2. Determine the phlebostatic axis (reference point) for the CVP measurement. This may be determined by several landmarks:
   a. Using the midclavicle, locate the fourth intercostal space and follow the space across the chest wall to the midaxillary line.
   b. Mark this site with an X.
   c. Align this site with zero on the CVP monometer when obtaining readings. This should be at the level of the right atrium.

3. Connect the monometer to the stopcock on the infusion line, using sterile technique.

4. Flush CVP line with the IV fluid before measurement.

5. Turn the stopcock so that the monometer fills with fluid. The stopcock port to the child is in the "Off" position.

6. Turn the stopcock so that the port is open between the child and the monometer.

7. Turn stopcock to resume fluid infusion.

8. Record the readings as well as the child's position and whether he or she was breathing spontaneously or crying.

9. Dressings are changed every 48 hours using sterile technique. Record the condition of the skin surrounding the insertion site. Record dressing changes.

RATIONALE/EXPECTED OUTCOME (EO)

EO: The child will have the CVP measured at the same reference point each time.

EO: The child's infusion line and manometer will be handled using sterile technique to prevent sepsis.

This will ensure patency of the catheter.

The fluid column will fall with fluctuations in inspiration and expiration. Once the fluid level has stabilized, the height of the fluid column at the peak of the respiratory oscillations will correspond to the CVP reading.

The most accurate reading is spontaneous breathing. If the child is on a ventilator, disconnect it momentarily, if the child can tolerate it. Positive pressure ventilation alters the CVP reading by decreasing venous return. If the child cannot tolerate being disconnected, indicate that the reading was obtained while on positive pressure ventilation.

EO: The child will have an accurate CVP reading recorded.

EO: The child's skin at the insertion site will remain intact without sign of infiltration or infection.

Patient/Family Education: Home Care Considerations

1. Teach the family the rationale for the catheter.

2. Teach the family function, care, and operation of the catheter, as well as site care and the actual CVP determination.

3. Reassure the child and family that if ventilatory support is removed during a manometer reading, it will not harm the child, and the ventilator will be returned without difficulty.

References

Massachusetts General Hospital. (1980). *Massachusetts General Hospital Manual of Nursing Procedures.* (2nd ed.). Boston: Little Brown and Company.

Stenzel, J.P., Green, T.P., Fuhrman, B.P., et al (1989). Percutaneous central venous catheterization in a pediatric intensive care unit: A survival analysis of complications. Critical Care Medicine, *17*(10), 984–988.

Pericardiocentesis

43

Definition/Purpose

Percutaneous introduction of a needle into the pericardial space is performed for the following reasons:

1. Emergency removal of intrapericardial fluid in the treatment of pericardial tamponade.
2. Elective removal of pericardial fluid in the presence of a chronic or recurrent pericardial accumulation leading to decreased cardiac output.
3. As a diagnostic procedure for direct analysis of pericardial fluid.

   This procedure is performed most safely in the operating room, cardiac catheterization laboratory, or intensive care unit.

Standard of Care

1. The child should be well-sedated before the procedure.
2. The procedure will be performed under sterile, aseptic conditions.
3. The child will be attached to an ECG monitor during and after the procedure.

Assessment

1. Assess the pertinent history and physical findings for any of the following:

   Congenital cardiac lesion

   Medications

   Recent exposure to illness

   Any previous surgical procedures

   Tachycardia

   Comparison of blood pressure in the upper and lower extremities

   Tachypnea

   Dyspnea

   Retractions

   Skin color

   Pulses

   Presence of murmur or thrill

   Blood count

   Pattern of feeding

   Weight loss or gain

   Current chest x-ray result.

2. Assess for history of iodine allergy because povidone-iodine is used for skin preparation.

3. Assess the psychosocial factors with relation to developmental level, coping mechanisms, previous experience with hospitalization, and the child's usual family routines.

4. Assess the family's knowledge of the diagnosis, prognosis, and future plans for care.

Nursing Diagnoses

The following is a list of possible diagnoses and could apply, depending on the child's age, clinical situation, and physical condition:

Anxiety

Decreased cardiac output

High risk for infection

High risk for injury

Impaired skin integrity

Planning

In planning to assist the physician in pericardiocentesis the following equipment must be assembled:

Povidone-iodine

Sterile drapes

Sterile gauze

Sterile gloves

1% lidocaine

3–5-mL syringes

22-gauge needles

20-gauge, $2\frac{1}{2}$-inch spinal needle

3-way stopcock

30–50 mL syringes

Sterile alligator clip

No. 15 scalpel blade and holder

ECG monitor

Specimen tubes

Interventions

PROCEDURE

1. Explain the procedure to the child (if appropriate) and to the family. Have guardian sign a consent form.

2. Sedate the child as ordered.

RATIONALE/EXPECTED OUTCOME (EO)

The child and family will cooperate with the procedure if they understand what to expect.

EO: The child and family will express their concerns to the staff and verbalize an understanding of the procedure.

Sedation is usually required and may necessitate capable airway management and ventilation to ensure the safety of the child.

EO: The child will be adequately sedated before the test begins.

PROCEDURE	**RATIONALE/EXPECTED OUTCOME (EO)**

3. Position the child supine at a 30°–45° angle to the horizontal plane. The extremities should be held by the assistant.

4. Attach the limb leads of an ECG monitor.

5. Put on sterile gloves.

6. The physician will clean and sterilize the precordium with povidone-iodine solution and drape the area with sterile towels.

7. The physician will infiltrate the area just below the xiphoid process with 1% lidocaine.

   The infiltration needs to penetrate through the muscle layer to achieve adequate anesthesia.

   EO: The child will have decreased pain at the site of the text.

8. Attach the spinal needle to the stopcock and a 30–50-mL syringe.

9. Connect the V lead of the electrocardiogram to the hub of the needle, using the alligator clip.

   This will graphically record any epicardial contact. Ventricular contact will show S–T elevations as well as premature ventricular contractions. Atrial contact will show P–R segmental elevations and atrial contractions.

   EO: The child will be free from complications with the test.

10. Turn ECG recorder to the V lead position.

11. The physician will make a 2-mm incision just below the xiphoid.

    This will facilitate penetration of the skin by the needle.

12. The physician will advance the needle through the incision at an angle 60°–70° from the horizontal of the abdomen, pointing cephalad and to the left of the midthoracic spine (Fig. 43-1).

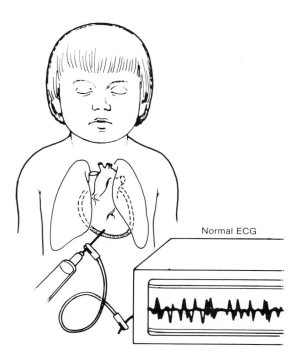

Normal ECG

Figure 43-1. Normal ECG.

PROCEDURE

RATIONALE/EXPECTED OUTCOME (EO)

13. Monitor ECG during the procedure. The needle is advanced slowly until pericardial fluid is obtained or evidence of myocardial contact is seen in the ECG (Fig. 43-2).

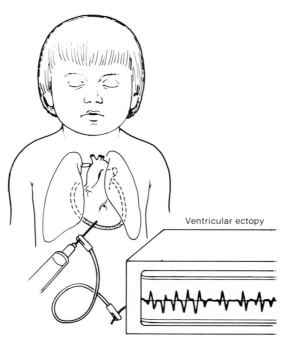

Figure 43-2. Ventricular ectopy.

14. When the fluid source is reached, a hemostat is clamped across the needle barrel at the skin surface.

This prevents further penetration by the needle.

15. The fluid is aspirated slowly.

Excess speed in removal of the fluid and decompression can result in pericardial shock or myocardial insufficiency.

EO: The child shows improvement in his or her clinical status (improvement in cardiac output).

16. After drainage is completed, the needle is removed and the puncture site covered with a sterile dressing.

Interpretation of Results:

a. If no fluid is obtained, fluid is usually loculated anterior.

b. If fluid is serous or serosanguineous, obtain the following tests: culture, gram stain, glucose, protein, and cell count (for uremic or purulent pericarditis).

c. If fluid is bloody, the sample is either intracardiac (if it clots) or from penetrating trauma in the pericardial space (if it does not clot).

PROCEDURE	RATIONALE/EXPECTED OUTCOME (EO)
17. Obtain a postprocedure chest x-ray as ordered.	Comparison can be made between the pre- and postprocedure film.
18. Observe the child closely with vital signs checked every 15–30 minutes and ECG monitoring. Monitor for the following complications:	*EO: The child's vital signs will be maintained within normal limits.*

Acute

    a. Pneumothorax
    b. Hemopericardium
    c. Myocardial penetration

Delayed

    a. Pericardial leakage (cutaneous fistula)
    b. Local infection
    c. Pericardial–peritoneal fistula
    d. Slowly developing pneumothorax
    e. Pneumopericardium
    f. Pericardial tamponade

EO: The child's skin at the puncture site will remain intact, without signs of infection.

19. Record the procedure in the medical record, along with how the child tolerated the procedure and any complications.

Patient/Family Education: Home Care Considerations

1. Reinforce the information given to the family by the physician. Correct any misconceptions.
2. Provide the names and phone numbers of persons to contact should problems develop (for example, shortness of breath, retractions, cyanosis, fever, cough, or weight loss).
3. Teach the parents to monitor the needle insertion site for drainage, redness, and pain, and to notify the physician if concerns develop.
4. Counsel the child and parents regarding the importance of continued long-term follow-up.

References

Civetta, J.M., Taylor, R.W., & Kirby, R.R. (1988). *Critical care.* Philadelphia: JB Lippincott Co.

Fleisher, G. & Ludwig, S. (1988). *Textbook of pediatric emergency medicine.* Baltimore: Williams & Wilkins.

Lanros, N.E. (1988). *Assessment and intervention in emergency nursing.* Norwalk, CT: Appleton & Lange.

Hematologic System Procedures

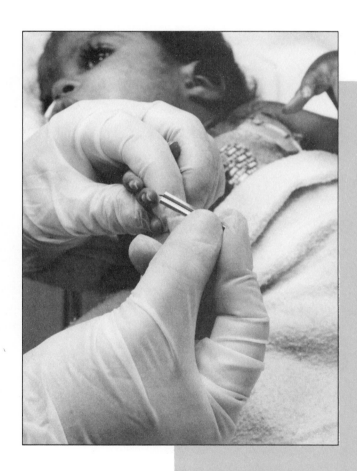

Unit VII

Blood Product Transfusion

44

Definition/Purpose

The transfusion of blood products into the venous system assists in maintaining hemodynamic equilibrium in the child. Transfusion therapy may be used to quickly restore blood volume following hemorrhage, burns, or injuries to blood vessels; to combat shock; to treat severe chronic anemia by increasing the oxygen-carrying capacity of the blood, or to maintain the coagulation properties of blood by supplying clotting factors.

Standard of Care

1. Unless the transfusion is an emergency, a consent for the transfusion must be signed by the child's parent or guardian before the infusion.
2. The nurse or physician who obtains the blood for typing and cross-matching must identify the child correctly and label the specimen accurately.
3. Two registered nurses must check the child's identification number with the number on the blood product, the physician's order with the blood product, and the compatibility of the child's blood with the blood product to be transfused, and that the appropriate consents have been signed.
4. The expiration date on the blood product must be checked before infusion.
5. If the blood components need to be refrigerated, they must be placed in a designated, monitored blood refrigerator.

Assessment

1. Assess the child's medical history for recent trauma, clotting disorders, chemotherapy, bone marrow suppression, fluid shifts or imbalances, previous transfusion and possible reactions to them, or any other finding that would complicate or contraindicate a transfusion.
2. Assess the child's height and weight to determine whether the prescribed amount and rate of transfusion are appropriate.
3. Assess clinical laboratory values to determine whether the type of blood product is appropriate.
4. Assess psychosocial factors relative to developmental stage; moral, ethical and religious principles; and the fear of contracting a disease from the blood product.
5. Assess the child's and family's knowledge of the potential benefits and risks of the therapy and their willingness to learn.

Nursing Diagnoses

The following is a list of possible diagnoses and could apply, depending on the child's age, clinical situation, and physical condition:

Anxiety

High risk for injury

Impaired gas exchange

Fluid volume excess

High risk for infection

Decreased cardiac output

Hypothermia

Planning

In planning to infuse a blood product the following equipment must be obtained:

Non-sterile gloves

Y-tubing with blood filter

Volume-regulated infusion pump (that is approved for blood infusion)

Appropriate blood product

50-mL bag of normal saline

Thermometer

Blood pressure equipment

Stethoscope

Interventions

PROCEDURE

1. Reinforce the physician's explanation about the proposed transfusion, the procedure, and the potential complications.

2. Acknowledge concerns and reassure the family that others have expressed similar feelings.

3. Obtain an informed consent for the transfusion.

4. Identify the child and verify the blood (type, Rh factor, donor number, expiration date) with another nurse or physician. Order only as much blood as can be infused in 4 hours (Table 44-1).

RATIONALE/EXPECTED OUTCOME (EO)

The child and family will be more cooperative if they understand the need for the transfusion and the procedure to be used.

EO: The child and family will have decreased anxiety regarding the transfusion.

EO: The child and family will understand the transfusion procedure.

Transfusions are legal matters requiring consent for treatment or documented refusal to receive blood components.

There is significant cell death after 4 hours at room temperature.

Table 44-1. Blood Components

Components	Description	Indications	Dose/Rate	Matching	Shelf Life	Filter	Tubing
Whole blood	Single-donor unadulterated blood	10–15% blood loss— Exchange transfusions	20 mL/kg initially, followed by any volume needed to stabilize child. As rapidly as necessary to reestablish volume.	Necessary	21 days at 5°C (41.0°F)	Micro-aggregate	Standard IV tubing suitable for infusion pump
Packed red blood cells	Concentrated RBCs with plasma, leukocytes, and platelets removed	Anemia; surgical blood loss; suppression of erythropoiesis	10–15 mL/kg (1 mL/ kg will increase hematocrit by 1%.) 5 mL/kg/hr; or 2 mL/kg/hr in CHF.	Necessary	Stored fresh—21 days; stored frozen—3 years	Micro-aggregate	Standard IV tubing suitable for infusion pump

(continued)

Table 44-1. (*continued*)

Components	Description	Indications	Dose/Rate	Matching	Shelf Life	Filter	Tubing
Washed RBCs	RBCs washed with saline removing 93% of leukocytes	Immuno-suppressed children; children with history of febrile transfusion reactions.	10–15 mL/kg (1 mL/kg will increase hematocrit by 1%.) 5 mL/kg/hr or 2 mL/kg/hr in CHF.	Necessary	Stored fresh: 21 days; stored frozen: 3 years	Micro-aggregate	Standard IV tubing suitable for infusion pump.
Platelet concentration	Platelets in a small amount of plasma	Thrombocytopenia (<20,000) Platelet count <50,000 in a child who requires surgery	1 unit for every 7–10 kg of body weight will increase the platelet count by 50,000. Administer each unit over 5–10 minutes.	Unnecessary	Up to 72 hrs after whole blood collection	Micro-aggregate	Standard IV tubing or platelet administration set.
Granulocytes	WBCs	Sepsis in severe neutropenia (<500 mm^3); unresponsive to antibiotics	10 mL/kg/day Slowly over 2–4 hours. Mild fever and chills are common.	Must be ABO compatible	Must be infused within 6 hours of collection	Standard blood filter or screen-type microaggregate filter.	Standard IV tubing.
Fresh frozen plasma	Portion of blood that contains clotting factors and proteins.	Hemorrhage; hypovolemic shock; DIC; liver disease.	Hemorrhage: 15–30 mL/kg Clotting: 10–15 mL/kg Hemorrhage: as fast as tolerated. Clotting: 2–3 hours.	Must be ABO compatible	Fresh—6 hrs after collection; fresh frozen—12 months at 20°C (68.0°F) or 2 hours after thawing.	Standard blood filter or micro-aggregate filter	Standard IV tubing.
Cryoprecipitate	Concentrated factor VII and fibrinogen (100 U factor VII/unit)	Hemophilia A; DIC; Von Willebrand's disease	1 bag/5 kg—Mild; 1 bag/2 kg—Severe. Repeat every 12–24 hours as rapidly as possible.	ABO compatibility preferred	12 months if frozen at 20°C (68.0°F) and up to 6 hours after thawing.	Standard blood filter or micro-aggregate filter	Standard IV tubing
Albumin	Blood protein	Hypoproteinemia; volume expander; burns	5% = 1 gm/kg = 20 mL/kg 25% = 1 gm/kg = 4 mL/kg 5% = 1–2 mL/minute 25% = 0.2–0.4 mL/minute	Unnecessary	5 years—Use at 2°C (35.6°F) filter 3 years—packaged at room temperature		Use tubing packaged with product.
Factor VIII concentrate	Concentrated powdered blood clotting Factor VII	Hemophilia A	20 U/kg—minor 40 U/kg—severe 2 mL/minute	Unnecessary	Refer to manufacturer's expiration date	Filter needle provided with package	Withdraw reconstituted solution from vial via filter needle; then administer via syringe

PROCEDURE	**RATIONALE/EXPECTED OUTCOME (EO)**
5. Gather equipment.	
6. Wash hands.	
7. Start peripheral IV if no previous IV access is available.	
8. Using the Y-tubing, connect the 50-mL bag of normal saline to one port and flush the line. Connect IV tubing to the child's venous access.	Dextrose solutions cause hemolysis; thus the use of normal saline.
9. Inspect catheter insertion site for signs of infiltration (swelling, redness, and warmth) or infection (pain and drainage) prior to starting the blood transfusion.	
10. Wearing gloves, connect the blood bag to the other Y-tubing port. Allow blood to warm to room temperature (not more than 30 minutes).	
11. Administer prescribed antihistamine when the child has a known history of transfusion reactions.	*EO: The child will not experience complications of blood product administration.*
12. Take baseline vital signs (temperature, pulse, respiration, and blood pressure)	
13 Using an infusion pump to regulate flow, stop the normal saline and begin the blood infusion at a low rate for 15 minutes.	Early detection of adverse reactions can be achieved by close clinical monitoring.
14. Identify possible transfusion reactions promptly:	*EO: The child will maintain adequate oxygenation of all body tissues.*
a. Monitor vital signs. Watch for increased, shallow, or labored respirations; stridor or wheezing; tachycardia; and decreased blood pressure.	Circulatory overload, especially in children with respiratory, renal, or cardiac disease, may develop if the child is unable to compensate for additional fluid.
b. Remain with child during first 15 minutes of transfusion.	
c. Note changes in skin color or mentation.	*EO: The child displays normal skin color. The child remains alert and free from changes in mental status.*
d. Auscultate lungs for rales, rhonchi, or muffled breath sounds.	
e. Assess for signs of pyrogenic reaction (fever, chills, nausea, vomiting, headache, abdominal pain, and hypotension). If there is no reaction after the initial 15 minutes, infuse at ordered rate.	Pyrogenic reactions can occur if the blood becomes contaminated with bacteria. *EO: The child will remain free from infection.*
15. Monitor vital signs every 15 minutes for the first 2 hours, and then every 30 minutes until the infusion is complete. Compare the readings to baseline vital signs.	Hemolytic reactions are caused by ABO and Rh incompatibilities. When a reaction occurs, there is an antibody–antigen response that causes red blood cells to obstruct blood flow to organs, including the lungs. *EO: The child will maintain vital signs within normal limits.* *EO: The child is free from discomfort associated with an allergic reaction.*
16. Initiate measures to correct transfusion reactions (Table 44-2):	
a. Stop transfusion and infuse normal saline. Notify physician.	
b. Position child for comfort and to decrease respiratory distress.	
c. Administer oxygen and monitor its effectiveness.	
d. Administer the prescribed medications.	
e. Continue to monitor vital signs.	

Table 44-2. Transfusion Reactions

Type	Prevention	Signs and Symptoms	Nursing Interventions
Hemolytic	Identify child and blood product to ensure match. Begin infusion slowly and remain with child for first 15 minutes. Reactions begin soon after initiation of transfusion.	Burning at infusion site Flushing Chest pain Headache Low back pain Shock	Stop transfusion. Treat shock (administer oxygen and fluids). Recheck blood slip. Obtain two blood samples: one for centrifuge (red plasma indicates hemolysis) one for the blood bank Obtain first voided urine to test for hemoglobinuria.
Allergic	Determine whether child has a history of allergic reactions to transfusions. Administer antihistamine minutes before starting infusion.	Urticaria Facial or glottal edema Pulmonary edema or asthma Anaphylaxis	Stop transfusion. Treat life-threatening reaction (to medications and intubation).
Febrile	Keep child warm during transfusion. Administer antipyretic medication to children known to have this reaction. Transfuse with leukocyte-poor RBCs or frozen washed packed cells.	Chills and fever Headache Flushing Tachycardia General discomfort	Stop transfusion. Treat symptoms.
Air embolism	Avoid introducing air into the system.	Cyanosis Dyspnea Shock Cardiac arrest	Treat shock or cardiac arrest immediately. Lower child's head and turn on left side; this will allow air to collect in RA, where it can be released slowly to the lungs.
Bacterial	Maintain aseptic technique. Do not allow blood to stand at room temperature for more than 45 minutes.	Shaking fever Hypotension Dry or flushed skin Abdominal or extremity pain Vomiting Bloody diarrhea	Stop transfusion. Administer antibiotics. Treat shock. Monitor vital signs Monitor fluid and electrolyte balance.
Circulatory overload	Give packed RBCs instead of whole blood. Administer infusion slowly.	Labored breathing Dry cough Pulmonary edema Rales at bases of lungs	Slow infusion. Raise the head of bed. Monitor vital signs. Administer diuretics.

PROCEDURE

   f. Record intake and output.
   g. Obtain first voided specimen for urinalysis.
17. Monitor for signs of hypothermia (chills, low temperature, and irregular heart rate). If child shows signs of hypothermia:
   a. Stop infusion and maintain IV line with normal saline.
   b. Warm blood product with electric warming coil.

RATIONALE/EXPECTED OUTCOME (EO)

Blood is stored at a cool temperature and should be used within 30 minutes of arrival from the blood bank. Small children can develop hypothermia if chilled blood is infused.

EO: The child will maintain a body temperature at pretransfusion level.

PROCEDURE	**RATIONALE/EXPECTED OUTCOME (EO)**
c. Warm child with additional blankets and over-the-bed heater.	
18. Assess child every 4 hours for signs of hyperkalemia (malaise, muscle weakness, mental confusion, diarrhea, nausea, irregular pulse, and paralysis). If child shows signs of hyperkalemia: a. Hold oral or IV potassium preparations. b. Record cardiac rhythm strip every 4 hours. c. Administer oral or rectal cation resins to remove excess potassium. d. Monitor CVP, pulmonary artery pressure, and cardiac output every 2–4 hours.	The composition of donor blood changes within 24 hours of collection. By the expiration date, the potassium levels have increased, with increased lysis of blood cells. Children with renal disease may be unable to excrete this potassium load and are at risk for hyperkalemia. *EO: The child will maintain normal potassium levels.*
19. When the desired amount of the blood component has infused, stop the transfusion, flush the line with normal saline, and either hang a maintenance fluid or discontinue the access site. The transfusion should be completed within 4 hours; after 4 hours, return remaining blood to the blood bank.	

Patient/Family Education: Home Care Considerations

1. Offer the family an explanation of precautionary measures employed by the blood bank to ensure safety of blood products.

2. Inform the family of the availability of support groups to donate blood or to initiate blood drives when large quantities of blood are required.

References

Barrel, M., Landier, W., Stlyffe, E. (1987). How to administer blood components to children. *Maternal-Child Nursing, 12*(3), 178–184.

Cullins, L. (1979). Preventing and treating transfusion reactions. *American Journal of Nursing, 79*(5), 935–936.

Mahoney, D.H., Jr. (1987). Blood component therapy: Redefined guidelines for pediatric patients. *Consultant, 27*(1), 130–138.

Taylor, B.N., Wagner, P.L., & Kraus, C.L. (1987). Development for a standard for time-effective patient assessment during blood transfusions. *Journal of Nursing Quality Assurance, 1*(2), 66–71.

Wise, B.V., & Nolan, L.L. (1990). A risk of blood transfusions for premature infants. *Journal of Maternal Child Nursing, 15*(2), 86–89.

Exchange Transfusion

45

Definition/Purpose

In 1924, before the etiology of hemolytic disease of the newborn was known, Hart and McDonald successfully performed the first exsanguination transfusion on an infant with icterus, hoping to remove toxins from the blood. During the first attempt at an exchange transfusion, 300 mL of blood was removed from the infant's anterior fontanelle while 336 mL of donor blood was simultaneously transfused into the saphenous vein in the ankle. It was not until 1946 that the technique was developed more fully. Techniques were described for the removal of blood from the radial artery or the umbilical artery and infusion into the saphenous or umbilical vein. Valentine, in 1962, used a method of a balanced drip exchange transfusion whereby heparinized donor blood is infused by continuous drip while an exsanguination drips from the umbilical vein. This procedure required 6–8 hours.

The method described here is one of several acceptably safe techniques for replacing a child's blood with fresh donor blood. An exchange transfusion, whether total or partial, is performed for the following reasons:

1. To remove excess bilirubin and prevent kernicterus
2. To treat anemia or polycythemia
3. To prevent jaundice in Rh sensitization
4. To remove circulatory toxic substances and poisons
5. To improve oxygenation in preterm infants
6. To replace sickled cells of children in painful vasoocclusive crisis.

Standard of Care

1. The exchange transfusion is performed by two staff members, physician and nurse; one to withdraw blood and administer the blood, and one to record the exchanges.
2. Follow the infection control recommendations for the handling of blood and blood products.
3. Dispose of supplies and withdrawn blood in designated containers.
4. The exchange transfusion will be carried out under sterile conditions.
5. Resuscitation equipment, oxygen administration equipment, and suction equipment should be close at hand.
6. Blood components to be infused will be checked according to hospital policy by two persons.

Assessment

1. Assess pertinent history for toxic ingestion, Rh and ABO incompatibility, polycythemia, infection, bruising, liver or metabolic disease, bowel obstruction, diabetic mother, sickle cell disease, breast-feeding, or response to phototherapy.
2. Assess physical findings of increasing jaundice, pallor, lethargy, tremors, poor feeding, hypotonia, or convulsions.

3. Assess the family's knowledge of the causes and treatment of the disease process and the follow-up care needed.

Nursing Diagnoses

The following is a list of possible diagnoses and could apply, depending on the child's age, clinical situation, and physical condition:

Pain

High risk for infection

Fluid volume excess

Altered tissue perfusion

High risk for injury

Ineffective thermoregulation

Planning

When preparing to assist with an exchange transfusion, the following equipment must be gathered:

Blood product to be infused (for example, packed red blood cells, fresh frozen plasma, or albumin)

Blood administration set

Blood warmer

Sterile gloves

50-mL syringes

3-way stopcock

Waste blood container

Calcium gluconate (10%; drawn up in a labeled syringe)

Blood sample tubes

Goggles

Masks

Sterile drapes

Sterile gowns

Caps

Interventions

PROCEDURE	**RATIONALE/EXPECTED OUTCOME (EO)**
1. Explain the procedure to the family. Obtain a consent for the procedure as well as for the transfusion of blood.	Follow hospital policy regarding obtaining legal consent for procedures and administration of blood products. *EO: The child and family will verbalize their concerns.*
2. Assemble needed equipment (Fig. 45-1).	
3. Attach the child to a cardiopulmonary monitor with the alarms set.	Hyperkalemia, hypocalcemia, air embolism, and hypothermia may be etiologic factors in cardiac arrest. *EO: The child will be adequately monitored during the procedure.*
4. Record baseline vital signs.	

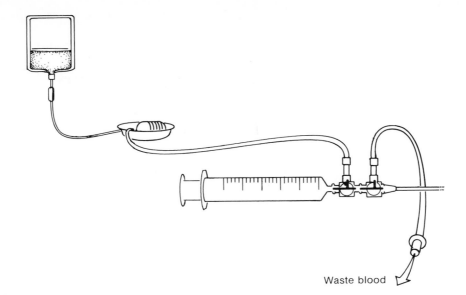

Waste blood

Figure 45-1.

PROCEDURE

5. If the child is small, and at risk of hypothermia, place him or her under a radiant warmer.

6. Position the child prone; restrain if needed.

7. Check blood components to be infused according to hospital policy.

8. Prepare the blood product by attaching the filter and appropriate tubing to pass the blood through the warmer.

9. Assist the physician in gowning and gloving.

10. Assist the physician in establishing intravenous access for withdrawal and infusion of blood.

11. Prime all tubing with blood and attach to access.

12. The initial increment of blood withdrawn from the child is sent to the lab for baseline studies. The volume of the initial increment and all successive increments is determined by the weight of the child.

13. The physician will connect a syringe to the stopcock and draw donor blood into the syringe after positioning the stopcock valves. Transfuse the blood into the child slowly.

14. Next, reverse the stopcock valves and aspirate the same volume of blood as transfused. Again, adjust the stopcock valves and empty this blood into the waste container.

15. Readjust the stopcock valves, draw donor blood into the syringe, transfuse it into the child, aspirate blood out, and empty into waste container.

RATIONALE/EXPECTED OUTCOME (EO)

Chilling of the child can result in apnea, increased caloric needs, and increased oxygen consumption.

EO: The child will maintain a normal body temperature.

EO: The child will experience minimal discomfort during the procedure.

Children can become hypothermic after transfusion of large quantities of cold bank blood. A lowering of body temperature can interfere with the normal function of the heart.

EO: The child will not be exposed to infectious agents during the transfusion due to contamination of blood product during administration.

EO: The child will maintain adequate tissue perfusion throughout the procedure (cardiopulmonary and cerebral).

The volume of blood to be exchanged per cycle should be 3–5 mL/kg.

EO: The child will remain normovolemic and well-hydrated.

This cycle is repeated over and over until the appropriate blood volume has been exchanged.

PROCEDURE	**RATIONALE/EXPECTED OUTCOME (EO)**

16. The nurse will record on the flow sheets the exact amounts of blood infused and wasted and the exact time frames for each cycle (Fig. 45-2).

MICHAEL REESE HOSPITAL AND MEDICAL CENTER

Department of Pediatric Nursing

Pediatric Partial Exchange Transfusion Form   Date: _____

TIME	BLOOD	INFUSED	BLOOD WITHDRAWN		TEMP	AP	RESP	B/P	NOTES	MEDS
		Total In		Total Out						
									Developed by: Reneta Stadnicki, RN Originated: January, 1983	

Figure 45-2.

17. Record vital signs on the record sheet every 15 minutes during the procedure. Be alert for signs of anaphylaxis.

18. Be aware of the potential need for calcium gluconate during the procedure.

The citrate of donor blood can depress calcium ion concentration sufficiently to produce tetany.

EO: The child will maintain a normal calcium blood level throughout the exchange transfusion.

If calcium is needed, infuse slowly.

Calcium increases the irritability of the heart muscle. Too rapid infusion will cause bradycardia.

PROCEDURE	**RATIONALE/EXPECTED OUTCOME (EO)**
19. Monitor blood glucose every 30 minutes during the exchange and every hour following the exchange.	The increased glucose in preserved blood produces an increased serum glucose concentration in the child. *EO: The child will maintain normal serum glucose levels during the transfusion to prevent an increase in insulin secretion which can lead to severe postexchange hypoglycemia.*
20. After the exchange transfusion is completed, send postexchange electrolytes, CBC, calcium, bilirubin, or hemoglobin electrophresis, etc., to the lab as ordered by the physician.	A toxic concentration of potassium accumulates in blood stored for longer than 1 week. Transfusion of such blood produces an increase in serum potassium. *EO: The child will be protected from potential injury due to electrolyte imbalances.*

21. Document on the flow sheet (see attached) and in the medical record:
  a. Time exchange was begun
  b. Time exchange was completed
  c. Total amount of blood withdrawn
  d. Total amount of blood infused
  e. Any changes in vital signs, neurologic, cardiac, or respiratory status
  f. Medications administered during the exchange
  g. Laboratory values obtained before, during, and after the exchange transfusion
	EO: The child's medical record will accurately reflect the procedure.

Patient/Family Education: Home Care Considerations

1. Educate the family as to the reason for the exchange transfusion, the procedure itself, and its benefits and risks.
2. Assist the family in adjusting to a diagnosis that requires long-term therapy and medical attention (such as sickle cell disease).
3. Encourage the child's participation in age-appropriate activities.
4. List resources available in the community to assist the family.

References

Gradolf, B. (1983). Sickle cell anemia in children. *Issues in Comprehensive Pediatric Nursing, 6,* 295–306.

Hathaway, G. (1984). The child with sickle cell anemia: Implications and management. *Nurse Practitioner, 9*(10), 16–22.

Landier, W.C., Barrell, M.L., & Styffe, E.J. (1987). How to administer blood components to children. *Maternal/Child Nursing, 12*(3), 178–184.

Page, S. (1989). Rh hemolytic disease in the newborn. *Neonatal Network, 7*(6), 31–41.

Phototherapy

46

Definition/Purpose

Hyperbilirubinemia, an elevation of serum bilirubin, is a condition characterized by jaundice of the skin, the sclera of the eyes, the mucous membranes, and the body fluids. It is caused by the deposition of bilirubin pigment that is released when the red blood cells undergo hemolysis. Phototherapy accelerates bilirubin turnover and excretion by photo-oxidation.

When total serum bilirubin levels reach 15–20 mg per 100 mL during the first week of life, hyperbilirubinemia is considered to be present. The significance of hyperbilirubinemia lies in the high incidence of kernicterus associated with serum bilirubin levels over 19–20 mg per 100 mL. At these levels, unconjugated bilirubin penetrates cells of the brain and brain stem, producing cellular dysfunction and profound damage characterized by lethargy, poor feeding, stiffening of the body, and a high-pitched cry.

Blue light of wavelength 425 to 475 has been found most effective in the photodegradation of bilirubin. Blue lights, however, can be unpleasant to work around. Nursery staff complain of headache, nausea, and vertigo when blue lights are used without ultraviolet screening filters; thus a sheet of Plexiglas G should be used as an effective ultraviolet screen.

Standard of Care

1. The infant's temperature will remain within normal limits throughout phototherapy.
2. The infant will remain hydrated throughout the therapy.

Assessment

1. Assess pertinent history of Rh or ABO incompatibility, polycythemia, infection, bruising, liver or metabolic disease, bowel obstruction, diabetic mother, or breast feeding.
2. Assess physical findings of jaundice, pallor, dark-concentrated urine, lethargy, hypotonia, poor suck, irritability, tremors, convulsions, or high-pitched cry. Assess laboratory findings for an elevated bilirubin level.
3. Assess the family's knowledge of the causes and treatment of hyperbilirubinemia, the follow-up care needed, and the psychosocial concerns of having a sick newborn.

Nursing Diagnoses

The following is a list of possible diagnoses and could apply, depending on the child's age, clinical situation, and physical condition:

Impaired skin integrity

High risk for injury

TREATMENT GRID

Serum bilirubin mg/100 mL	Hours of life of infant			
	<24	24–48	49–72	>72
<5	O	O	O	O
5–9	P	P	O	O
10–14	E	P	P	P
15–19	E	E	P	P
20+	E	E	E	E

O, observe infant
P, phototheraphy
E, exchange transfusion

If the following are present, treat as the next higher bilirubin category:
A. Birth weight <1500 g
B. Perinatal asphyxia
C. Respiratory distress
D. pH <7.25
E. Temperature <35°C
F. Serum protein <5 g/100 mL
G. CNS deterioration

Figure 46-1. Adapted from Levin, D., Morriss, F., & Moore, G. (1979). A practical guide to pediatric intensive care. St. Louis: C. V. Mosby, p. 265.

Sensory/perceptual alterations

Ineffective thermoregulation

Fluid volume deficit

Altered parenting

Planning

When planning to care for a baby needing phototherapy, the following equipment should be gathered:

Radiant warmer or isolette

Phototherapy light source

Eye shields

Diaper

Face mask

Interventions

PROCEDURE	**RATIONALE/EXPECTED OUTCOME (EO)**
1. Explain the phototherapy procedure to the patients.	The parents will express concerns to the staff.
2. Remove all clothing from the infant.	Phototherapy produces the greatest effect on the infant when a large surface area is exposed to the light. *EO: The child's maximum surface area will be exposed to the light.*
3. Place a face mask over the genital area as a diaper. Remove plastic or metal nosepiece.	When the male infant is placed so that the testes are exposed to the light, a diaper covers the area to prevent damage to these organs. *EO: The child's genital area will be protected from the light.*
4. Cover the infant's eyes with eye patches. Keep nasal	Eye shields protect the infant's eyes from the lights. In-

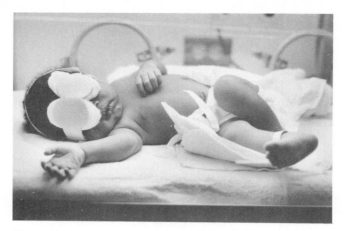

Figure 46-2.

PROCEDURE

passages unobstructed with patches (Fig. 46-2).

5. Place the infant in a neutral thermal environment using a radiant warmer or an isolette. A cap may be used to prevent heat loss from the head.

6. Place lights approximately 18 inches from the infant (Fig. 46-3).

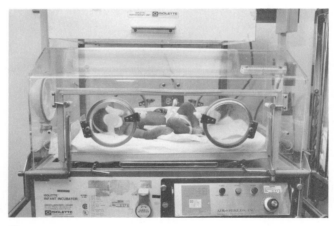

Figure 46-3.

7. Document the color and condition of the skin on admission and every 8 hours (or as necessary).

8. Monitor direct and indirect bilirubin levels per agency schedule; notify physician of results.

9. Position on side or prone; change position every 2 hours; monitor skin condition.

RATIONALE/EXPECTED OUTCOME (EO)

fants are obligate nose breathers; thus do not allow patches to cover nose.

EO: The infant's eyes will be protected from the lights.

Maintain axillary temperature of 36.5°–37.0°C (97.6–98.6°F) to avoid cold or heat stress. Exposure of the infant's skin to air may compromise thermoregulation.

EO: The infant's temperature remains stable within acceptable range.

"Bronze baby syndrome" is a brownish or greenish discoloration of the skin that occurs if phototherapy is used in the presence of underlying liver disease.

Serum bilirubin levels usually fall 1–3 mg/dL after 8–12 hours.

This will enhance circulation and decrease the potential for pressure damage.

EO: The infant's skin will remain intact.

PROCEDURE	**RATIONALE/EXPECTED OUTCOME (EO)**
10. Keep skin clean and dry.	
11. Record number and quality of stools.	Side effects of phototherapy include loose green stools due to accelerated intestinal transit time.
12. Monitor skin turgor and mucous membranes for signs of dehydration.	Phototherapy increases bowel motility, which could result in loose stools. Bilirubin and enzymes excreted in the stool can be irritating to the skin. Phototherapy also increases insensible water loss.
	EO: The infant maintains good skin turgor. The infant has moist mucous membranes and flat fontanelles.
13. Monitor intake and output and specific gravity.	*EO: The infant voids at least 1 mL/kg/hr with urine specific gravity of less than 1.010.*
14. Administer feedings (bottle or breast feeding) as soon as possible. Offer water between feedings.	
15. Turn lights off and uncover eyes at every feeding or bath to inspect scleral color.	Eye shields are necessary, but they restrict the infant's interaction capabilities.
	EO: The infant makes eye contact when shields are removed.
16. Talk to and touch infant during nursing care.	*EO: The infant responds to voice and touch by quieting.*
17. Encourage parents to visit and participate in the infant's care.	The need for phototherapy restricts the amount of time the infant can be in contact with the parents.
	EO: The infant and parents show attachment behaviors.
18. If the mother is still hospitalized, take the infant to the mother's room for feeding or use in-room phototherapy (if acceptable).	*EO: The infant is held and talked to by the parents.*
19. Hold infant during feedings.	The phototherapy treatment restricts the normal bonding process unless efforts are made to actively involve the parents.
20. Keep parents informed of infant's treatment and progress to allay their fears.	
21. Allow parents to express their feelings.	

Patient/Family Education: Home Care Consideration

1. Encourage parents to visit and care for the infant as they are able. Evaluate the care they deliver and offer positive reinforcement or be a role model for appropriate behavior.
2. Teach parents the signs of jaundice and urge them to report them to the health team (yellowing skin, sclera, mucous membranes, or body fluids).
3. Give parents phone numbers and names to call in case of questions, illness of the infant, or recurrence of the jaundice.

References

Avery, G. (1987). *Neonatology: Pathophysiology and management of the newborn*. 3rd ed. Philadelphia: J.B. Lippincott Company.

Dortch, E., & Spottiswoode, P. (1986). New light on phototherapy: Home use. *Neonatal Network, 4*(2), 30–34.

Sbrana, G., Donzelli, G. P., & Vecchi, C. (1987). Phototherapy in the management of neonatal hyperbilirubinemia: Efficacy with light sources emitting more than 500 nanometers. *Pediatrics, 80*(3), 395–398.

Wilkerson, N. N. (1989). Treating hyperbilirubinemia. *Journal of Maternal Child Nursing, 14*(1), 32–36.

Blood Collection

47

Definition/Purpose

A child seldom enters the hospital without having some type of blood test performed. The physician's and nurse's roles in the collection of blood samples include such decisions as:

1. Selecting the tests that are important in diagnosis and treatment
2. Deriving maximum data from a single sample
3. Collecting the required amount in the least traumatic manner for the child and family
4. Obtaining the results of the test and explaining the implications to the family.

Three sources of blood may be used for diagnostic purposes: venous, capillary, and arterial.

- Venous—Blood samples can be obtained by venipuncture, the percutaneous introduction of a needle attached to a syringe into the lumen of a vein. The site for venipuncture should be safe, easily accessible, and of sufficient size to contain a volume of blood adequate for the specimen sought. Veins that are visible or palpable are easier and safer sites than veins located solely by anatomical relationships.

- Capillary—Collection of blood from a puncture wound or small incision of the skin is one of the oldest methods of obtaining a specimen. Because this method is less frightening and painful to the child and more simple to perform, it is preferred if the specimen obtained is satisfactory for the test desired. Sites most adaptable to the collection of capillary blood include the heel (for infants under 2 years of age), or the finger (for the older child).

- Arterial—Under certain circumstances it may be necessary to obtain a sample of arterial blood for oxygen concentration as well as other indicators of respiratory status. The preferred sites for arterial puncture are the radial, dorsalis pedis, posterior tibial, or temporal artery in infants. The brachial artery can also be used; however, whenever possible, the radial artery is preferred to the brachial artery because it has an open anastomosis via the palmar arch with the ulnar artery, and puncture-induced arteriospasm usually will not cause ischemia distal to it.

Standard of Care

1. Maintain good handwashing techniques.
2. Wear gloves whenever contact with the child's blood is anticipated.
3. Dispose of needles and other sharp instruments in designated containers without recapping.
4. Bag and label specimens to protect other personnel from injury and exposure.
5. The amount of venous and arterial blood needed depends on the tests ordered and the laboratory equipment used. Consult laboratory manual for recommendations.
6. Record the amount of blood withdrawn on the output record. Premature and small, critically ill infants can lose dangerously large amounts of their blood volume through blood collections for testing if these are not monitored.

Assessment

1. Assess the child's pertinent history for previous experience with blood collection.
2. Assess the physical findings for location of good veins, sites of previous collections, child's preference for right- or left-handed, and the type of specimen needed (arterial versus venous).
3. Assess the psychosocial and developmental factors related to coping mechanisms for painful procedures, age and developmental level, and what comforts the child.
4. Assess the child's and family's knowledge of the reason for the blood collection and the anticipated frequency of collections.

Nursing Diagnoses

The following is a list of possible diagnoses and could apply, depending on the child's age, clinical situation, and physical condition:

Fear

High risk for infection

High risk for injury

Impaired skin integrity

Pain

Planning

When planning to collect a blood specimen, the following equipment must be assembled:

Syringe

Needle (either a scalp vein needle or a standard straight needle)

Tourniquet or rubber bands

Specimen container

Alcohol pad or povidone-iodine pad

Nonsterile gloves

Adhesive bandages

Dry gauze pads

Lancet (for capillary sticks)

Capillary tubes

Sodium heparin

Specimen bag

Ice (for arterial specimen)

Interventions

PROCEDURE	RATIONALE/EXPECTED OUTCOME (EO)
VENIPUNCTURE	
1. Select the site for the venipuncture.	The site should be safe, easily accessible and of sufficient size to contain a volume of blood adequate for the specimen sought.
2. Explain to the child and family at which site you are going to attempt to obtain the blood sample. Answer their questions and concerns.	*EO: The child and family will express their fears and anxieties through asking questions.*

PROCEDURE

3. Apply a tourniquet around the selected extremity.

4. Cleanse the skin with alcohol or povidone-iodine according to your hospital infection control policy.

5. Attach the needle to the syringe and check for patency. Put on gloves.

6. The needle and syringe are aligned in the direction of the vein. Inform the child (if appropriate), when the skin puncture will occur.

7. With the needle at a 30° angle to the skin surface, the skin is punctured directly over the vein.

8. Advance the needle underneath the skin into the vessel.

9. The required amount of blood is aspirated.

10. Release the tourniquet.

11. Place a dry gauze over the puncture site with pressure as the needle is removed.

12. Expel the blood into the specimen container.

13. Apply adhesive bandage over puncture site.

14. Label specimen and place in bag.

15. Document collection of specimen in the medical record.

Venipuncture in Scalp (used in infants)

16. Place the child in the supine position. The head is immobilized to the side by an assistant.

17. The area to be used is shaved of hair (Fig. 47-1). Explain to the family that the hair will grow back.

RATIONALE/EXPECTED OUTCOME (EO)

Distention of the vein aids location by palpation.

EO: The puncture site will not become a focus for infection.

The plunger should move within the barrel of the syringe, expelling air through the needle.

The vein is not entered in this first maneuver.

This is evidenced by aspiration of blood into the syringe.

Continue pressure over the puncture site for 3 minutes to prevent a hematoma from forming.

EO: The child's skin will remain intact.

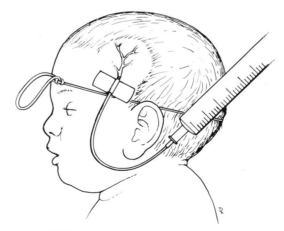

Figure 47-1.

18. Two rubber bands are fastened together. One is used to encircle the head from the eyebrows to the occiput.

The attached rubber band is used as a handle to lift the tourniquet rubber band away from the head at the end of the procedure.

PROCEDURE	**RATIONALE/EXPECTED OUTCOME (EO)**

PROCEDURE

19. The area is cleansed with an antiseptic solution. Put on gloves.

20. Apply traction to the skin around the vein with the free hand.

21. The tubing of the needle should not be connected to the syringe.

22. Insert the needle through the skin to the side of the vein and slowly advance into the vein.

23. Attach the syringe to the needle hub and gently apply negative pressure.

24. Collect the amount of blood needed, remove the rubber band tourniquet by cutting it, hold pressure over the site for 2–4 minutes.

25. Label specimen. Place in bag. Document collection in record.

Capillary Puncture (Foot)—used in infants

26. Wrap the entire foot in a warm wet towel for 5–10 minutes prior to the puncture.

27. Clean the area with antiseptic solution. Put on gloves.

28. Hold the heel with the thumb and index finger, milking the heel until it appears flushed.

29. Forcefully introduce the lancet through the skin into the subcutaneous tissue and quickly remove from the incision (Fig. 47-2).

RATIONALE/EXPECTED OUTCOME (EO)

This prevents the spread of microorganisms.

EO: The puncture site will not become a focus of infection.

This will help immobilize the vein.

This eliminates a closed system with a syringe that might prevent backflow of blood once the vein is entered.

Because the size of the veins are small, the appearance of blood in the tubing may lag 1–3 seconds behind the venipuncture; therefore the vein must be entered slowly to avoid puncturing both walls and causing a hematoma.

Too much pressure can collapse small veins.

EO: The child's vein will be entered, blood collected, and the needle removed in a safe, efficient manner.

EO: The blood specimen will be sent to the laboratory for testing.

This produces hyperemia at the puncture site.

EO: The child's capillary bed will dilate.

Let area dry completely before puncture. A damp area may dilute the blood sample or hemolyze it, causing distorted values.

EO: The puncture site will not become infected. The puncture site will be completely dry before a blood sample is obtained.

Because of the course of the plantar arteries and veins, the medial aspect of the plantar surface of the heel is the preferred site. The more medial surface of the heel pad should be avoided as a precaution against scar formation that may prove painful when the infant begins to walk.

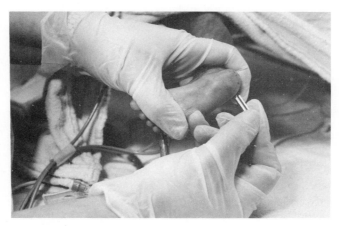

Figure 47-2.

PROCEDURE	**RATIONALE/EXPECTED OUTCOME (EO)**
	EO: The child will have the capillary puncture performed in a safe manner taking into account scar formation and future problems that could develop.
30. Gently squeeze the area. When an adequate volume of blood appears on the skin surface, permit the blood to flow into the collecting tube.	Excessive squeezing will lead to hemolysis, thus increasing potassium values.
	EO: The child's blood will not hemolyze from excessive squeezing of the heel.
31. When collection is complete, apply pressure to the area with a dry gauze for 2–3 minutes.	*EO: The puncture site will stop bleeding in 2–3 minutes with pressure applied.*
32. Label specimen. Place in bag. Document collection in record. (A finger puncture in the distal aspect of the finger pad may be done in children over the age of 2 years. The procedure is the same as the heel stick.) (Fig. 47-3).	

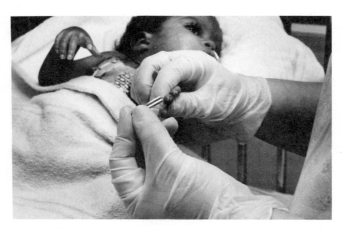

Figure 47-3.

Arterial Puncture

33. Clean the site with a povidone-iodine swab.	
34. Also clean the blood drawer's index and second fingers with antiseptic solution so that the artery may be palpated. (Sterile gloves may also be worn to palpate.) Rinse syringe with heparin, being sure to expel all heparin before drawing blood.	For blood gases, the specimen must be collected anaerobically and must be anticoagulated with a small amount of heparin placed in the syringe before collection of the blood.
	EO: The syringe will be prepared so that the blood will not clot.
35. *For older children:* Insert the needle (bevel up) at a 45°–60° angle, piercing both walls of the artery. Slowly withdraw the needle, applying negative pressure with the syringe. Reentry into the artery lumen is signaled by the appearance of bright red blood in the syringe. *For small infant:* Enter the skin with needle bevel down at a 10° angle. After the needle enters the skin, apply negative pressure with the syringe. Advance the needle toward the pulsation. Arteriopuncture will be signaled by bright red blood in the syringe.	*EO: The child will have blood drawn in the most age-appropriate manner.*

PROCEDURE	**RATIONALE/EXPECTED OUTCOME (EO)**

36. When the blood is collected, place a dry gauze over the site. Apply firm pressure while removing the needle and for 5 minutes after the needle is removed.

A tear or large hole in a vessel may result in a massive hematoma; therefore, use small-gauge needles and apply pressure once the needle is removed.

EO: The child will have blood drawn without causing injury to the blood vessels.

37. As before, label specimen, place in bag with ice, and document collection in record. The specimen must reach the laboratory in a timely manner.

38. Dispose of blood-drawing supplies in properly marked containers.

Patient/Family Education: Home Care Considerations

1. Educate the family as to the reason for the blood collections, the procedure itself, and the anticipated frequency.

2. Reinforce the information given to the family by the physician regarding test results.

References

Hunt, C.E. (1973). Capillary blood sampling in the infant: Usefulness and limitations of two methods of sampling compared with arterial blood. *Pediatrics, 57,* 501.

Moss, G., & Staunton, C. (1970). Blood flow, needle size and hemolysis. *New England Journal of Medicine, 282,* 967.

Bone Marrow Aspiration

48

Definition/Purpose

Marrow is a soft tissue that fills the medullary cavity of the long bones, the large haversian canals, and all spaces between the trabecula of spongy bone. It is an organ the size of the liver and produces 1010 red cells and half that number of platelets and granulocytes per hour. Two varieties of marrow are recognized. When fat cells predominate, the color is yellow and the tissue is called *yellow marrow*. When blood cells predominate, the color is red and the tissue is known as *red marrow*. In infants, the marrow is contained in the medullary cavity of long bones, where it continues to be produced, but in decreasing quantities, until puberty.

Small samplings of marrow may be obtained for hematologic testing by inserting a needle percutaneously through the cortex of a bone into the medullary cavity. This technique is easy to perform and can be repeated when medically indicated. The specimen can be dried, stained, and examined immediately.

Several sites are satisfactory for the procurement of bone marrow specimens. Table 48-1 lists the acceptable anatomic sites for bone marrow aspiration and indicates the age ranges for which the procedure is acceptable.

Table 48-1. Acceptable Anatomic Sites

Site	Age to Which Adaptable
Anterior iliac crest/Posterior iliac crest	Any age
Femur	0–2 years
Tibia	0–2 years
Spinous vertebral process	2 years or older
Sternum (more dangerous than other sites because of its proximity to vital structures in the mediastinum)	6 years or older

(Adapted from Hughes, W., & Buescher, E. *Pediatric Procedures.* Philadelphia: W.B. Saunders Co.)

One must, however, take into consideration the age of the child. Specimens from long bones of children over 2 years of age may not be satisfactory because of hematopoiesis, whereas both the anterior and posterior portions of the iliac crest contain active cellular elements at any age (Fig. 48-1).

Standard of Care

1. The aspiration will be performed using sterile technique.
2. The puncture site will be free of bleeding and hematoma.
3. The child will be monitored for early signs of complications following the procedure.

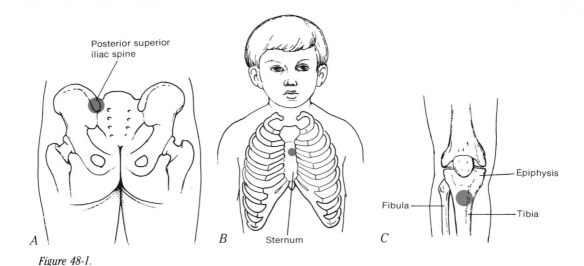

Figure 48-1.

Assessment

1. Assess the child's pertinent history and physical findings for the course of the current illness, prior treatment including bone marrow aspirations and infections, childhood illnesses, signs of anemia, leukopenia, or thrombocytopenia.
2. Assess the child for an allergy to iodine.
3. Assess the child's developmental level, coping mechanisms, and ability to accept explanations regarding procedures.
4. Assess the child's and family's previous experience with hospital procedures, as well as their level of knowledge and readiness to learn.

Nursing Diagnoses

The following is a list of possible diagnoses and could apply, depending on the child's age, clinical situation, and physical condition:

Fear

Anxiety

High risk for infection

Impaired skin integrity

Pain

Planning

When planning to assist the physician in a bone marrow aspiration, the following equipment must be gathered:

Povidone-iodine solution

Gauze pads

1% lidocaine

25-gauge needle

1–2-mL syringe

2–20-mL syringes

Microscope slides

Sterile gloves

Bone marrow needle

Glass coverslips

Interventions

PROCEDURE	**RATIONALE/EXPECTED OUTCOME (EO)**

1. Assemble all necessary equipment.

2. Explain the procedure to the child (if age-appropriate), and to the family members. Obtain a signed consent.

   A prepared, well-informed child and family will tend to cooperate with the procedure.

   EO: The child and family will verbalize their fears, as well as an understanding of the need for aspiration.

3. Position the child according to the anticipated site of aspiration:

   EO: The child will be positioned to provide maximum exposure to the area of aspiration.

   a. Anterior iliac crest—lateral recumbent or supine
   b. Posterior iliac crest—prone or lateral recumbent with head flexed and knees drawn up to abdomen
   c. Distal third of thigh—Supine with sandbag underneath
   d. Sternum—Supine with arms at sides and feet together
   e. Tibia—Supine position with sandbag under proximal third of lower leg
   f. Vertebral process—Prone with feet together and arms at side.

4. The physician will put on sterile gloves and cleanse the area with povidone-iodine. Sterile drapes will be applied.

   EO: The child will not develop an infection at puncture site.

5. The puncture point will then be infiltrated with 1% lidocaine by the physician.

   The soft tissue and skin will be anesthetized.

   EO: The child will not experience any unnecessary discomfort.

6. The bone marrow needle is then inserted through the skin at an angle of about 90° until the bone is reached. When bone is encountered, increased pressure is applied to push the needle through the cortex. Slight back-and-forth rotation may be required.

   Entrance into the marrow cavity is revealed by a decrease in resistance.

7. The physician will remove the obturator and attach the syringe to the needle. Aspiration is achieved by a rapid sustained pull on the syringe plunger for 1–2 seconds. This will cause a sharp pain.

   The marrow will bubble into the syringe. Do not aspirate for more than 2 seconds, because it will cause pain and will draw blood into the marrow, thus diluting the specimen.

   EO: The child will have marrow aspirated and sent for appropriate testing.

8. The specimen may be handled in several ways. The hematologist will determine how the specimen needs to be preserved.

9. The obturator is then replaced into the needle and the needle is removed.

10. Hold pressure on the puncture site for 5 minutes.

    This will prevent bleeding and hematoma formation, especially if the child is thrombocytopenic.

    EO: The child will have no bleeding from the puncture site.

11. The child is then helped to return to a comfortable position.

12. Monitor the child for complications related to the puncture:

    EO: The child will be monitored for signs and symptoms of a developing complication from the aspiration:

    a. Hemorrhage
    b. Cardiac tamponade

    From a sternal puncture

PROCEDURE   **RATIONALE/EXPECTED OUTCOME (EO)**

    c. Osteomyelitis

    d. Fracture of tibia

    e. Infection

    f. Pneumothorax.   From inadvertent entry into the pleural cavity during a sternal puncture.

13. Document the bone marrow aspiration location, the child's tolerance of the procedure, and the specimens obtained in the medical record.

EO: The child's medical record will indicate that a bone marrow aspiration was attempted.

Patient/Family Education: Home Care Considerations

1. Educate the family as to the reason for the marrow aspiration, the procedure itself, and the anticipated frequency.

2. Reinforce the information given to the family by the physician; correct any misconceptions.

References

Crosby, W.H. (1970). Bone marrow: More questions than answers. *New England Journal of Medicine, 283*(19), 991.

Hamner, S.B. & Miles, M.S. (1988). Coping strategies in children with cancer undergoing bone marrow aspiration. *Journal of the Association of Pediatric Oncology Nurses, 5*(3), 11–15.

O'Rourke, A. (1986). Bone marrow procedure guide. *Oncology Nursing Forum, 13*(1), 66–67.

Pfaff, V.K., Smith, K.E., & Gowan, D. (1989). The effects of music: Assisted relaxation on the distress of pediatric cancer patients undergoing bone marrow aspiration. *Childrens' Health Care,* Fall 232–236.

Neurologic System Procedures

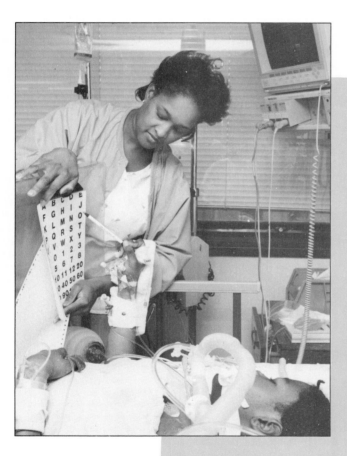

Unit VIII

Lumbar Puncture

49

Definition/Purpose

A lumbar puncture, or "spinal tap," is performed by introducing a needle into the subarachnoid space of the lumbar spinal canal. The needle is inserted through a stylet into the interspace between the third and fourth lumbar vertebrae.

The lumbar puncture may be performed to:

1. Measure CSF pressure
2. Examine the spinal fluid
3. Introduce medication, air, or radiopaque contrast material into the subarachnoid space.

The lumbar puncture can aid in the diagnosis of intracranial or intraventricular hemorrhage if blood is present in the fluid. The fluid can be sent for culture, Gram's stain, cell count, glucose and protein tests to aid in the diagnosis of inflammation or infection. Also antibiotics, chemotherapy, or anesthesia may be introduced into the subarachnoid space to treat infection and malignant cells or to decrease pain. Lastly, air or contrast media are used to outline subarachnoid structures and to pinpoint CSF obstructions or leaks.

Standard of Care

1. This entire procedure will be carried out under strict aseptic technique.
2. An assistant is always needed to restrain the child. The child, even if lethargic, should be held firmly to prevent unexpected movement during the procedure.

Assessment

1. Assess the pertinent history and physical findings for signs of increased intracranial pressure. Signs of increased intracranial pressure include:
   a. Decreased level of consciousness
   b. Unilateral or bilateral pupil dilation or sluggish response to light
   c. Tachycardia, severe bradycardia, hypertension with widened pulse pressure
   d. Apnea or abnormal breathing pattern
   e. Decorticate or decerebrate posturing
   f. Abnormal or absent reflexes
   g. Bulging fontanelle
   h. Vomiting or diarrhea
   i. Sunset eyes
   j. Increased head circumference (OFC) in the infant with open fontanelles or sutures

If any of these are present in the infant, the lumbar puncture should proceed with caution, and only when the CSF sample is absolutely necessary to treat the infant's disease. If these signs are present in the older child with fused cranial sutures, the lumbar puncture may be postponed since the sudden release of CSF and pressure by the puncture can result in herniation of the medulla through the foramen magnum.

2. Assess the age, developmental level, and coping strategies of the child.

3. Assess the family's knowledge of the reasons for the test, outcomes, and potential adverse reactions to the test.

Nursing Diagnoses

The following is a list of possible diagnoses and could apply, depending on the child's age, clinical situation, and physical condition:

Fear

Anxiety

High risk for infection

High risk for injury

Impaired skin integrity

Pain

Planning

To assist in the preparation of a lumbar puncture, the following equipment must be assembled:

4 povidone-iodine swabs

Sterile drape(s)

3-mL syringe with 25-gauge needle

3-way stopcock

Spinal fluid pressure monometer

2 lumbar puncture needles

Adhesive bandage

3 fluid collection tubes

(All of the above are usually contained in prepackaged spinal tap tray.)

Sterile gloves

Ampule of 1% lidocaine

Interventions

PROCEDURE

1. Explain the lumbar puncture procedure to the family and to the child, (if appropriate). Obtain a written consent form for the procedure from the parent or guardian.

2. The nurse places the child in the knee-to-chest position, either seated or reclining, with neck flexed toward the knees (Fig. 49-1).

Recumbent Position

The assistant may restrain the patient by directing one arm under the flexed knees and grasping the child's wrists. This restrains both the upper and lower extremities. The assistant's other arm is

RATIONALE/EXPECTED OUTCOME (EO)

EO: The child and parents will express concerns and fears to the staff.

This position provides maximal separation of the vertebral bodies.

EO: The child will be positioned to provide optimal alignment for the procedure to be completed safely.

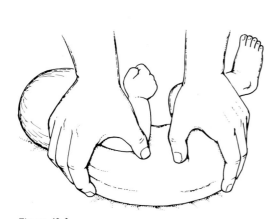

Figure 49-1.

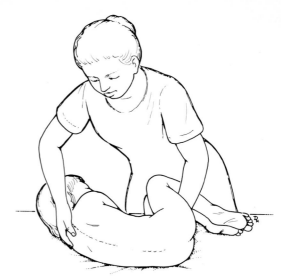

Figure 49-2.

PROCEDURE	**RATIONALE/EXPECTED OUTCOME (EO)**

placed posteriorly around the patient's neck and shoulders (Fig. 49-2).

Sitting Position

The older child may sit voluntarily on the table, with elbows resting on knees and back arched. A pillow can be placed in front of the chest and the child instructed to grasp it. The small infant must be held in a sitting position by the assistant. By flexing the thighs on the abdomen, the assistant is able to grasp the elbow and knees in both hands, thus flexing the spine in the appropriate angle (Fig. 49-3).

The sitting position is feasible only in the small infant who is unable to struggle or in the older child who will cooperate without restraint.

Some modification of position may be necessary if the child is intubated or has fractures.

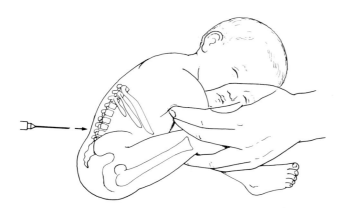

Figure 49-3.

3. Once the child is positioned, the back is draped and the puncture area is identified and scrubbed with povidone-iodine.

The entire procedure is performed using strict aseptic technique.

EO: The child will not acquire a focus of infection at the puncture site.

4. The physician will then infiltrate Xylocaine intradermally around the area of the puncture.

This provides local anesthesia to the site.

EO: The child will express minimal discomfort.

PROCEDURE

5. The needle and stylet are next firmly inserted by the physician into the subarachnoid space.

6. When the needle is in proper position and a free drip of CSF is established, the spinal pressure manometer is attached to the needle hub by means of a 3-way stopcock. Fluid is allowed to fill the manometer. The column is measured in millimeters.

7. Before the lumbar puncture is completed, a measurement of the CSF closing pressure is made. The opening and closing pressures may be used to calculate an Ayala's index:

$$Ayala's\ Index = \frac{quantity\ of\ fluid\ removed \times closing\ pressure}{initial\ pressure}$$

   Normal range is 5.5–6.5
   Greater than 7.0 is indicative of the presence of a large CSF reservoir (hydrocephalus). An index of 5.0 or less indicates subarachnoid obstruction.

8. When all samples are collected and measurements completed the needle is withdrawn and an adhesive bandage is placed over the puncture site.

9. Throughout the procedure, the nurse will monitor the child for complications:
   a. Brain stem herniation, although unusual, is the most serious complication. Others include:
      • Decreased responsiveness
      • Tachycardia or bradycardia
      • Sluggish or unequal pupil reaction to light
      • Hypertension
      • Abnormal breathing due to positioning during the procedure (and not to herniation)
      • Abnormal posturing
   b. Penetration of a nerve—most frequently leg pain
   c. Breakage of the needle in an uncooperative patient

10. After the procedure, continue to observe the child for the above complications as well as severe headache and bleeding from the puncture site. Keep the child lying flat for 1 hour after the procedure. Moni-

RATIONALE/EXPECTED OUTCOME (EO)

The normal pressure in the relaxed patient is 50–200 mm. Each heartbeat creates a fluctuation of 2–5 mm and each respiration 4–10 mm. The effect of compressing the veins of the neck (Queckenstedt's test) for 10 seconds raises the spinal pressure to 250–300 mm. It should return to normal with cessation of pressure. Absence of a rise indicates a spinal fluid block.

EO: The child will have opening and closing pressures obtained.

Color of CSF:
a. Clear—normal
b. Red (bloody)—intracranial hemorrhage or a traumatic tap without hemorrhage (usually clears with flow of fluid)
c. Cloudy—infection
d. Yellow (xanthochromic)—hyperbilirubinemia or hemolyzed RBCs.

EO: The child will have all CSF samples collected and evaluated.

EO: The child remains free from personal injury.

EO: The child will experience minimal side effects from the procedure.

Leakage of CSF through the puncture hole in the meninges causes the headache pain.

EO: The skin at the puncture site will remain intact.

PROCEDURE   **RATIONALE/EXPECTED OUTCOME (EO)**

tor vital signs, level of consciousness, and motor activity every 15 minutes for 1 hour and then every 30 minutes for another hour.

Patient/Family Education: Home Care Considerations

1. Reinforce the information regarding the results of the lumbar puncture given by the physician to the family. Correct any misinformation and fill in gaps of needed information.

2. Explain to both the child (if appropriate) and the family the need for bedrest to help prevent or decrease the incidence of headache.

References

Bass, B., & Vandervoort, M.K. (1988). Postlumbar puncture headache. *Canadian Nurse, 9*(3), 15–17.

McGrath, P.A., & Deveber, L.L. (1986). Helping children cope with painful procedures. *American Journal of Nursing, 86*(11), 1278–1279.

Cisternal Puncture

50

Definition/Purpose

A *cisternal puncture* is performed by introducing a needle in the exact midline at the depression between the occiput and the upper border of the spinous process. This procedure is not commonly used today, but it is performed when there is blockage in the spinal tract.

The cisternal puncture may be performed to measure CSF pressure, examine the spinal fluid, and introduce medication, air, or radiopaque contrast material into the subarachnoid space.

The volume of CSF varies with the body size of the child. A 2-kg newborn has a total of 10–15 mL of CSF if delivered vaginally or 30–60 mL if delivered by cesarean section. (Compare this to the 100–150 mL of CSF that a 70 kg adolescent may have.)

Standard of Care

1. This entire procedure will be carried out under strict aseptic technique.
2. An assistant is always needed to restrain the child. The child, even if lethargic, should be held firmly because a slip in technique may cause the needle to be introduced into the medulla.

Assessment

1. Assess the pertinent history and physical findings for signs of increased intracranial pressure:
   a. Decreased level of consciousness
   b. Unilateral or bilateral pupil dilation or sluggish response to light
   c. Tachycardia, severe bradycardia, or hypertension with widened pulse pressure
   d. Apnea or abnormal breathing pattern
   e. Decorticate or decerebrate posturing
   f. Abnormal or absent reflexes
   g. Bulging fontanelle
   h. Vomiting or diarrhea
   i. Sunset eyes

   If these are present in the infant, the cisternal puncture should proceed with caution only if the CSF sample is absolutely necessary to treat the child's disease.

2. Assess the age, developmental level, and coping strategies of the child.
3. Assess the family's knowledge of the reason for the test, outcomes, and potential adverse reactions to the test.

Nursing Diagnoses

The following is a list of possible diagnoses and could apply, depending on the child's age, clinical situation, and physical condition:

Anxiety

Fear

High risk for infection

High risk for injury

Impaired skin integrity

Pain

Planning

To assist in the preparation of a cisternal puncture, the following equipment must be assembled:

4 povidone-iodine swabs

Sterile gloves

Sterile drapes

3-mL syringe with 25-gauge needle

3-way stopcock

Spinal fluid pressure manometer

2 Lumbar puncture needles

Adhesive bandage

3 fluid collection tubes

(All of the above are usually contained in prepackaged spinal tap tray.)

Ampule of 1% lidocaine

Soap and razor

Intervention

PROCEDURE	RATIONALE/EXPECTED OUTCOME (EO)
1. Explain the cisternal puncture procedure to the family and to the child (if age-appropriate). Obtain written consent for the procedure from the parent or guardian.	*EO: The child and parents will express concerns and fears to the staff.*
2. Shave the occiput and neck.	
3. Position the child on his or her side, with the neck moderately flexed (as if for a lumbar puncture). Alignment of the vertebral column should be maintained.	This position provides maximal separation of the vertebral bodies. *EO: The child will be positioned to provide optimal alignment for the procedure to be safely completed.*
4. Drape the neck and scrub with povidone-iodine.	The entire procedure is performed using strict aseptic technique. *EO: The child will not acquire a focus of infection at the puncture site.*
5. The physician will infiltrate intradermally around the area of the puncture with Xylocaine.	This provides local anesthesia to the site. *EO: The child will express minimal discomfort.*
6. Wearing sterile gloves, the physician palpates the uppermost cervical spine. The needle is introduced in the midline just above this level, and is directed upward and forward in the direction of the external auditory meatus (Fig. 50–1).	The direction of the needle is along a straight line from the base of the occiput, through the external auditory meatus, to the glabella.

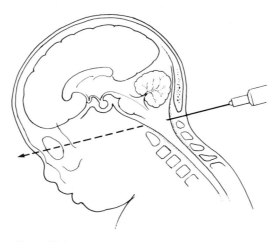

Figure 50-1.

PROCEDURE	**RATIONALE/EXPECTED OUTCOME (EO)**
7. As the needle is advanced slowly by the physician, the stylet should be removed frequently until the cisterna is reached.	The dura is dense in this area and can be detected when pierced. The cisterna magna is at a depth of 1–2 cm in the infant and about 4–4.5 cm in the adolescent.
8. Once CSF appears, the fluid pressure and specimens can be obtained (as described for the lumbar puncture).	*EO: The child will have opening and closing pressures obtained. The child will have all CSF samples collected.*
9. When all samples are collected and measurements completed, the needle is withdrawn and an adhesive bandage is placed over the puncture site.	
10. Throughout the procedure, the child must be monitored for by the nurse for complications. (See Lumbar Puncture.)	Arterial damage may result in hemorrhage into the cistern or fourth ventricle.
	EO: The child remains free of personal injury. The child will experience minimal side effects from the procedure.
11. After the procedure, continue to observe the child for complications as described for lumbar puncture.	

Patient/Family Education: Home Care Considerations

1. Reinforce the information regarding the results of the cisternal puncture given by the physician to the family. Correct any misinformation and fill in gaps of needed information.
2. Explain to both the child (if appropriate) and the family the need for bedrest to help prevent or decrease the incidence of headache.

Reference

Menkes, J.H. (1990). *Textbook of child neurology.* Philadelphia: Lea and Febiger.

Ventricular Puncture

51

Definition/Purpose

A *ventricular puncture* is important as an emergency procedure and occasionally as a diagnostic procedure. It is a dangerous procedure and should be done only for proper indications and with great care. As long as the anterior fontanelle or coronal suture is patent to admit a needle, it may be used for ventricular puncture. If the fontanelle is closed, a needle may be introduced through a coronal suture line in children up to 2 years old. The procedure is useful in the differentiation of the causes of hydrocephalus.

Standard of Care

1. The procedure will be carried out under strict aseptic technique.
2. An assistant is always needed to restrain the child.

Assessment

1. Assess the history and physical findings for signs of increased intracranial pressure. (See Chap. 49 for the signs of increased ICP.)
2. Assess for allergies, especially iodine.
3. Assess the age, developmental level, and coping strategies of the child.
4. Assess the family's knowledge of the reason for the test, outcomes, and potential adverse reactions.

Nursing Diagnoses

The following is a list of possible diagnoses and could apply, depending on the child's age, clinical situation, and physical condition:

Fear

Anxiety

High risk for infection

High risk for injury

Impaired skin integrity

Pain

Planning

To assist in preparation for a ventricular puncture, the following equipment must be assembled:

Ampule of 1% lidocaine

4 povidone-iodine swabs

Sterile drape(s)

3-mL syringe with 25-gauge needle

3-way stopcock

Spinal fluid pressure monometer

2 lumbar puncture needles

Adhesive bandage

3 fluid collection tubes

(All of the above are usually contained in prepackaged spinal tap tray)

Sterile gloves

Soap and razor

Long (10 cm) spinal needle

Povidone-iodine

Xylocaine

Interventions

PROCEDURE	**RATIONALE/EXPECTED OUTCOME (EO)**
1. The physician will explain the ventricular puncture procedure to the family and obtain written consent.	*EO: The parents will express concerns and fears to the staff.*
2. The child is placed in the supine position and restrained on a restraining board or with the help of other caretakers.	*EO: The child will be positioned to provide optimal alignment and access to the area.*
3. Shave a wide area over and around the anterior fontanelle (Fig. 51-1).	

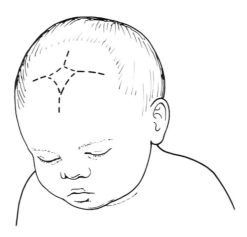

Figure 51-1.

4. The physician will don sterile gloves. Scrub the area with povidone-iodine and drape the field posteriorly and laterally, leaving the face uncovered.	This will prevent an infection at the puncture site. *EO: The child will not acquire a focus of infection at the puncture site.*
5. In older children, the physician will infiltrate the scalp with xylocaine in the midpupillary line at, or slightly anterior to, the coronal suture. In infants, the scalp is infiltrated in the midpupillary line over the fontanelle.	This provides local anesthesia to the site. *EO: The child will express minimal discomfort.*
6. The physician will introduce the needle through the scalp, fontanelle, and dura into the subdural space.	

PROCEDURE	**RATIONALE/EXPECTED OUTCOME (EO)**
7. The stylet is removed to check for subdural fluid collections.	
8. The needle is then directed toward the medial canthus of the ipsilateral eye and the anterior aspect of the zygoma.	
9. After enough fluid has been collected, the needle is withdrawn slowly while the fluid continues to drip.	When the drip stops, the physician places a fingertip at the edge of the skin. The distance from the finger to the bevel end of the withdrawn needle gives a measure of the cortical thickness. *EO: The child's ventricle will be successfully tapped.*
10. For elective shunt taps a 23-gauge butterfly is introduced by the physician through the dome of the pumping device after it has been prepped and draped.	The pressure can be measured and fluid can be aspirated for laboratory tests. If a shunt blockage is probable, it will not be possible to aspirate fluid.

11. Throughout and after the procedure, the child must be monitored by the nurse for complications:
 a. Brain stem herniation
     Decreased responsiveness
     Tachycardia and bradycardia
     Sluggish or unequal pupil reaction to light
     Hypertension
     Abnormal breathing
     Abnormal posturing
	EO: The child will experience minimal side effects from the puncture.

b. Hemorrhage	It is possible to tear pial vessels or bridging veins and cause subdural bleeding.
c. Continued leak of CSF after the procedure	Cotton soaked in collodion will seal the hole, or a skin suture will prevent leakage.
d. Infection	Sterile technique must be used to prevent pathogens from entering the ventricles.

Patient/Family Education: Home Care Considerations

1. Reinforce the information regarding the results of the ventricular puncture given by the physician to the family. Correct any misinformation and fill in gaps of needed information.
2. Explain to the family the need for constant monitoring and attention to the potential side effects.

Reference

Menkes, J.H. (1990) *Textbook of child neurology.* Philadelphia: Lea and Febiger.

Subdural Puncture

52

Definition/Purpose

The subdural space is a noncommunicating space that lies between the pia-arachnoid and the dura mater. The cerebral vessels traverse the subdural space with little support. Serious head trauma can cause rupture of these vessels and development of a subdural hematoma because this compartment has no channel of escape. This space does allow for some cerebral expansion without cerebral compression, but the critical capacity is small. Evacuations of subdural blood or fluid in young infants should be attempted when such collections cause symptoms (such as seizures and unilateral paresis) from increased intracranial pressure.

Standard of Care

1. The entire procedure must be carried out under aseptic technique.
2. Continuous monitoring of cardiac status is essential.

Assessment

1. Assess the pertinent history and physical findings for signs of increased intracranial pressure. (See Chapter 49, Lumbar Puncture, for signs of increased intracranial pressure.)
2. Assess the age, developmental level, and coping strategies of the child and family.
3. Assess the family's knowledge of the reasons for the test, outcomes, and potential complications.

Nursing Diagnoses

The following is a list of possible diagnoses and could apply, depending on the child's age, clinical situation, and physical condition:

High risk for infection

High risk for injury

Impaired skin integrity

Pain

Planning

To assist in the preparation of a subdural puncture, the following equipment must be assembled:

Soap and razor

Povidone-iodine solution

Sterile gloves

Ampule of 1% lidocaine or TB syringe with needle

10-mL syringe

19- or 20-gauge, 2 × 2 cm spinal needle

Collecting test tubes with stoppers (sterile)

2 sterile towels

Interventions

PROCEDURE	**RATIONALE/EXPECTED OUTCOME (EO)**
1. Prepare the infant in the supine position after performing the appropriate measures for resuscitation and stabilization.	
2. The assistant holds the head face-up with one hand on either side of the face.	This position provides maximal visualization of the puncture area. *EO: The child will be positioned to provide optimal alignment for the procedure to be completed.*
3. Shave the scalp around the lateral boundaries of the anterior fontanelle (the anterior two thirds of the head).	The entire procedure is performed using strict aseptic technique. *EO: The child will not acquire a focus of infection at the puncture site.*
4. The physician will put on sterile gloves.	
5. The site is prepared with povidone-iodine.	
6. One sterile towel will be placed under the child's head and a second one across the posterior half of the skull.	
7. The physician will palpate the coronal suture at the lateral aspect of the anterior fontanelle.	
8. The physician will make a skin wheal with 1% lidocaine over the selected site. Wait at least 5 minutes for infiltration and anesthesia.	This provides local anesthesia to the site. *EO: The child will exhibit minimal discomfort.*
9. The physician will insert a 19- or 20-gauge needle into the skin at a right angle to the surface, stretching it slightly to obtain a Z-track. The needle is advanced between the edges of the coronal suture until the feeling of resistance lessens (Fig. 52-1).	A Z-track will prevent leakage of fluid when the needle is removed.

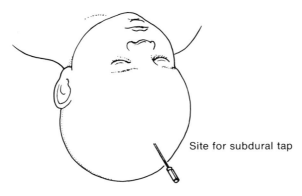

Site for subdural tap

Figure 52-1.

PROCEDURE	**RATIONALE/EXPECTED OUTCOME (EO)**
10. The stylet is removed by the physician and the fluid or blood is allowed to drain into collection tubes. 10 mL can be safely evacuated.	*EO: The child will have all fluid collected and evaluated.*
11. When collection is complete, the physician withdraws the needle in the same line as insertion and applies a dry gauze pad over the site.	
12. Throughout the procedure, the child must be monitored by the nurse for complications:	
a. Bleeding	The needle tip may lacerate tiny blood vessels and cause bleeding into the subdural space.
b. Infection	Infection may result from an improperly prepared operative field or contaminated needles.
c. Herniation	If more than 10–20 mL of fluid is removed at one time, intracranial pressure will decrease too rapidly and cause herniation.
	EO: The child will experience minimal side effects from the procedure.

13. After the procedure, the child should be monitored for changes in intracranial pressure:
   a. Change in level of consciousness.
   b. Change in pupil size and response to light.
   c. Changes in blood pressure, heart rate, respiratory rate, and pattern.
   d. Changes in muscle tone, motor function, and reflexes.
All of the above need to be monitored hourly (or more often if the condition warrants). Document findings in the medical record and notify the physician of changes in the condition.	

Patient/Family Education: Home Care Considerations

1. Reinforce the information regarding the results of the procedure given by the physician to the family. Correct any misinformation and fill in gaps of needed information.

2. Explain the need for continuous monitoring of the child once he or she is discharged. Help the family coordinate follow-up appointments, radiologic studies, and other necessary post-procedure care.

References

Fleisher, G. & Ludwig, S. (1988). *Textbook of pediatric emergency medicine.* Baltimore: Williams & Wilkins.

Menkes, J.H. (1990). *Textbook of child neurology.* Philadelphia: Lea and Febiger.

Transillumination of the Head

53

Definition/Purpose

Transillumination has become a quick and noninvasive means of using a light source to diagnose abnormal fluid or air collections in various parts of the body. In infants, transillumination of the head is a useful procedure to evaluate for hydrocephalus and subdural fluid collections. The same procedure can be used on any body part to aid in blood vessel location, detection of pneumothorax, pneumoperitoneum, or hydrocele.

Standard of Care

1. The operator should apply the light source to an area on his or her own skin and note how long it takes for the skin temperature to become uncomfortable. This is the maximum time for transilluminating any given area of the child's skin.

Assessment

1. Assess the pertinent history and physical findings for signs of hydrocephalus or subdural collection of fluid:
   a. Increased head circumference
   b. Bulging anterior fontanelle
   c. Separated sutures
   d. Sunset eyes—eyes depressed and increased amount of sclera visible
   e. Vomiting, irritability, and listlessness
   f. Papilledema
   g. Cranial bruits
   h. Increased area of transillumination
   i. Disturbances in muscle tone and reflex response
   j. Respiratory irregularities
   k. Increasing systolic blood pressure with widening pulse pressure
   l. Bradycardia.
2. Assess for extracranial, cranial, and intracranial factors that may influence the result of the transillumination:

Extracranial:

   a. Thickness of scalp and subcutaneous fat layer in older children
   b. Collection of subcutaneous fluid
      Caput succedaneum
      Cephalohematoma
      Infiltration of intravenous infusion fluid

Cranial:

A cranial thickness of 2.5 mm with overlying skin does not transmit light. The skull reaches this thickness between 6–12 months of age.

Intracranial:

Thickness of cortical mantle fluid accumulation between the skull and the cortical surface.

3. Assess the age and developmental level of the child.
4. Assess the family's knowledge of the reasons for the test, outcomes, and possible adverse reactions to the test.
5. Assess the family's acceptance of the child's level of functioning and prognosis.

Nursing Diagnoses

The following is a list of possible diagnoses and could apply, depending on the child's age, clinical situation, and physical condition:

Anxiety

High risk for injury

Planning

To transilluminate a body part, the following equipment must be obtained:

Flashlight with a fitted rubber ring or transilluminator.

Interventions

PROCEDURE

1. Explain the transillumination procedure to the family.

2. Darken the room.

3. Support the head of the infant with one hand and apply the light source snugly to the area of the head to be examined.

4. Rotate the light source and note the size of the light corona around the source.

   Repeat this procedure within the same area on the opposite side of the head and compare the light ring sizes. Repeat the procedure at 5–6 sites on each side of the cranium and over the anterior and posterior fontanelles.

RATIONALE/EXPECTED OUTCOME (EO)

EO: The family will have an opportunity to ask questions and express concerns and fears to the staff.

If the light source is not held tightly against the skin, light can escape from the edges and obscure the full extent of transillumination.

EO: The child's head will be transilluminated without any irritation to the skin due to the heat of the light.

Any asymmetry suggests abnormality; also, transillumination can be symmetrical but excessive. Be aware that false positives may be seen in a child with mild cortical atrophy. In an infant with hydranencephaly, hydrocephalus, or subdural effusions, the glow from the flashlight can be seen on the opposite side of the skull.

The above figure demonstrates a severe hydrocephalus in which cerebral transillumination results in illumination across the midline symmetrically, and even through the retinas.

Patient/Family Education: Home Care Considerations:

1. Assist the family in their understanding of the interpretation of the test and options for treatment.
2. Teach the family members the technical skills (if any) as well as behavioral techniques needed in caring for the child (for example, scheduling, routines, and equipment).
3. Provide telephone numbers of physicians, information regarding community agencies and day care.

References

Menkes, J. H. (1990). *Textbook of child neurology.* Philadelphia: Lea and Febiger.

External Ventricular Drain (EVD)

54

Definition/Purpose

An external ventricular drain (EVD) is used by neurosurgeons to relieve intracranial pressure in children with posterior fossa tumors and cerebral trauma needing temporary shunting. It is also used in the treatment of ventriculitis due to an infection in a previously placed shunt that is unresponsive to antibiotic therapy. In the latter case, the infected shunt is removed and an EVD is placed and remains in place until the infection can be eradicated and a new internal shunt inserted.

The temporary use of EVD and antibiotics for the treatment of shunt infections is safe and offers many advantages. Because of the direct access to the cerebrospinal fluid, cultures can be obtained, intraventricular drug therapy can be administered, and antibiotic levels in the CSF can be measured. Intracranial pressure can also be closely monitored.

In hydrocephalus or space-occupying lesions, the CSF within the cranial vault is under high pressure. By inserting a catheter into the ventricle, an outlet is provided for CSF flow. A collection chamber with a graduated height scale is attached to the external drain to allow for drainage of CSF under sterile conditions and at an ordered pressure.

Standard of Care

1. Sterile technique must be adhered to at all times when preparing, entering, or changing the system.
2. Sterile technique should be employed when redressing the drain's exit site.

Assessment

1. Assess the pertinent history for congenital or acquired defects requiring shunting procedures, onset of symptoms, medications currently taken, and any allergies to medications.
2. Assess physical findings for altered level of consciousness, signs and symptoms of increased intracranial pressure, and signs of infection (sepsis) due to ventriculitis.
3. Assess developmental factors for age, coping strategies, and favorite activities that can be maintained with a drain in place.
4. Assess the child's and family's knowledge of the expected treatment, outcome, and potential complications.

Nursing Diagnoses

The following is a list of possible diagnoses and could apply, depending on the child's age, clinical situation, and physical condition:

Anxiety

Fear

High risk for infection

High risk for injury

Impaired skin integrity

Diversional activity deficit

Fluid volume deficit

Pain

Planning

When planning to care for a child with an EVD, the following equipment must be gathered:

IV pole

Sterile gloves

Povidone-iodine swab

20-gauge 1½-inch needle on 20-mL syringe

2 4 × 4s

Interventions

PROCEDURE	**RATIONALE/EXPECTED OUTCOME (EO)**
1. Explain to the child and family the need for the EVD and the care and immobility necessary after insertion.	Offer explanations at an appropriate level for the child and family, and let them express concerns and fears. They may express feelings of guilt for the underlying condition as well as not being able to prevent the infection.
2. Provide reassurance and information about the infection process so the family does not feel responsible for the child's current state.	*EO: The child and family will express their concerns and have their questions answered, thus decreasing their fear and anxiety.*
3. The child will go to the operating room for removal of an existing shunt and insertion of an EVD. (See Pre- and postoperative care.)	
4. Upon arrival back to the unit, along with routine postoperative care, the drainage system connected to the intraventricular cannula must be securely mounted to an IV pole or the head of the bed at the desired height for the desired intracranial pressure (ICP) (Fig. 54-1).	The ICP is controlled by the height of the collection bag above the proximal tip of the catheter. Proper placement of the bag is critical. To maintain an ICP at 15 cm/H$_2$O, the 15 cm mark on the height scale connected to the bag should be located at the approximate level of the catheter tip in the ventricle. It is critical that neither the child nor the collection bag be raised or lowered accidently. Thus, if the child's ICP is less than 15 cm/H$_2$O, there will be no drainage; if the ICP is greater than 15 cm/H$_2$O, the system will drain to maintain the ordered set pressure. The one-way valve in the drainage tubing is designed to prevent reflux; it is not a pressure-regulating device.
	EO: The child will have the drainage bag positioned at the prescribed height for adequate relief of ICP.
5. Check the entire system to be sure all stopcocks or clamps are in the "On" position.	CSF will not drain from the ventricles while the tubing is occluded.
6. Check the CSF level in the drainage bag every 2 hours and record. For low increment measurement, separate the front and back of the bag to allow fluid to collect at the bottom.	Markings on the bag provide approximate volumes of CSF collected.

7. When the drainage bag becomes ¾ full, fluid must be removed from the bag. Two methods may be used:
  a. The drainage bag can be completely replaced:
    • Close the clamps.
	The drainage bag should not be allowed to fill completely, as this will inhibit CSF drainage.
	EO: The drainage system will be emptied at appropriate intervals using sterile technique.

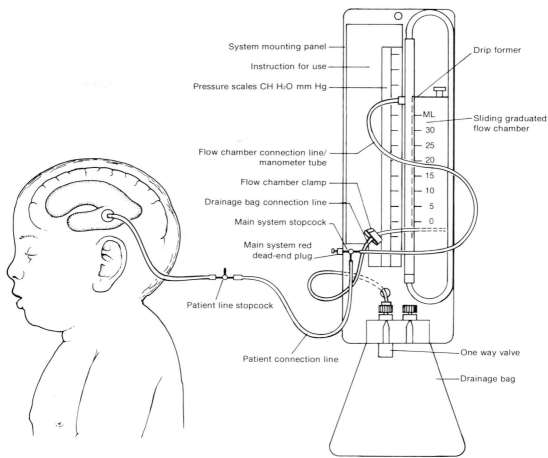

System mounting panel

Instruction for use

Pressure scales CH H₂O mm Hg

Drip former

ML
30
25
20
15
10
5
0

Sliding graduated flow chamber

Flow chamber connection line/ manometer tube

Flow chamber clamp

Drainage bag connection line

Main system stopcock

Main system red dead-end plug

Patient line stopcock

Patient connection line

One way valve

Drainage bag

Figure 54-1.

PROCEDURE

- Put on sterile gloves.
- While holding a sterile 4 × 4 in each hand, grasp the drainage tubing above and below the disconnection point.
- Remove the collection bag and discard along with 4 × 4.
- Connect new bag.
- Wash junction point with povidone-iodine swab and let dry.
- Remount drainage bag at correct height.
- Open all clamps.

b. The drainage bag can be drained:
- Put on sterile gloves.
- Swab the withdrawal port with povidone-iodine swab.
- Insert a 20-gauge or smaller 1½ inch needle with syringe attached into the withdrawal site.
- Open the tube clamp and withdraw fluid.
- When all fluid is withdrawn, reclamp the tube at withdrawal site and remove needle.

Always record the amount, color, and consistency of the CSF.

RATIONALE/EXPECTED OUTCOME (EO)

EO: The child's CSF drainage will be measured and examined for abnormalities.

PROCEDURE	**RATIONALE/EXPECTED OUTCOME (EO)**

8. The physician determines the amount of activity. When changing the child's position, clamp the tubing. The child may be up for short periods of time with the tubing clamped or with the drainage bag remounted at the ordered level and unclamped.

In the recumbent position, ICP is lower and increases with sitting or standing.

EO: The child will safely be able to change position and participate in diversional activities.

9. Record intake and output every 8 hours and total for 24 hours. Assess the child's hydrational state. (See Hydrational Assessment.) The physician may order intravenous replacement of CSF with normal saline.

CSF contains sodium chloride, protein, glucose, and potassium. A large amount of drainage that is not replaced can result in electrolyte and fluid imbalances.

EO: The child will be hydrated and free from electrolyte and fluid deficit.

10. Monitor the cannula insertion site for redness, swelling, pain, drainage, or dislodgement of the cannula.

Although the indication for the EVD is usually a shunt infection, infection is a common complication of the system caused by skin contaminants. Also, the presence of a foreign body may trigger a ventriculitis or meningitis. Lesions developing from a breakdown of tissue may also serve as a focus of infection.

EO: The child will not develop a superimposed infection from a contaminated system or a skin breakdown. The child's skin will remain intact around the cannula.

11. Observe the child every 2 hours (or more frequently) for signs and symptoms of changing intracranial pressures due to shunt failure:
    a. Check pupil response to light.
    b. Check bilateral strength.
    c. Check range of motion of extremities.
    d. Check for purposeful movements.
    e. Check level of consciousness.
    f. Check for nuchal rigidity.
    g. Check for increased scalp tension at the anterior fontanelle.
    h. Check for congestion of scalp veins.
    i. Check for altered blood pressure, bradycardia, nausea, vomiting, headache, apnea, and seizures.

Although a child with EVD may seem normal, his or her condition can change rapidly.

Too rapid decompression, as well as distention of the ventricles, can cause tentorial herniation resulting in increased ICP.

EO: The child will be monitored for changing neurologic status.

Patient/Family Education: Home Care Considerations

1. Teach parents the signs and symptoms of cerebral infection.
2. Teach parents the signs and symptoms of increased intracranial pressure.
3. Teach the parents and child how the EVD works, the importance of remaining in the same position, and what type of activities the child can participate in while the EVD is in place.

References

Baxter Healthcare Corporation. (1988). *Heyer-Schulte hermetic external CSF drainage system.* Deerfield, IL: Baxter Healthcare Corporation.

Scheinblum, S., & Hammond, M. (1990). The Treatment of children with shunt infections: Extraventricular drainage system care. *Pediatric Nursing, 16*(2), 139–143.

Yogev, R. (1985). Cerebrospinal fluid shunt infections. *Pediatric Infectious Disease, 4*(2), 113–117.

Intracranial Pressure Monitor

55

Definition/Purpose

The cranium contains the brain, blood vessels, and cerebrospinal fluid (CSF). These three components are noncompressible and occupy a fixed space. The brain occupies 80% of the intracranial space, and blood vessels and cerebrospinal fluid occupy approximately 10% each. The intracranial volume is equal to the sum of the volumes of the brain, cerebral blood, and the cerebrospinal fluid within the cranium. The intracranial pressure is the pressure exerted by these substances. The normal pressure is 80–180 mm H_2O (0–15 mm Hg).

Mild or gradual increases in intracranial volume can produce a compensatory decrease in the volume of the other intracranial contents: the brain can be compressed or displaced; CSF can be displaced from the subarachnoid space or reabsorbed more rapidly; or the blood volume can be decreased. Once the limits of intracranial compensation have been reached, even a small increase in intracranial volume will produce a significant rise in intracranial pressure. When intracranial pressure is high, cerebral blood flow is reduced, leading to brain ischemia, cerebral edema, and brain death.

The child with increased intracranial pressure demonstrates an altered level of consciousness, pupil dilation with decreased reactivity to light, and alterations in vital signs. The infant may be uninterested in feeding and may vomit frequently. The anterior fontanelle is full and tense, with the scalp veins distended and the eyes deviated downward ("sunset eyes"). The child may also demonstrate decreased motor function as well as abnormal reflexes or posturing (Table 55-1).

Table 55-1. Signs and Symptoms of Increased Intracranial Pressure in Children

	Infants	Children
	Early Signs	
Lethargy	X	X
Irritability		X
Headache		X
Anorexia or vomiting	X	X
Tense bulging fontanelle	X	
High-pitched cry	X	
Diplopia or blurred vision		X
Papilledema		X
Increased head circumference	X	
Separation of cranial sutures	X (If ICP elevation persistent)	X (If chronic ICP elevation)
	Late Signs	
Altered LOC	X	X
Tachycardia, then bradycardia	X	X
Systolic hypertension with widened pulse pressure	X	X
Altered respiratory rate or pattern	X	X
Pupil dilation and sluggish response to light	X	X
Decerebrate or decorticate posturing	X	X

Determining an accurate ICP at any given time depends upon the method of measurement. A presumptive diagnosis of increased ICP can be made based on the clinical presence of the above signs and symptoms of increased ICP. These criteria, however, are not entirely reliable. Efforts to directly measure ICP were first described in 1866. In 1960, Lundberg outlined criteria for ideal ICP monitoring. The criteria called for a monitor that would minimize the risk of infection, CSF leakage, and trauma as well as provide continuous, reliable pressure readings. No system has yet been developed to meet all the criteria (Table 55-2).

Intracranial pressure monitoring along with clinical assessment provides the most useful information about the child's condition.

Table 55-2. Comparison of ICP Monitoring

	FIC*	FF**	E***
Placement	Subarachnoid Intraventricular Intraparenchymal	Subarachnoid Intraventricular	Epidural
Infection risk	No static fluid column—decreased risk	Static fluid column—Increased risk	No static fluid column—Decreased risk
CSF drainage	Able to drain—continuous ICP monitoring	Able to drain—noncontinuous ICP reading	No drainage
Artifact	None	Very likely	None
Waveform	Needs dedicated equipment	Uses bedside monitor for waveform and alarm	Needs dedicated equipment

* Fiber-optic transducer-tipped catheter (FTC)
** Fluid-filled (FF)
*** Epidural (E)

Standard of Care

1. Strict aseptic technique is used when handling the dressings, tubings, and monitoring cables related to ICP monitoring.

Assessment

1. Assess the pertinent history and physical findings for the presence of congenital defects, onset of symptoms, mechanism of injury, medications, allergies, level of consciousness, vital signs, changing head circumference, seizures, blurred or double vision, bulging fontanelle, high-pitched cry, presence or absence of gag reflex, and change in motor functions.
2. Assess psychosocial and developmental factors for coping strategies, family interaction patterns, habits and routines, favorite objects, and acceptance of the child's condition.
3. Assess the patient's and family's knowledge of the treatment and its expected outcome; the family's readiness and willingness to learn about the illness; and their acceptance of the condition.

Nursing Diagnoses

The following is a list of possible diagnoses and could apply, depending on the child's age, clinical situation, and physical condition:

Altered tissue perfusion

Ineffective breathing pattern

Ineffective airway clearance

Impaired physical mobility

Ineffective family coping

Fear

Fluid volume excess or deficit

Impaired skin integrity

Impaired gas exchange

Planning

In planning to care for a child with increased intracranial pressure, the following equipment is needed:

Flashlight

Reflex hammer

Thermometer

Stethoscope

Blood pressure monitoring device (usually for arterial invasive monitoring)

Hypothermia blanket

Interventions

PROCEDURE	**RATIONALE/EXPECTED OUTCOME (EO)**
1. Monitor neurologic status every 1–2 hours or more frequently, with comparison to previous findings: • LOC • Pupillary size, symmetry, reactivity, and deviation • Response to stimuli • Motor and sensory function	Subtle changes in neurological signs can indicate deterioration or improvement in status. These changes can only be detected by frequent monitoring and comparison. *EO: The child maintains or improves neurologic status.*
2. Monitor vital signs every 15 min–1 hr.	Intracranial hypertension is noted by decreased pulse and increased blood pressure with widening pulse pressure.
3. Monitor temperature continuously, especially if a hypothermia blanket is being used.	Elevated body temperature increases oxygen consumption, which aggravates increased ICP.
4. If a hypothermia blanket is used, remove the blanket when the child's temperature reaches 1–2 degrees above normal.	The child's temperature will continue to drift downward even after the hypothermia blanket has been discontinued. *EO: The child's vital signs will remain within normal limits for age.*
5. Monitor intake and output and specific gravity hourly. Notify physician of urinary output of less than 0.5 mL/kg/hr or greater than 2 mL/kg/hr.	SIADH (Syndrome of Inappropriate secretion of AntiDiuretic Hormone) can occur with brain disorders, stress, surgery, or medications, and causes excretion of large amounts of dilute urine. *EO: The child excretes 1 mL of urine/kg/hr.*
6. Administer fluids, within fluid restrictions.	Fluid restriction aids in decreasing extracellular fluid. Increased ICP can be decreased by control of fluid intake. *EO: The child maintains electrolytes within normal limits.*
7. Monitor electrolytes, BUN, and creatinine.	
8. Weigh child daily on the same scale, at the same time, and in the same clothing.	Changes in weight are an indication of fluid balance.

PROCEDURE	RATIONALE/EXPECTED OUTCOME (EO)

PROCEDURE

9. Monitor skin turgor and mucous membranes every 1–2 hours.

10. Monitor respiratory rate, depth, and pattern every 30–40 minutes.

11. Monitor circulatory status (for example, skin color, pulse, and blood pressure) every hour. Monitor arterial blood gases and report findings to physician.

12. Administer oxygen as ordered by the physician.

13. Encourage deep breathing. Avoid coughing, percussion, and postural drainage.

14. Auscultate chest for breath sounds.

15. Suction the oropharynx; if intubated, hyperventilate by giving 6–8 breaths of 100% oxygen with the Ambu bag before and after suctioning. Limit suctioning to 10–15 seconds.

16. Place child in a semi-Fowler position with head elevated 30°. Avoid prone position, exaggerated neck flexion, and extreme hip flexion of 90°.

17. Monitor ICP continuously and record readings as the child's condition warrants. Calculate the CPP. Place a strip of the ICP waveform in the medical record.

18. If ventriculostomy drainage is anticipated, maintain the drainage bottle above the insertion site, as ordered by the physician.

19. Maintain strict asepsis at all times when manipulating the system and dressings.

20. Organize nursing care to allow the child optional rest periods around periods of low ICP.

21. Give mouth care every 2–4 hours.

22. Check eyes for corneal irritation. Irrigate eyes every 2 hours with artificial tears, normal saline, or other fluid as ordered.

23. Reposition every 2 hours. Check for redness and pressure areas.

24. Use an eggcrate mattress, bed board, and other protection for bony prominences.

RATIONALE/EXPECTED OUTCOME (EO)

EO: The child will demonstrate moist mucous membranes, adequate skin turgor, and systemic perfusion.

Abnormal respirations are associated with increased ICP.

An irregular pattern of breathing or an inability to clear pulmonary secretions causes acid–base disturbances, which alter oxygenation and increase ICP.

These treatments increase intra-abdominal and intrathoracic pressure, thus interfering with drainage of blood vessels from the head.

EO: The child will demonstrate effective air exchange and be free from respiratory complications.

This provides adequate oxygenation so that carbon dioxide will not build up and aggravate increased ICP.

Semi-Fowler position with head elevation provides for drainage from the cranial vault and decreases intracranial pressure. Avoiding these positions means avoiding increased intra-abdominal and intrathoracic pressure, which would interfere with drainage from the venous vessels of the head and brain.

Cerebral perfusion pressure (CPP) is the amount of pressure needed in the cerebral vasculature to supply oxygen and nutrients to the brain. CPP is calculated by subtracting the mean ICP from the mean arterial blood pressure. Normal CPP is 60–90 mm Hg (50 mm Hg is minimum for cerebral perfusion).

EO: The child will maintain adequate cerebral perfusion.

Placing the drainage bottle too low below the insertion site provides for too rapid removal of CSF and can lead to brain herniation. Placing the bottle too high prevents drainage from occurring.

This helps prevent infection.

EO: The child will not have a focus of infection at the catheter site.

The child in a coma is at risk for corneal abrasions because of an absent corneal reflex.

Hypothermia may be used to slow metabolism and decrease cerebral blood flow. This places the child at risk for skin breakdown.

EO: The child will be free from skin breakdown.

EO: The child is free from injury.

PROCEDURE	**RATIONALE/EXPECTED OUTCOME (EO)**
25. Monitor for seizure activity and notify physician if it occurs.	
26. Monitor elimination status. Check for diarrhea or constipation.	Diarrhea may indicate intolerance to enteral feedings. Constipation may be a result of inactivity.
27. Reorient the child to the environment. Allow for favorite objects to be placed in the bed.	*EO: The child is oriented to the environment.*
28. Play the child's favorite music and tapes of the family's voices. When present, encourage the family to talk to the child.	*EO: The child will be soothed by familiar sounds and voices.*

Patient/Family Education: Home Care Considerations

1. Keep the family informed of the child's progress, prognosis, and plan of treatment.

2. Encourage verbalization and questions about the current status of the child and future projected needs.

3. Correct any misinformation that the family may have.

4. Identify support groups and resources available to the family.

References

Drummond, B.L. (1990). Preventing increased intracranial pressure: Nursing care can make the difference. *Focus on Critical Care*, *17*(2), 116–122.

Fridlund, P.H., Vos H., & Daily, E.K. (1988). Use of fiber-optic pressure transducer for intracranial pressure measurements: A primary report. *Heart and Lung*, *17*(2), 111–120.

Hickman, K., Mayer B., & Muwaswes, M. (1990). Intracranial pressure monitoring: Review of risk factors associated with infection. *Heart and Lung*, *19*(1), 84–90.

Jackson, P. (1983). Assessing increased intracranial pressure in infants and young children. *Critical Care Update*, *10*(9), 8–15.

McElroy, D., & Davis, G. (1986). SIADH and the acutely ill child. *Maternal/Child Nursing*, *11*(3), 93–96.

Ommaya Reservoir

56

Definition/Purpose

The Ommaya Reservoir, first introduced in 1963 for the treatment of meningitis, is a dome-shaped device with a catheter protruding from the base. The dome rests between the scalp and the skull, while the catheter fits through the burr hole into the ventricle. The dome is made of a biologically inert material which eliminates rejection problems and permits at least 200 accesses with a 20-gauge or smaller needle (Fig. 56-1).

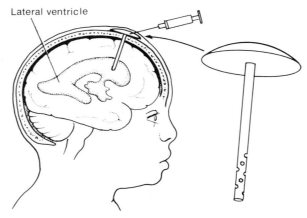

Lateral ventricle

Figure 56-1.

Once in place, the Ommaya Reservoir can be used for administration of chemotherapy, antibiotics and analgesics, withdrawal of cerebral spinal fluid for examination, and intracranial pressure monitoring. For children, the major advantage is the decreased pain and anxiety related to repeated lumbar punctures. Also, with correct placement of the reservoir, there can be certainty of where the medication is being administered. Ommaya and Posner reported better distribution of medication delivered intraventricularly versus intrathecally. Use of the Ommaya Reservoir maintains more consistent levels of chemotherapy with a longer remission from disease.

Standard of Care

1. Access to the reservoir is accomplished under sterile conditions.
2. Before the insertion of the reservoir, the following are suggested:
   a. Obtain a head CT to visualize any tumors and the ventricular size.
   b. Allow several days after the last lumbar puncture to permit reexpansion of the ventricles.
   c. Avoid areas where tumors are present.

Assessment

1. Assess the pertinent history for the symptoms leading to the diagnosis, the date diagnosis was made, and recent signs of intracranial hypertension or infection.

2. Assess the physical findings for signs of intracranial hypertension or infection.
3. Assess for a history of allergies to iodine.
4. Assess the psychosocial concerns and developmental factors, such as coping mechanisms, previous hospital experiences, and the usual routines and daily activities of the family. Also assess the child's and family's level of understanding and their willingness to learn.

Nursing Diagnoses

The following is a list of possible diagnoses and could apply, depending on the child's age, clinical situation, and physical condition:

Anxiety

Fear

High risk for infection

Altered tissue perfusion (cerebral)

High risk for injury

Planning

When planning to care for a child with a reservoir, the following equipment must be gathered:

Lumbar puncture tray

25-gauge needle

Povidone-iodine

Medication to be administered in a syringe

Sterile glove

Interventions

PROCEDURE	**RATIONALE/EXPECTED OUTCOME (EO)**
Preoperative	
1. Explain to the child and family the positive and negative aspects of the reservoir. Answer their questions.	The family must have adequate knowledge about the reservoir to feel they can make a decision in the child's best interest. *EO: The child and family will experience less fear and anxiety if they have their questions answered.*
Postoperative	
2. Inspect the surgical wound for infection (redness, swelling, tenderness, or drainage).	The reservoir is a link from the outside to the central nervous system. Without proper technique for accessing the device, or when the child is granulocytopenic, infection can occur. *EO: The child's wound will not become infected.*
3. Assess the child for a general infection of the reservoir (for example, fever, headache, or stiff neck).	*EO: An infection of the reservoir will be identified and treated.*
4. Assess the child's neurologic status.	Neurologic status may be at risk with the placement of the reservoir as evidenced by seizures, hemiparesis, de-

| **PROCEDURE** | **RATIONALE/EXPECTED OUTCOME (EO)** |

creased level of consciousness, and disseminating necrotizing leukoencephalopathy (characterized by confusion, spasticity, ataxia, or coma).

EO: The child maintains or improves neurologic status.

5. Obtain baseline vital signs.

Accessing the Reservoir

6. Assemble equipment.

7. Assist the child into a comfortable position, usually lying flat.

Trendelenburg position may be necessary for gravitational benefits.

8. Assess patency of the reservoir by depressing the dome and watching for easy refill. **Do not** depress the dome if the child's neurological status has changed.

The function of the reservoir can cause problems if the catheter becomes misplaced or blocked. Tissue damage can result from movement of the catheter or medication inserted in the incorrect location.

9. Prepare a sterile field.

10. The physician will put on sterile gloves.

11. The physician will clean the area over the dome with povidone-iodine (if no allergy reported).

The hair over the dome will not be allowed to grow back. This area is easily covered by the remaining hair.

12. Using sterile technique, the physician will insert the needle through the scalp and into the dome.

CSF should flow back into the needle. It should not be forcefully removed.

13. If an intracranial pressure reading needs to be obtained, it should be done at this time, prior to withdrawal or insertion of fluid.

Withdrawal of fluid would decrease the pressure; insertion of fluid would increase the pressure.

EO: The child's ICP will be measured.

14. The physician will withdraw enough CSF for testing. Withdrawing 3 mL of extra CSF for flush is also necessary. If CSF cannot be gently withdrawn, the catheter may be clogged or misplaced.

The capacity of the reservoir is 1.5 mL; therefore, withdraw an additional 3 mL for flushing after medication administration.

15. Dilute medication with preservative-free saline. The physician will insert the medication.

16. The physician will flush the reservoir with the extra CSF and remove the needle.

EO: The child will have medication inserted through the reservoir in a safe manner.

17. Instruct child to lie quietly for 15–30 minutes after the procedure.

18. Monitor the child every 15 minutes for one to two hours, then every four hours for changes in neurologic status or vital signs. Report changes to the physician immediately.

EO: The child's vital signs and neurologic status will be monitored after the medication administration.

Patient/Family Education: Home Care Considerations

The child and the family should be instructed on the following points:
1. The child should avoid bumps to the reservoir area. Play must be noncontact.
2. Any sign of infection should be brought to the physician's attention. Incisional infection may include excessive redness, tenderness, discharge, or swelling. Reservoir infection may include fever, headache, neck stiffness, and a change in mental status.
3. After 7–10 days, the sutures will be removed and the child's hair can then be washed regularly to decrease the chance of infection.
4. Teachers and school nurses should be made aware of the presence of the reservoir.

References

Cornwell, C. (1990). The Ommaya Reservoir: Implications for pediatric oncology. *Pediatric Nursing, 16*(3), 249–251.

Esparza, D.M., & Weyland, J.B. (1982). Nursing care for the patient with an Ommaya Reservoir. *Oncology Nursing Forum,* September, 17–20.

Leavens, M.E., Hill, C.S., Çech, D.A., et al. (1982). Intrathecal and intraventricular morphine for pain in cancer patients. *Journal of Neurosurgery, 56,* 241–245.

Fluid and Electrolyte Balance

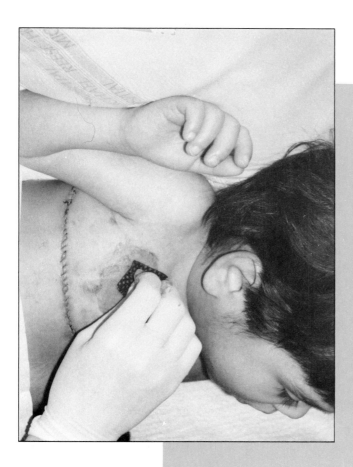

Unit IX

Intravenous Therapy

57

Definition/Purpose

The choice of an intravenous solution depends on the specific purpose for which it is intended. Generally, intravenous fluids are administered to achieve one or more of the following goals:

1. To provide water, electrolytes, and nutrients to meet daily requirements
2. To replace water and correct electrolyte deficits
3. To provide a route for intravenous drug administration.

Solutions are categorized as isotonic, hypotonic, or hypertonic, according to whether their osmolality is the same, less than, or greater than that of blood. Electrolyte solutions are considered isotonic if the total electrolyte content is approximately 310 m Eq/L. They are considered hypotonic if the total electrolyte content is less than 250 m Eq/L and hypertonic if the total electrolyte content exceeds 375 m Eq/L. The nurse must keep in mind that the osmolality of plasma is 300 mm Osm/L. Some common water and electrolyte solutions are listed in Table 57-1 with comments about their use.

Table 57-1. Composition of Frequently Used Parenteral Fluids

Electrolytes

Solution	Element	Amount		Nursing Implications
Dextrose solutions (D5W, D10W, D50W) D5W—osmolality of 252 mOsm/L	None	—		Isotonic solution that that supplies 170 cal/L (D5W) or 1700 cal/L (D50W) and free water to aid in renal excretion of solutes. Solution may aggravate hypokalemia. Do not administer with blood.
Normal saline (0.9 sodium chloride) Osmolality of 308 mOsm/L	Sodium Chloride	154 154	m Eq/L m Eq/L	Isotonic solution used to treat an extracellular volume deficit. Does not supply free water for excretory purposes. Supplies an excess of Na^+ and Cl^-; can cause fluid volume excess and hyperchloremic acidosis if used in excess volumes, especially in patients with compromised renal function.
Lactated Ringer's solution (Hartmann's solution) Osmolality 274 mOsm/L	Sodium Potassium Calcium Chloride Lactate	103 4 3 109 28	m Eq/L m Eq/L m Eq/L m Eq/L m Eq/L	Isotonic solution that contains multiple electrolytes in the same concentration as found in plasma. Used in the treatment of hypovolemia, burns, and fluid lost as bile or diarrhea. Does not supply free water for renal excretory purposes. Check urine flow before administering solutions containing potassium.
Plain Ringer's solution Osmolality: 274 mOsm/L	Sodium Potassium Calcium Chloride	147 4 4.5 155.5	m Eq/L m Eq/L m Eq/L m Eq/L	Isotonic solution that contains multiple electrolytes with chloride in excess of normal plasma. Used to correct dehydration.
3% NaCl (hypertonic saline) Osmolality: 1026 mOsm/L	Sodium Chloride	513 513	m Eq/L m Eq/L	Grossly hypertonic solution used only in critical situations to treat hyponatremia. Administer small volumes at slow rates.

(continued)

Table 57-1. (*continued*)

Electrolytes

Solution	Element	Amount		Nursing Implications
Dextrose with saline D5/.45 NaCl	Sodium	77	m Eq/L	Slightly hypertonic solution when compared to plasma. Provides electrolytes plus 170 cal/L. Used for fluid replacement and correction of dehydration and sodium depletion.
	Chloride	77	m Eq/L	
D5/.9 NaCl	Sodium	154	m Eq/L	
	Chloride	154	m Eq/L	
Dextran 40 10% injection with 0.9 NaCl	Sodium	77 500	m Eq/ mL	Provides plasma volume expansion. Used for early fluid replacement when blood or blood products are unavailable. Allergic reaction possible.
	Chloride	77 500	m Eq/ mL	

In most instances, the parenteral administration of fluids is best carried out by infusing them directly into the venous system. Many sites are readily available for venoclysis, however, the largest visible vein is not necessarily the preferred one. One must consider the comfort of the patient, position and extent of restraint, the vessel's ability to maintain a needle, the solution to be injected, and possible hazards and complications from the selected site. Accessible veins for venoclysis are illustrated in Fig. 57-1.

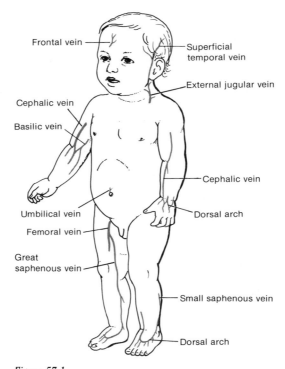

Figure 57-1.

Veins of the Scalp

These veins are used only in infants. In order of preference, they are the frontal, superficial temporal, posterior auricular, supraorbital, occipital, and posterior facial. Arteries follow closely the course of the superficial veins of the scalp. Arterial and venous vessels may be differentiated by the following means:

- Pulsations can be palpated in an artery.
- A vein is palpated as a furrow beneath the skin, an artery is a more firm and distended vessel.

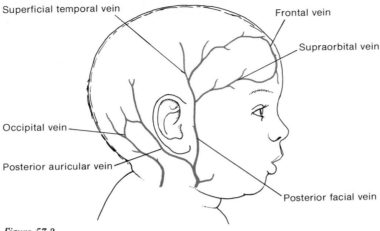

Figure 57-2.

- Arteries are deep, whereas veins are more superficial and can be visualized (Fig. 57-2).

Veins of the Forearm and Antecubital Fossa

Veins and arteries are in close proximity in the antecubital space. About 10% of individuals have an aberrant artery in this space that may be mistaken for a vein. Thus, care must be taken to avoid cannulating an artery. The most frequently used veins are the cephalic, the basilic, and the median basilic (Fig. 57-3).

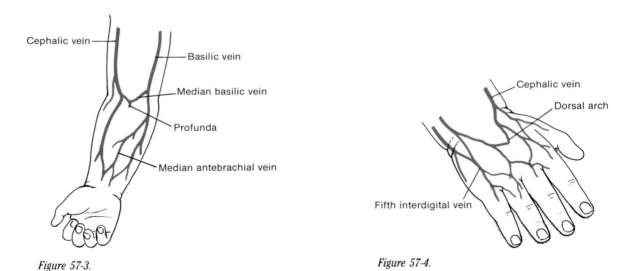

Figure 57-3.

Figure 57-4.

Veins on the Dorsum of the Hand

Tributaries of the cephalic and basilic veins are potential sites for infusion in infants and children. It has been suggested that the fifth interdigital vein in infants is fairly constant and easier to locate than the other veins (Fig. 57-4).

Veins on the Dorsum of the Foot

The median and lateral margin veins of the foot are suitable sites for both infants and children (Fig. 57-5).

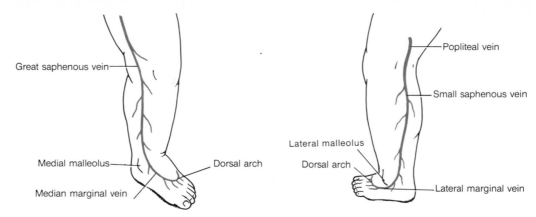

Figure 57-5.

Great Saphenous Vein of the Ankle

This vein lies between the medial malleolus and the anterior tibial tendon (see Fig. 57-5).

Three main types of venipuncture devices are available: steel scalp vein needles, indwelling plastic catheters inserted over a steel needle, and indwelling plastic catheters inserted through a steel needle. Scalp vein or butterfly needles are short steel needles with plastic wing handles. They are easy to insert but infiltrate easily because they are small and nonpliable. Short plastic catheters require the additional step of advancing the catheter into the vein following venipuncture. Because they are less likely to infiltrate, these devices are preferred over scalp vein needles (Fig. 57-6). Plastic catheters inserted through a

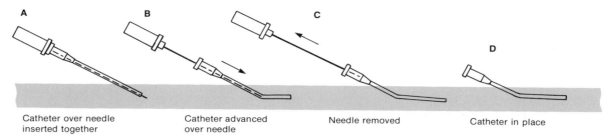

Figure 57-6. Insertion of catheter over a needle.

hollow needle are usually called intracatheters. They are available in long lengths and are well-suited for central lines. They are, however, more difficult to place than the other two devices and are usually inserted solely by the physician (Fig. 57-7).

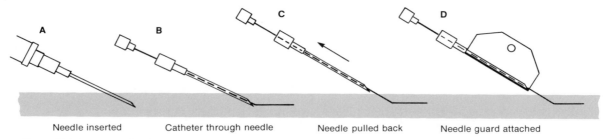

Figure 57-7. Insertion of catheter through a needle.

Standard of Care

1. Change intravenous solutions every 24–48 hours, depending on institution policy.
2. Change intravenous tubings every 48–72 hours.
3. Change site of infusion every 72 hours. (This may not be feasible in pediatric patients because of limited access sites.)

Assessment

1. Assess pertinent history and physical findings for previous experiences with IVs, location of good veins for infusion, sites of previous IVs and infiltrations, preference for right or left arm, hydrational status, age, and weight.
2. Assess the child's coping mechanisms for painful procedures, the child's previous experience with restricted activities, and the child's normal habits and routines.
3. Assess the family's knowledge of IV therapy and their level of acceptance and readiness to learn.

Nursing Diagnoses

The following is a list of possible diagnoses and could apply, depending on the child's age, clinical situation, and physical condition:

Fluid volume excess

Fluid volume deficit

Impaired physical mobility

Fear

Diversional activity deficit

Pain

Planning

When planning to insert an intravenous catheter, the following equipment must be assembled:

Infusion set, solution, filter (.22 μm), drip chamber, and tubing

Appropriate size infusion device

3- or 5-mL syringe filled with normal saline

Materials for restraints

Soap and razor to shave scalp hair (on infant)

Tourniquet (rubber band)

Povidone-iodine swabs

Alcohol swabs

Tape and armboard

Sterile gloves

Infusion pump

1% lidocaine (1 mL in syringe with 25-gauge needle attached)

Antibiotic ointment

Interventions

PROCEDURE	**RATIONALE/EXPECTED OUTCOME (EO)**

1. Prepare the child as appropriate to age and development.

IV insertion is a painful and unfamiliar procedure to the child and parent.

EO: The child will be appropriately prepared for the IV insertion.

2. Discuss why the IV is necessary and the probable length of IV treatment.

The child, in most cases, has no choice whether or not an IV will be inserted and usually does not want one.

EO: The child will experience a minimal amount of fear.

Infant. Provide information to parent. Handle the infant gently, and speak softly. Avoid inserting IV into the same arm the child uses for thumbsucking. Cuddle the infant immediately after IV insertion. Do not feed the infant immediately prior to insertion.

EO: The infant has the IV inserted with minimal trauma. The infant quiets and comforts soon after completion of the procedure. Vomiting and aspiration are possibilities with an agitated infant.

Toddler to Preschooler. Prepare the child immediately prior to the procedure. Give simple explanations in concrete terms, and allow the child to see and touch equipment. Explain that you will help the child hold still and that it is OK to cry; emphasize that the IV is not punishment. Cuddle the child immediately after insertion.

EO: Toddlers and preschoolers have a limited attention span and are likely to become anxious if prepared too soon.

School-Age. Prepare child ahead of time, but on the day of insertion. Give the child choices as appropriate (For example, right or left arm, and the type of tape). Give positive reinforcement after completion of the procedure.

The school-age child fears body multilation and needs time to master new skills and experiences.

EO: The older child describes and plays out the procedure.

Adolescent. Prepare the teenager several hours to a day before the procedure. Approach discussions on a more adult level; discuss fears related to procedure. Included teenager in decisions (for example, site, use of an armboard, and tape).

The adolescent needs time between preparation and insertion to absorb explanations and ask questions.

EO: The adolescent verbalizes fears and attempts self-control during the insertion.

3. Calculate fluid requirements; check if they coincide with the physician's order and with the diagnosis (Table 57-2).

The amount of fluid may be decreased in patients with neurologic, cardiac, or renal problems and increased in patients who are dehydrated or in sickle cell crisis.

EO: The child will maintain appropriate fluid volume for age, size, diagnosis, and status.

4. Use infusion device to monitor the flow rate.

A controller infuses fluid using gravity, whereas a pump will infuse fluid against a certain amount of pressure.

Table 57-2. Calculation of Maintenance Fluids: Body Weight Formula

Weight	Concentration
Newborns (up to 72 hours old)	60–100 mL/kg
≤10 kg	100 mL/kg (May be increased to 150 mL/kg if renal or cardiac function normal)
11–20 kg	1000 mL for the first 10 kg plus 50 mL/kg for each kg over 10 kg
21–30 kg	1500 mL for the first 20 kg plus 25 mL/kg for each kg over 20 kg

PROCEDURE

RATIONALE/EXPECTED OUTCOME (EO)

5. Gather equipment.
6. Choose site and type of device. A warm compress over the area may help distend the veins.

Careful site selection will increase the likelihood of successful venipuncture and preservation of the vein. Asepsis is essential to prevent infection.

7. Wash hands.
8. Put on sterile gloves.
9. Scalp vein insertion:
   a. Bundel or "mummy" infant for the insertion.
   b. Have another nurse aid the operator by manually positioning the infant's head.
   c. Locate the site and then shave the hair.
   d. Prepare the site by scrubbing with povidone-iodine swab for 60 seconds in a circular motion, moving outward from the puncture site. Allow 1–2 minutes to dry. If the child is allergic to iodine, scrub with a 90% alcohol swab.
   e. Apply a rubber band tourniquet (Fig. 57-8).

Explain to the parent that this site permits greater freedom of movement, less chance of dislodging the IV, and easier insertion. This area should be large enough to permit taping of the needle. Strict asepsis and careful site preparation are essential to prevent infection.

EO: The child will have an infusion device inserted free from complications and with minimal trauma.

The tourniquet distends the vein and makes it easier to enter.

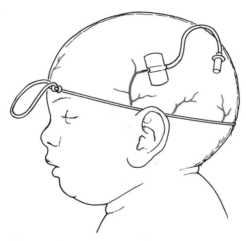

Figure 57-8.

f. Prepare the needle by attaching the syringe with normal saline to the needle and forcing out a few drops of saline.
g. Select a segment of vein that is fairly straight; the needle should be placed in the direction of blood flow.
h. Grasp the needle by the winged tabs, bevel up.

i. Anchor the vein with a finger of the free hand by stretching the skin.
j. Hold the needle parallel to the long axis of the vein.
k. Introduce the needle into and through the skin, but do not penetrate the vein.

This determines the patency of the needle.

Bevel-up position produces less trauma to the skin and vein.
Applying traction to the vein helps to stabilize it.

The two-stage procedure decreases the chance of thrusting the needle through the wall of the vein as the skin is entered.

PROCEDURE

l. The needle is then gently advanced into the vessel until blood appears in the tubing. Do not advance needle once blood is seen.

m. Release the tourniquet.

n. Check the patency of the system by infusing 2–3 mL of saline from the syringe into the vein.

o. Tape the system in place using the method shown in Figure 57–9.

RATIONALE/EXPECTED OUTCOME (EO)

The needle cannot be advanced without piercing the distal wall of the vein.

This method increases the stability of the needle tip in the vein.

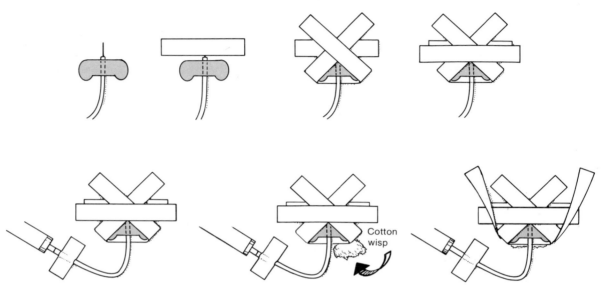

Figure 57-9.

p. Attach the hub of the needle tubing to the adapter of the infusion set tubing.

q. Set the appropriate rate on the infusion pump and begin infusion. Document site, size of needle and time of insertion in chart. Also document drip rate.

10. Catheter-over-needle (angiocath) insertion

a. Restrain the child for insertion; a second nurse may be needed to aid the child in controlling himself during procedure.

b. Select an adequate length of vein.

c. Apply the tourniquet.

d. Cleanse the site with either povidone-iodine or alcohol (as above).

e. Put on sterile gloves.

f. Anesthetize the selected skin entry site by injecting it with an intradermal bleb of 1% lidocaine. Wait 1–3 minutes for the agent to take effect.

g. With your free hand, steady the child's extremity and pull skin taut over the vessel.

h. Holding needle bevel-up and at a 45° angle, pierce the skin.

This will decrease the pain on insertion.

PROCEDURE

      i. Decrease angle or the needle and enter the vein either directly from above or from the side.

      j. Advance the needle ¼ in after back flow of blood is visible.

      k. Hold the needle hub and slide catheter over the needle.

      l. Remove the needle; hold catheter hub in place.

    m. Release the tourniquet and attach the infusion device.

      n. Tape cannula in place.

      o. Apply antibiotic ointment over insertion site and cover with an adhesive bandage.

      p. Label the dressing with type of catheter, date of insertion; and your initials.

      q. Document the site, cannula type, and time in medical record.

11. Use an armboard of appropriate size for child.

12. Restrain the child's extremities as necessary. Explain the reason for restraint to the parents. Release the child from restraints every 2 hours.

13. Assess restrained extremities for pulses, movement, sensation, temperature, and color every hour.

14. Use medicine cup or drinking cup cut in half and padded to protect the IV site from the child's touch.

15. Check for pressure areas every 2 hours (especially if using foot veins).

16. Offer diversional activities appropriate to age and development.

17. Monitor vital signs, and maintain accurate intake and output. Weigh the child daily, at the same time, on the same scale, and in the same clothes. Assess for edema (for example, fontanelle, dependent, periorbital).

18. Explain to child and parents the importance of keeping infusion constant. Caution them not to regulate the IV.

19. Monitor the IV site every 1–2 hours:

      a. Check temperature of site

      b. Check symmetry of limbs or head

      c. Touch the site above the catheter to see if it is soft or taut.

      d. Check for "bogginess" in the scalp by pressing on the head.

      e. Ask the child if it hurts; note nonverbal signs of pain.

20. Dilute medications in the appropriate amount of fluid to prevent phlebitis.

21. Discontinue infusion if infiltration has occurred. El-

RATIONALE/EXPECTED OUTCOME (EO)

Advancing the needle ensures that the plastic catheter has entered the vein.

Antimicrobial ointments decrease the risk of infection.

Documentation is essential to facilitate care and for legal purposes.

Physical restraining devices are used to keep the child from moving.

EO: The child is free from neurovascular impairment.

EO: The child maintains a patent IV.

When restrained, the child has limited freedom of movement. IV administration is an artificial method of delivering fluids that bypasses the body's regulatory mechanism, thus making it easy to over- or underhydrate the child.

EO: The child maintains normal blood pressure, heart rate, and urine for his or her age and weight. The child has good skin turgor.

The child and parents need information and teaching in order to deal appropriately with the IV equipment.

EO: The child is free from pain associated with continuous IV therapy.

Phlebitis may cause pain at the site.

EO: The child experiences quick resolution of the infiltration.

PROCEDURE	RATIONALE/EXPECTED OUTCOME (EO)
evate the limb, and apply a warm moist compress. Report to appropriate person(s). Document infiltration in the medical record.	
22. Take the child for walks to the playroom; let the child sit in the hallway where there is more activity.	The equipment and restraining devices used for an IV limit a child's freedom of movement. *EO: The child will receive adequate stimulation to meet growth and development needs.*
23. Have developmentally appropriate toys and games in the bed.	
24. Encourage activity that does not require use of the extremity that has the IV.	
25. Teach the child and parents how to move the IV pole, unplugging the infusion pump for walks and then plugging it back in to recharge.	
26. For school-age children and adolescents, set up a study schedule and encourage them to keep up with their school work.	

Patient/Family Education: Home Care Considerations

1. Discuss with the child and the parents why the infusion is necessary and its expected duration.
2. Teach reasons for restraints (for example, to avoid touching the site and to immobilize the area).
3. Explore methods to maintain mobility.
4. Explain to the parents that an infant or child with an IV still needs to be held, and teach them methods for picking up and holding an infant with an IV.
5. Ask parents to call the nurse if the IV is not infusing, for example, it is not dripping, the alarm is sounding on the pump, or the site is painful, red, swollen, or warm to touch).
6. Explain to the parents of adolescents that rebellion may show itself in lack of cooperation with the therapy. These patients may rebel, if they feel threatened. They require consistent limits, which must be clearly communicated to the patient, parents, and staff.

References

Abbott, P., & Schlacht, K. (1984). Pediatric IVs: A special challenge. *Canadian Nurse, 80*(10), 24–26.

Blatz, S., & Paes, B.A. (1990). Intravenous infusion by superficial vein in the neonate. *Journal of Intravenous Nursing, 13*(2), 122–128.

Sheckfuss, B. (1985). Pediatric IV care. *NITA, 8*(1), 75–82.

Heparin Lock

58

Definition/Purpose

Heparin lock needles are used for interrupted intravenous infusions. These are standard infusion devices modified so that after the infusion is completed, the intravenous solution can be discontinued but the venous access maintained. After the infusion is completed, the heparin lock needle is filled with a heparinized saline solution to prevent clotting. The obvious advantage to this type of intravenous device is that the patient has to be attached to an intravenous fluid line only when infusions are being administered, and therefore has increased mobility.

Standard of Care

1. The heparin lock is to be flushed every 8–12 hours (according to institution policy) if continuous intravenous fluids are not being administered, or after each infusion of medication or fluids.
2. The infusion site should be changed every 72 hours; however, this may not be possible because the child has limited access sites.

Assessment

1. Assess the pertinent history and physical findings for previous experience with IVs and heparin lock needles.
2. Assess the child's coping mechanisms for painful procedures and normal habits and routines that would be aided by the use of a heparin lock.
3. Assess the family's knowledge of IV therapy and their level of acceptance and readiness to learn.

Nursing Diagnoses

The following is a list of possible diagnoses and could apply, depending on the child's age, clinical situation, and physical condition:

Impaired physical mobility

Fear

Diversional activity deficit

Pain

Planning

When planning to insert and maintain a heparin lock, the following equipment is needed:

Heparin lock needle of the appropriate size

Povidone-iodine swabs

Alcohol swabs

Heparin flush solution (10 U/mL) in TB syringe with 25-gauge needle attached, or a prefilled syringe

Tourniquet

Tape

Sterile gloves

Syringe with 2 mL normal saline and a 25-gauge needle attached.

Interventions

PROCEDURE	RATIONALE/EXPECTED OUTCOME (EO)
1. Explain to the child and parent(s) the need for venous access and the advantages of the heparin lock.	*EO: The child and parents will understand the need for the venous access.*
2. With the appropriate restraint in place, prepare the skin and insert the needle using the steps described in the procedure Intravenous Medications (Chap. 24) (Fig. 58-1).	*EO: The child will have the infusion device free from complications and with minimal trauma.*

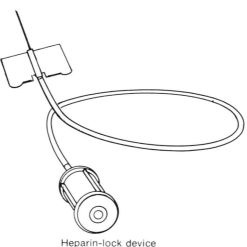

Heparin-lock device

Figure 58-1.

3. Secure the needle in place.	
4. Clean the rubber flange with povidone-iodine swab, and insert the 25-gauge needle connected to the TB syringe into the flange.	
5. Flush out the blood that has accumulated in the tubing from insertion with 0.5–0.8 mL of heparinized solution.	This will prevent clotting of blood in the needle and tubing.
6. Remove the needle from the flange while still putting pressure on the plunger of the syringe.	This will prevent a negative pressure from forming in the needle and allowing blood to back up and clot in the device.
7. To administer medications or IV fluids through the heparin lock, clean the flange with povidone-iodine or alcohol, insert a 25-gauge needle connected to a syringe of normal saline into the flange, aspirate for a blood return, and then flush with 2 mL of normal saline before and after administration of medica-	A number of IV fluids and medications are not compatible with heparin. Flushing the needle and tubing will decrease the likelihood of a reaction. *EO: The child will have IV fluids and medications administered free of complications (such as drug reactions, infiltrations, and skin irritation).*

PROCEDURE

tions or IV fluids. If there is no blood return, remove the needle and reinsert a new one.

8. Chart the amount of heparin given, and the time and condition of the IV site in the patient's permanent medical record. Also record amount of saline flush on intake and output (I & O) sheet.

RATIONALE/EXPECTED OUTCOME (EO)

EO: The child will show no evidence of discomfort at or around the IV site.

Patient/Family Education: Home Care Considerations

1. Explain to the child and parents why the venous access is necessary and how the heparin lock device functions.
2. Explain safe methods for the child to maintain mobility and perform age-appropriate tasks.
3. Tell the child and parents to call the nurse if blood backs up in the tubing or if the child complains of pain at or around the IV site.

References

Ashton, J. Gibson, V., & Summers, S. (1990). Effects of herapin versus saline solution on intermittent infusion device irrigation. *Heart and Lung, 19*(6), 608–612.

Çyganski, J.M., Donahue, J.M., & Heaton, J.S. (1987). The case for the heparin flush. *American Journal of Nursing, 87*, 796–797.

Dunn, D.L., & Lenihan, S.F. (1987). The case for the saline flush. *American Journal of Nursing, 87*, 798–799.

Right Atrial Catheter

59

Definition/Purpose

The right atrial catheter is an indwelling silicone catheter that is intended for long-term administration of total parenteral nutrition, medications, and blood products, and to draw venous blood samples. The catheter is tunneled through the subcutaneous tissue of the chest and exits between the nipple and the sternum. Two incisions are made, one below the clavicle (the entrance site) and the second between the nipple and the sternum (the exit site). A tunnel is made through the subcutaneous tissue between the two incisions. The catheter is pulled through the tunnel and inserted into the vein. The catheter is then advanced into the right atrium. A Dacron cuff lies midway between the entrance and exit sites to help anchor the catheter and act as a protective barrier to prevent ascending infection (Figs. 59-1 and 59-2). The catheters may be single, double, or multiple lumen, depending on the intended use and the patient's needs.

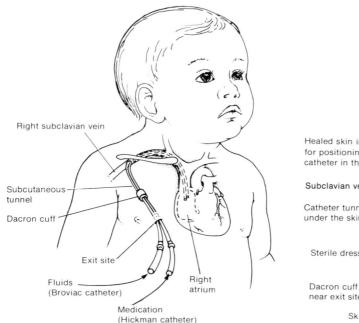

Figure 59-1. Double lumen catheter.

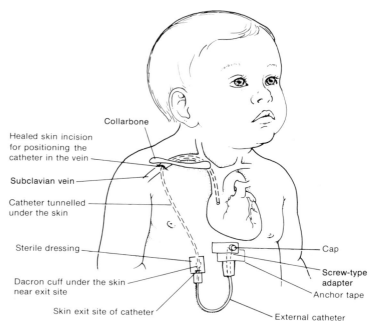

Figure 59-2. Single lumen catheter.

Standard of Care

1. It is recommended to have two people to change the dressing of a moving child; one of these should be a registered nurse. A trained parent may also assist the RN in changing the dressing.
2. The transparent semipermeable membrane is to be changed by an RN or trained

parent every 48–72 hours or prn when the dressing becomes nonocclusive. A gauze dressing should be changed every 48 hours.

3. The injection cap will be changed once a week by an RN or trained parent.

4. Right atrial catheters will be irrigated with a heparinized saline solution (10 U/mL) every 12 hours. They will also be irrigated after the administration of medications or blood and the withdrawal of blood samples, with 3 mL of solution or less depending on the size of the child.

5. Medications will be administered through the right atrial catheter by an RN. The pharmacy should be consulted regarding dilution of medications and over what length of time the medication needs to be administered.

6. Multidose vials of medications should be avoided. However, multidose vials can be used for 24 hours after the initial dose if the vials have been dated and timed.

7. Total parenteral nutrition (TPN) fluid is changed every 24 hours. Dextrose solutions above 10% are considered TPN and are changed every 24 hours. Ten-percent (and below) dextrose solution is changed every 48 hours.

8. All fluids infused through the right atrial line are filtered by a .22-μm inline filter. (Exceptions to this are intralipids and certain medications that are inactivated by the filter).

9. The intravenous tubing is changed every 48 hours.

10. A continuous infusion of fluid through the right atrial catheter will be heparinized at a rate of $\frac{1}{2}$–1 U/mL of fluid to prevent clotting (if the child's condition permits).

11. Place a line clamp at bedside, on clothing, or on the line of every child with a right atrial catheter.

Each institution has specific procedures for the care of these catheters. Use the above standards of care as guidelines but follow the procedures that your institution has outlined.

Assessment

1. Assess pertinent history and physical findings to determine the need for long-term total parenteral nutrition, chemotherapy, antibiotics, blood product replacement, or frequent blood sampling.

2. Assess psychosocial and developmental factors that would predict acceptance of the catheter, such as body image, fear, anxiety, effect of the disease on self-concept, and the family's interaction.

3. Assess the patient's and family's knowledge of the function, care, and operation of the catheter and their readiness and willingness to learn.

Nursing Diagnoses

The following is a list of possible diagnoses and could apply, depending on the child's age, clinical situation, and physical condition:

Anxiety

High risk for injury

High risk for infection

Body image disturbance

Impaired skin integrity

Planning

When caring for a child with a right atrial catheter, assemble the following equipment:

Dressing Change

Dressing change kit (sterile gloves, acetone or alcohol swabs, povidone-iodine swab, povidone-iodine ointment)

Transparent semipermeable membrane

Steri-strips

Two 2 × 2 split gauze dressings (for 2 × 2 dressing)

1-inch tape

Application of Injection Cap

Sterile gloves

Mask

10 mL heparin flush (10 U/mL) in syringe with 23-gauge needle attached.

Injection cap

3 povidone-iodine swabs

Sterile barrier

Smooth-edged clamp

1-inch tape

Irrigation of Catheter

5 mL heparin flush (10 U/mL) in syringe with 23-gauge needle attached

Povidone-iodine swabs

Sterile gloves

Medication Administration

Syringe with 23-gauge needle containing medication

5 mL heparin flush (10 U/mL) in syringe with 23-gauge needle attached

2 povidone-iodine swabs

Sterile gloves

Acquisition of Blood Samples

Appropriate lab tubes, transmittals, and ice (if needed)

3 povidone-iodine swabs

5 mL heparin flush (10 U/mL) in syringe with 23-gauge needle attached

1 5-mL syringe with 23-gauge needle attached

1 appropriate-size syringe with 23-gauge needle attached for blood

Sterile gloves

Repair of Catheter

Mask

Sterile gloves

Suture removal kit (including sterile scissors)

1 14-gauge 2-inch angiocath

1 16-gauge 2-inch angiocath

1 18-gauge 2-inch angiocath

1 smooth-edged clamp

1 tongue blade

4 povidone-iodine swabs

1 sterile barrier

5-mL syringe containing heparinized saline solution with 23-gauge needle

Tape

Injection cap

Interventions

| **PROCEDURE** | **RATIONALE/EXPECTED OUTCOME (EO)** |

Preoperatively

1. Assess what the child and parents know about the catheter; elicit their concerns, fears, and questions.

The child and parents will have concerns about the insertion procedure. Providing information can promote a feeling of control and decrease anxiety.

EO: The child and parents will verbalize a decreased level of anxiety.

2. Provide information. Explain the procedure using pictures, drawings, and written information to describe location and uses.

3. Provide the child and family with a catheter of the type that is to be inserted. Allow the entire family to see and touch the catheter.

EO: The child and parents will indicate an understanding of insertion procedure, use of the catheter, and expected postoperative routine.

4. Explain routine procedures that will follow insertion of the catheter (for example, inspection of insertion site, frequent monitoring of vital signs, dressing changes).

Postoperatively

1. Maintain the dressings at the entrance and exit sites for the first 24 hours. Observe area around sites for bruising and tenderness along the tunnel.

The sites may produce serosanguineous drainage for several days, especially if the child is thrombocytopenic.

EO: The child's catheter will remain patent, in place, and free from complications to allow proper, safe administration of nutrition and medications.

2. Assess at least every 4 hours for signs of venous thrombosis (such as tenderness and edema of the shoulder, neck, and arm on the side of the catheter); also for unexplained difficulty infusing IV fluids; edema; subcutaneous fluid along the tunnel, or leakage around the catheter.

Hemorrhage or thrombosis may result after the catheter is placed.

Exit Site Care: Dressing Change (Transparent)

1. Check hospital protocol regarding exit site dressing change procedures. Use aseptic technique at all times. Assess entrance and exit sites for signs of infection with each dressing change, and report minor temperature elevations, tachycardia, tachypnea, or hypotension.

Neutropenic patients have a poor immune response; thus, they are more prone to infections. Once a foreign body is introduced into the child's body, the risk of infection increases.

EO: The child is afebrile.

2. Gather equipment.

3. Place child in a supine position.

4. Set up a sterile field on a flat surface for the dressing

PROCEDURE	**RATIONALE/EXPECTED OUTCOME (EO)**

change kit. Put on mask. Open transparent dressing and drop on the sterile field.

5. Completely remove old dressing and discard (Fig. 59-3).

EO: The child's skin integrity remains intact.

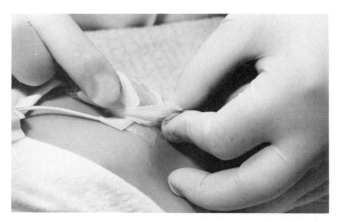

Figure 59-3.

6. Have an assistant restrain the child and hold catheter elevated at the hub so that the catheter does not touch the child's chest.

7. Wash hands.

8. Put on sterile gloves.

9. Open povidone-iodine swab stick and vigorously cleanse the skin once, starting at the exit site, moving outward in a circular motion, and cleansing the entire area where the dressing will be placed (Fig. 59-4). (Do not recleanse any area with the same swab.) Allow to air-dry.

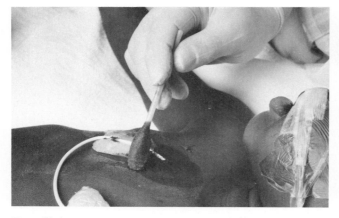

Figure 59-4.

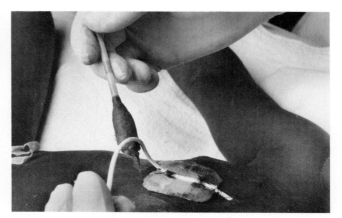

Figure 59-5.

10. Using another povidone-iodine swab stick, cleanse the length of the catheter that will be housed under the dressing, from the exit site outward toward the hub (Fig. 59-5).

PROCEDURE

11. Apply a small dab of povidone-iodine ointment to the exit site.

12. Apply the transparent dressing over the exit site and over the catheter. Do not coil the catheter under the dressing. The dressing should cover the exit site and approximately half of the catheter. The hub should be outside the dressing (Fig. 59-6A,B,C).

RATIONALE/EXPECTED OUTCOME (EO)

EO: The child has no drainage, inflammation, or redness at the exit site.

Coiling the catheter increases the risk of infection at the exit site.

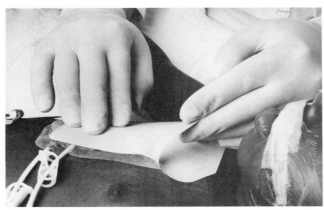

A

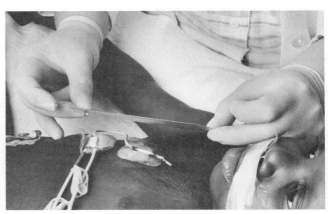

B

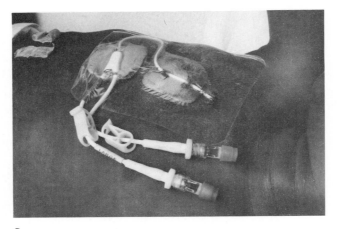

C
Figure 59-6.

13. Remove gloves.

14. Cut a notch in the middle of one Steri-strip. Place this Steri-strip under the catheter as it exits the dressing and overlap it onto the dressing. This will secure the dressing at the catheter exit site.

15. Secure the catheter with additional tape to prevent tension on the line.

16. Document the dressing change in the permanent medical record, noting date and time of change, the child's tolerance, and any abnormalities.

Exit Site Care: Dressing Change (2 × 2 Dressing)

1. For 2 × 2 gauze dressing, follow steps 1–12 above.

PROCEDURE	**RATIONALE/EXPECTED OUTCOME (EO)**
2. Place split 2 × 2s over catheter in opposite directions.	
3. Place tape over 2 × 2s to make an occlusive dressing.	
4. Coil catheter and tape securely.	
5. Document as above (step 16).	

Application of Injection Cap

PROCEDURE	**RATIONALE/EXPECTED OUTCOME (EO)**
1. Put on mask.	
2. Wash hands.	
3. Draw up 10 mL of heparin flush into a syringe with a 23-gauge needle attached.	
4. Open sterile barrier. Open the injection cap package and drop onto the sterile field. Open three povidone-iodine swabs and drop onto the sterile field.	When the catheter is not connected to continuous IVs, or one of the lumens is not connected, the lumen is capped like a heparin lock, enabling the child to move around freely while maintaining a closed sterile system. *EO: The integrity of the catheter will be maintained.*
5. Clamp catheter over protective tape.	
6. Put on gloves.	
7. Using one swab in each hand, grasp the plastic ridge of the hub in one hand and unscrew the old injection cap or IV tubing from the end of the catheter with the other hand.	
8. The old injection cap or IV tubing should be discarded quickly, along with the swab.	
9. Pick up the new injection cap and screw it on the end of the catheter.	
10. Take povidone-iodine swab and wipe off rubber tip of injection cap.	
11. Insert needle of heparin flush into rubber tip of injection cap. Unclamp catheter. Draw back on syringe to get air bubbles out of catheter and cap, but not enough to get blood into the syringe.	*EO: The child is free from air embolism.*
12. Inject the heparin solution. After 3 mL of solution has been injected, continue injecting, but remove the needle.	This prevents a vacuum effect at the distal end of the catheter, which would permit small amounts of blood to collect in the tip and occlude the catheter. *EO: The child has a catheter that will irrigate without difficulty.*
13. Remove gloves and mask.	
14. Tape the cap securely to the catheter hub.	
15. Document cap change in permanent record and place sign on bed as to the date of the next cap change.	

Irrigation of the Catheter

PROCEDURE	**RATIONALE/EXPECTED OUTCOME (EO)**
1. Draw up 5 mL of heparin flush into a syringe with a 23-gauge needle attached.	The catheter may become occluded by clot formation if not properly irrigated. The frequency of irrigation and the concentration of heparin may vary, depending on the child's vulnerability to the effects of heparin.

PROCEDURE	**RATIONALE/EXPECTED OUTCOME (EO)**

2. Set up a sterile field by opening sterile gloves on a flat surface.

3. Open povidone-iodine swab and drop onto sterile field.

4. Remove the protective sheath from the needle that is connected to the prefilled syringe and place the needle and syringe on the sterile field.

5. Put on gloves.

6. Wipe rubber tip of injection cap with povidone-iodine swab.

7. While holding the injection cap securely, insert the needle of the heparin flush into the rubber tip of the cap.

8. Draw back on syringe to get visible air bubbles out of the catheter and cap, but not enough to get blood into syringe.

EO: The child has a catheter with a good blood return prior to irrigation.

9. Inject the heparin solution. After 3 mL of solution is injected, continue injecting, but remove the needle.

If catheter is multi-lumen, each lumen must be irrigated.

Administration of Push Medications

1. Wash hands.

EO: The child's medications will be administered safely through the catheter.

2. Set up sterile field by opening sterile gloves on a flat surface.

3. Open povidone-iodine swabs and drop onto sterile field.

4. Remove the protective sheath from both needles connected to flush and medication syringes and place the needles and syringes on the sterile field.

5. Put on gloves.

6. Wipe rubber tip of injection cap with povidone-iodine swabs.

7. If the medication is compatible with heparin, insert the needle from the medication syringe into bull's-eye of injection cap. Draw back on syringe to get visible air bubbles out of the catheter, but not far enough to get blood into the syringe. Inject medication. Remove the needle and syringe from the injection cap. Wipe the cap with another povidone-iodine swab and flush catheter with a 3 mL heparin flush. If the medication is not compatible with heparin, flush the catheter before and after injecting the medication with normal saline and then heparinize catheter as the final step.

Consult an appropriate source for information on the safety of the IV push medication and its compatibility with heparin.

8. Document administration of medication.

Acquisition of Blood Samples

1. Wash hands.

2. Set up sterile field by opening sterile gloves on a flat surface.

EO: The child's blood is safely withdrawn from the catheter for laboratory tests.

PROCEDURE	**RATIONALE/EXPECTED OUTCOME (EO)**

3. Open povidone-iodine swabs and drop onto sterile field.

4. Remove the protective sheaths from all needles connected to syringes and place needles and syringes on sterile field.

5. Put on gloves.

6. Clean the rubber tip end of the injection cap with a povidone-iodine swab.

7. Insert needle from the empty 5-mL syringe into the injection cap. Draw a discard sample of 3–5 mL of blood. Withdraw the needle.

    This prevents dilution of the blood sample with saline and heparin or IV fluid.

8. Wipe injection cap again with povidone-iodine swab.

9. Insert needle from empty lab syringe and withdraw sample as ordered. Withdraw the needle.

    If using multi-lumen catheter, withdraw sample through the proximal lumen. Hickman catheters have an internal lumen large enough to allow for blood access or infusion. The Broviac catheter's internal diameter is smaller than the Hickman's; therefore, using the Broviac to draw blood is not recommended.

10. Flush catheter as outlined above. Document the amount of blood drawn and the child's response to the procedure.

11. If blood flow through the catheter is not brisk, ask the child and parents what usually facilitates blood withdrawal; or have the child try one or a combination of the following:

    The catheter may be lodged against the wall of the atrium.

    a. Change position (roll to side, sit upright, or lie flat).

    b. Take a deep breath or cough.

    c. Raise one or both arms overhead or lower arms.

    d. Perform Valsalva maneuver.

Repair of Damaged Catheter

1. Immediately clamp the catheter between the break and the patient, if the catheter leaks or is damaged.

    Prevent catheter damage by following these guidelines:
    Use smooth-edged clamps on the catheter.
    Do not use scissors to remove old dressings.
    Use ½–1-inch needles (no longer) for irrigations.
    Clamp over protective tap and rotate sites routinely.

    EO: The child's damaged catheter will be repaired using sterile technique.

2. Obtain needed equipment and set up sterile field.

3. Place the following on the sterile field:
Heparinized saline solution in syringe
Povidone-iodine swabs
Angiocatheters
Sterile scissors (from suture removal kit)
Injection cap.

4. Wash hands.

5. Put on gloves and mask.

6. Scrub approximately 2 inches of the line with pov-

PROCEDURE	**RATIONALE/EXPECTED OUTCOME (EO)**
idone-iodine swabs, starting at the site of the damage and wiping away from it in both directions.	
7. Using sterile scissors, cut through the newly prepped area of the catheter, leaving a smooth, even lumen.	
8. Withdraw stylus of angiocath approximately $\frac{1}{8}$ inch *prior* to insertion. Insert the largest possible angiocatheter into the remaining catheter and remove the stylus.	This will prevent a puncture to the catheter and further damage.
9. Follow the irrigation procedure and replace the injection cap or reconnect the IV fluids.	
10. Tape connections securely. Tape the newly repaired site to a tongue blade.	This will prevent the catheter from bending at the site of repair.
11. Document procedure and child's response. Notify the physician of the repair.	

Psychological Issues

1. Include the child and parents in the care of the catheter.	Having a catheter in place may be psychologically disturbing and may alter the child's body image related to physical appearance. *EO: The child and parents participate in catheter care.*
2. Provide a mirror so the child can look at the exit site.	*EO: The child and parents view the exit site.*
3. Arrange for the child and parents to visit with someone who has a right atrial catheter in place.	
4. Provide emotional support for their feelings.	*EO: The child and parents express concerns about physical appearance with catheter in place.*
5. Assess how the child and parents expect the catheter to affect the child's illness, recovery , and body; do not challenge their perceptions.	*EO: The child identifies ways of adapting to changed body image.*
6. Provide information as requested.	

Patient/Family Education: Home Care Considerations

1. Teach the child and parent the signs of site infection (for example, redness, warmth, inflammation, drainage, and tenderness).
2. Teach emergency actions for damaged catheter, dislodged injection cap, or accidental IV disconnection.
3. Instruct child and parents and have a return demonstration on site care and irrigation procedure.
4. Instruct parents to contact the physician whenever the catheter becomes clotted or dislodged; provide parents with a telephone reference list for assistance when problems occur.
5. If a flow control pump will be used in the home, demonstrate its correct operation.
6. Have child and parents administer medications or TPN using the procedures previously described.
7. Ensure that the teacher or school nurse knows safety measures for the care of the catheter; encourage parents to assist the teacher in preparing for the child's return to school.

References

Dufour, D.F. (1990). Information for teachers of children with central venous catheters. *Journal of Pediatric Oncology Nursing, 7*(1), 37–38.

Marcoox, C., Fisher, S., & Wong, D. (1990). Central venous access devices in children. *Pediatric Nursing, 16*(2), 123–133.

Meeske, K., & Davidson, L. (1988). Teacher's reference to right atrial catheters. *Journal of Pediatric Nursing, 3*(5), 351–353.

Nahata, M.C., King, D.R., Powell, D.A., et al. (1988). Management of catheter-related infections in pediatric patients. *Journal of Parenteral and Enteral Nutrition, 12*(1), 58–59.

Powell, C., Fabri, P.J., & Kudsk, K.A. (1988). Risk of infection accompanying the use of single lumen vs. double lumen subclavian catheters: A prospective randomized study. *Journal of Parenteral and Enteral Nutrition,* February, 127–129.

Young, G. P., Alexeyeff, M., Russell, D., et al (1988). Catheter sepsis during parenteral nutrition: The safety of long-term opSite dressings. *Journal of Parenteral and Enteral Nutrition,* April, 365–370.

Declotting Catheters with Urokinase

60

Definition/Purpose

When a central venous catheter or venous port becomes occluded, every attempt must be made to restore its patency. These catheters sometimes become occluded when the child changes position, so an attempt should first be made to have the child sit or lie differently or raise the arms above the head. If this technique does not work, the occlusion is most likely the result of a medication precipitate, a foreign body, a fibrin sheath, or a blood clot.

Approximately 80% of catheter occlusions in children are the result of blood clots. A clot develops when thrombin, an enzyme made from prothrombin, converts fibrinogen to fibrin, a collagen. The fibrin is what forms the clot. Normally, activated plasminogen forms plasmin, an enzyme that dissolves the clot in a process called fibrinolysis. This response to clotting does not take place in the lumen of a catheter or venous port; thus, a thrombolytic agent must be instilled to restore patency. This agent, *urokinase*, stimulates the conversion of plasminogen to plasmin, triggering fibrinolysis. Urokinase, unlike streptokinase, another thrombolytic agent, has a low incidence of allergic reactions and produces less systemic bleeding.

Standard of Care

1. The entire declotting procedure will be performed under strict aseptic technique.
2. The child's vital signs—temperature, pulse, respiration, and blood pressure—will be monitored every 30 minutes during the procedure and every 2 hours after the procedure for a total of 4 hours.
3. Urokinase can be instilled into the catheter twice within 2 hours. After 2–3 hours, the likelihood of declotting the catheter is slim.

Assessment

1. Assess pertinent history of previous occluded catheters or ports with the child and parent, and the treatment administered at that time.
2. Assess the reason the child has a central line and the propensity to hemorrhage or to have an allergic reaction.
3. Assess the child's and family's knowledge of the function, care, and complications related to the central line.
4. Assess the causes for a clotted central line (for example, inadequate heparinization of intravenous fluid infusing through the catheter, inadequate intravenous flow due to low infusion rate, or improper heparinization of capped line), and formulate a corrective plan.

Nursing Diagnoses

The following is a list of possible diagnoses and could apply, depending on the child's age, clinical situation, and physical condition:

Fear

Anxiety

High risk for injury

Planning

In order to declot a catheter, the following equipment must be assembled:

4 5-mL syringes

3 1½-inch 23-gauge needles

1 smooth-edged clamp

Sterile gloves

Sterile barrier

Mask

4 povidone-iodine swabs

2 5000 IU/mL vials of urokinase

1 10-mL vial of normal saline

1 10-mL vial of heparin flush (10 U/mL).

Interventions

PROCEDURE

1. Prepare the child and parent for the declotting procedure.

2. Check the child's vital signs—temperature, pulse, respiration, and blood pressure.

3. Put on mask.

4. Wash hands.

5. Assemble equipment on the sterile barrier, drawing up 3 mL of urokinase in one 5-mL syringe, 5 mL of normal saline in a second 5-mL syringe, and 5 mL of heparin flush in a third 5-mL syringe.

6. Clamp the catheter (Fig. 60-1).

RATIONALE/EXPECTED OUTCOME (EO)

EO: The child and parents will express their concerns to the staff.

Smaller syringes may create too much pressure and rupture an occluded line.

EO: The child will remain free from injury.

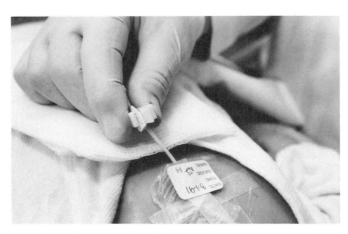

Figure 60-1.

PROCEDURE

7. Put on sterile gloves.
8. Disconnect intravenous tubing or injection cap from the central line.
9. Attach an empty 5-mL syringe to the catheter, unclamp it, and attempt to aspirate blood from the line (Fig. 60-2).

RATIONALE/EXPECTED OUTCOME (EO)

If blood is easily aspirated, the line is patent and should be irrigated with normal saline and either connected to the infusion fluid or capped and heparinized.

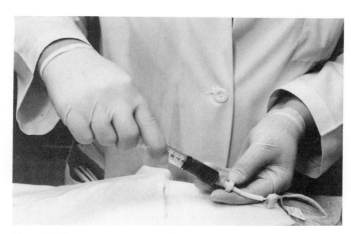

Figure 60-2.

10. If there is no blood return, reclamp the catheter and attach the 5-mL syringe with urokinase to hub.
11. Unclamp the catheter. Gently inject 2 mL of urokinase (5000 u/mL) into the catheter. If instillation meets resistance, use a repetitive push–pull action to maximize solution mixing within the catheter without creating excessive pressure.
12. Reclamp the catheter and allow the urokinase to remain in the line for 15–30 minutes.
13. Monitor the child for adverse reactions to the systemic urokinase:
    a. Inspect skin and mucous membranes to detect signs of bleeding.
    b. Report any signs and symptoms of hemorrhage (for example, decreased blood pressure, tachycardia, pallor, diaphoresis, or anxiety).
    c. Examine all urine and stool for gross evidence of bleeding; hematest urine and stool.
    d. Be alert to CNS symptoms resulting from intracranial hemorrhage (for example, headache, blurred vision, and decreased level of consciousness)
14. Remove urokinase syringe; replace with the empty 5-mL syringe.
15. Unclamp the catheter and attempt to aspirate blood from it. If there is no blood return, attempt aspiration at 5–10 minute intervals two more times. If catheter patency has not been reestablished by this

Occluded catheters may not accept a full 2 mL of solution. If strong resistance is felt, do not force the 2 mL into the catheter.

EO: The child has no bruising, petechiae, or bleeding, has normal vital signs for his or her age, and is free from pallor, diaphoresis, and anxiety.

PROCEDURE	**RATIONALE/EXPECTED OUTCOME (EO)**

time, the catheter should be clamped and the uro-kinase allowed to dwell for 30–60 minutes.

16. After the allotted time, unclamp the catheter and aspirate.

A second instillation of urokinase should be tried if catheter patency is not restored in 1–2 hours.

17. Once blood return is achieved, aspirate 4–5 mL of blood.

This will ensure the removal of any residual clot and urokinase.

18. Clamp catheter, remove syringe with blood, and connect the syringe with normal saline to hub.

19. Unclamp the catheter and irrigate with saline.

20. Clamp catheter, remove used syringe, and either connect the hub with infusion tubing and start infusion, or recap the line and heparinize.

EO: The child and parent(s) will indicate understanding of the results of the declotting procedure:
a. The integrity of the catheter is restored.
b. The integrity of the catheter is not restored and the catheter will need to be removed.

21. Document the declotting procedure and the child's response in the medical record.

Patient/Family Education: Home Care Considerations

1. If the catheter becomes clotted at home, review the heparinization technique with the family to determine if improper technique could have contributed to the occlusion. If this is the case, reteach the heparin flush procedure.

2. If the catheter becomes clotted in the hospital, explain the probable cause to the family and what corrective action will be taken to prevent further problems.

References

Bagnall, H.A., Gomperts, E., & Atkinson, J. (1989). Continuous infusion of low-dose urokinase in the treatment of central venous catheter thrombosis in infant and children. *Pediatrics, 83*(6), 963–966.

Brown, L.H., Wontroba, I., & Simonson, G. (1989). Reestablishing patency in an occluded central venous access device. *Critical Care Nurse, 9*(5), 114–118; 120–121.

Chan, M.K. (1987). Technique for restoring patency of occluded central venous catheters and infusion devices. *Pedidose News,* Chicago: Children's Memorial Hospital Pharmacy Service.

Cunliffe, M., & Polomano, R.C. (1986). How to clear catheter clots with urokinase. *Nursing '86, 16*(12), 40–43.

Wach, T. (1990). Urokinase administration in pediatric patients with occluded central venous catheters. *Journal of Intravenous Nursing, 13*(2), 100–102.

Total Parenteral Nutrition (Hyperalimentation and Intralipids)

61

Definition/Purpose

Total parenteral nutrition, sometimes called hyperalimentation, is the infusion of solutions containing dextrose, amino acids, lipids, minerals, vitamins, electrolytes, and trace elements into the blood to restore or maintain adequate nutrition in children who are unable to meet their needs via the gastrointestinal tract. Hypertonic solutions are administered via a right atrial catheter or central venous line. Less concentrated solutions may be given via a peripheral vein.

Standard of Care

1. Hypertonic infusates (greater than 10–12% dextrose) must be administered through a central venous catheter to avoid peripheral inflammation and thrombosis.
2. An infusion pump must be used to maintain a constant and correct flow of TPN.
3. TPN solution should be infused for no more than 24 hours per bottle.
4. Additives should not be infused into the TPN bottle or tubing. Medications to be administered should be given through a peripheral route, in the case of a single lumen central line, or through another lumen, as in the case of a multilumen central line. In situations when a peripheral route cannot be started, antibiotics or other life-saving drugs or blood products may have to be administered via the central line. When this is the case, the physician must write a specific order, stating that the medication is to be given through the central line. Any questions regarding compatibility of solutions and medications should be directed to the pharmacist.
5. Caloric requirements of the sick infant or child can be calculated according to these general guidelines:
   Infants: 120–150 cal/kg/day plus 130 mL of water/kg/day
   Toddlers or Older Children: 40–50 cal/kg/day plus 20 mL of water/kg/day.
   Adolescents: 40–50 cal/kg/day plus 20 mL of water/kg/day

Assessment

1. Assess the health history, with emphasis on problems that interfere with normal nutrition (for example, congenital defect, chemotherapy, burns, surgery, and respiratory compromise necessitating prolonged ventilatory support); the anticipated duration of treatment, and previous experience with TPN.
2. Assess for other chronic illnesses that may affect the treatment (for example, renal or cardiac disease or diabetes mellitus).
3. Assess the child's physical stature (height, weight, and head circumference) and plot on growth curve.
4. Assess the child's fluid status (skin turgor, edema, and moisture of mucous membranes); ability to ingest oral fluids; usual elimination patterns; the presence of draining wounds; and anticipated caloric needs.
5. Assess the psychosocial concerns and developmental factors that may affect the

initiation of TPN (for example, age, developmental level, daily activities, and resources to perform home parenteral nutrition).

6. Assess the child's and family's knowledge and acceptance of the health problem necessitating TPN, their understanding of the process of TPN, and their willingness to learn.

Nursing Diagnoses

The following is a list of possible diagnoses and could apply, depending on the child's age, clinical situation, and physical condition:

Altered nutrition, less than body requirements

High risk for injury

High risk for infection

Altered oral mucous membranes

Social isolation

Altered growth and development

Ineffective individual coping

Ineffective family coping

Planning

To administer TPN, assemble the following equipment:

TPN bottle

IV tubing with Luer lock connection

0.22-μm in-line filter

Infusion pump

Povidone-iodine swabs

Mask

Sterile gloves

Smooth-edged clamp

Tape

Sterile barrier

21-gauge straight needle

Interventions

PROCEDURE	**RATIONALE/EXPECTED OUTCOME (EO)**
1. Explain the rationale for TPN to the child and family. Explain how the procedure will be performed.	The child and family who understand the treatment for the health problem will be better able to participate in care and to support each other. *EO: The child and family will verbalize a need for TPN and cooperate with treatment.*
2. When the TPN fluid is delivered from the pharmacy, check the bottles against the order sheet. Do not hang the fluid if solution amounts or composition differ from the order.	This will ensure that the proper solution was prepared. *EO: The child will be free from injury associated with TPN.*

PROCEDURE

3. Check the solution for precipitates. Return it to the pharmacy if precipitates are present.

4. Refrigerate TPN until needed. Remove from refrigerator one hour before infusion.

5. Use strict aseptic technique when handling the catheter (See Chap. 59, Right Atrial Catheter).

6. Place sterile barrier on countertop. Put on mask.

7. Drop appropriate IV tubing and filter on sterile field.

8. Open povidine-iodine swabs and drop onto sterile field.

9. Put on sterile gloves.

10. Attach tubing to the TPN bottle and prime it, using caution not to contaminate distal end of tubing. Take off gloves (Fig. 61-1).

RATIONALE/EXPECTED OUTCOME (EO)

This may indicate incompatibility of components in the bottle.

Children receiving TPN may be malnourished and at greater risk of infection. Also, hypertonic glucose solution is an excellent culture medium for bacteria and yeast. Poor aseptic technique may result in contamination of the catheter or solution.

EO: The child will be free from infection.

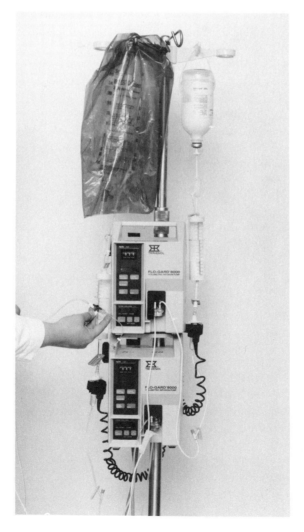

Figure 61-1.

PROCEDURE	**RATIONALE/EXPECTED OUTCOME (EO)**
11. Take bottle with tubing and filter to bedside. Clamp catheter with smooth-edged clamp. Put on sterile gloves. Disconnect old tubing and attach new tubing.	Disconnection of IV tubing attached to a central line without proper clamping may result in an air embolism or formation of clot at the distal end of the catheter.
12. Set pump for correct drops per min. Unclamp catheter and begin new infusion.	If child becomes short of breath, or has chest pain, coughing or cyanosis, clamp the catheter and position the child on his or her left side to keep air from going into pulmonary circulation, left heart, and atrial circulation.
	EO: The child is free from shortness of breath and chest pain.
13. Wipe off junction points of IV bag and tubing and IV tubing and catheter with povidone-iodine swabs.	The povidone-iodine will dry and form a seal at the connection points.
14. Remove gloves and mask.	
15. Tape all catheter connections securely to avoid disconnections.	
16. Check temperature every 4–6 hours and report evaluations above 37.8°C (99.6°F).	Persistent fevers may mean bacteremia, secondary to an infected catheter.
	EO: The child is afebrile.
	EO: The child has no redness, swelling, or discharge at the catheter insertion site.
17. Culture any purulent drainage from any part of the body.	
18. Monitor catheter insertion site hourly for signs of phlebitis and infiltration.	Infiltration of the solution (hyperosmolar) can cause tissue necrosis.
19. Do not increase rate to catch up if solution infuses too slowly; do not decrease rate rapidly if infusion is too fast.	Because TPN contains high glucose concentrations, insulin production is increased. If TPN rate is adjusted rapidly, blood sugar may fluctuate up or down, causing hypo- or hyperglycemia.
20. Check blood sugar or urine sugar/acetone every 4 hours for the first 48 hours and then every 8 hours. Observe for manifestations of hypoglycemia (for example, pallor, sweating, nausea, headache, blurred vision, and shakiness) or hyperglycemia (weakness nausea, thirst, and polyuria).	*EO: The child will maintain a serum glucose between 80–120 mg% or urine sugar of less than 3+.*
21. Measure height and weight daily on the same scale, as well as head circumference (in infants), and plot on a growth chart.	*EO: The child will grow along his or her own growth curve.*
22. Record intake and output; note unusual fluid losses, such as vomiting, diarrhea, or ostomies. Record specific gravity every 8 hours.	Urine volume should equal the amount of fluids infused minus insensible and extrarenal loss; use as a guideline to check for diuresis secondary to glucosuria.
	EO: The child will maintain a urine specific gravity below 1.015.
23. Administer intralipids as ordered using an infusion pump. Do not filter. Piggyback into TPN distal to filter using a 21-gauge needle into a rubber port.	The fat particles are too large to pass through a filter.
24. Take baseline vital signs and repeat every 10 minutes during the first 30 minutes of infusion to monitor for side effects of intralipids (for example, chills, fever, flushing, chest or back pains, vomiting, headache, and vertigo). Discontinue infusion if side effects occur.	*EO: The child will be free from injury associated with intralipids.*

PROCEDURE	**RATIONALE/EXPECTED OUTCOME (EO)**
25. Inspect oral mucous membranes every 8 hours.	TPN is hyperosmolar and may cause dehydration, thus drying the mucous membranes. These children may also be NPO and receive no oral stimulation from eating. *EO: The child will maintain oral mucous membrane integrity.*
26. Provide oral hygiene every 2–4 hours; massage gums.	
27. Provide an opportunity for infants to continue to develop their sucking reflex; offer a pacifier.	
28. Be an empathic and supportive listener for the child and family.	
29. Monitor for signs of depression and hopelessness.	
30. Work with overprotective family members to encourage the child to be independent.	Eating is a time to meet the body's need for nutrition and a time for social interaction. The child, unable to eat, may experience a grief process and become socially isolated. The catheter and IV tubing put restrictions on movement that limit exploration of the environment to attain developmental tasks. *EO: The child and family use effective coping behaviors to deal with the alteration in diet.* *EO: The child and family resume their normal schedule of activities, making changes as needed to protect the catheter.*
31. Educate the child and family regarding the treatments and long-term needs. Encourage parents to leave the child with other responsible persons and to take time for themselves.	
32. Ensure that parents have the address of a national or local support organization.	

Patient/Family Education: Home Care Considerations

1. Teach family or those who will administer TPN at home:
   a. Rationale for TPN
   b. Dressing change technique
   c. Symptoms to report to the physician
   d. Irrigation technique and injection cap changing technique
   e. Infusion setup via a pump
   f. Safety measures—
      - Keep pump out of reach of young children to prevent rate changes by the child.
      - Keep pump alarms on at all times.
      - Keep an intercom in child's room to monitor child and to be able to respond quickly to alarms.
      - Keep clamps readily accessible, in case catheter and tubing become disconnected.
      - Tuck catheter under clothing to prevent pulling at catheter and dressing.
2. Teach family to monitor intake and output and blood and urine glucose.
3. Teach family to weigh the child every other day on the same scale at the same time, in the same clothes.
4. Teach family to infuse solution at night while child is sleeping to decrease the interruption during the waking hours.

5. Refer family to support groups as necessary.

6. Ensure that child has an appointment for a return visit to the physician.

References

Barfoot, K. (1986). Home care of the child receiving nutritional support: A global approach. *Journal of the National Intravenous Therapy Association, 9*(3), 226–229.

Bender, J., & Faubion, W. (1985). Parenteral nutrition for the pediatric patient. *Home Healthcare Nurse, 3*(6), 32–39.

Brans, Y.W. (1990). Tolerance of fat emulsions in very low birthweight neonates: Effect of birthweight on plasma lipid concentrations. *American Journal of Perinatology, 7*(4), 114–117.

Frentner, S. (1987). Abdominal wall defects: Omphalocele and gastroschisis. *Neonatal Network, 6*(3), 29–41.

Orr, M.J., & Allen, S.S. (1986). Optional oral experiences for infants on long-term total parenteral nutrition. *Nutrition in Clinical Practice, 1*(12), 288–295.

Zlotkin, S., Stallings, V., & Pencherz, P. (1985). Total parenteral nutrition in children, *Pediatric Clinics of North America, 32*(2), 381–400.

Intraosseous Infusion

62

Definition/Purpose

Intraosseous infusion is defined as access to a child's general circulation via the bone marrow. First developed in the 1930s, intraosseous infusion is recommended for emergency administration of fluid and drugs. Since the bone marrow circulation communicates directly with the general circulation, fluids administered into marrow are immediately absorbed. The circulation times of intraosseous and IV fluid injections are the same. IV access is still preferred, but in situations when venous access is difficult, bone marrow infusions should be considered early in resuscitative efforts as an alternative to surgical techniques.

Among its advantages, bone marrow infusion results in a secure access to the circulation that is difficult for an uncooperative child to dislodge. The technique is also preferred over IV infusion in severely burned patients because the small bone-marrow blood vessels act as a filter to prevent pulmonary emboli.

Blood products, saline, plasma, glucose, Ringer's lactate, dopamine, dobutamine, and various antibiotics have been administered through intraosseous routes. Nearly any drug administered by IV infusion can be administered by intraosseous infusion.

The bony sites adaptable to intraosseous infusion in infants and small children are the tibia, the femur, and the iliac crest. Because the sternum is thin and underdeveloped in the child, this site should be used in adolescents only.

Standard of Care

1. Intravenous access should be achieved during the first 5 minutes of a resuscitation. It involves the use of multiple standard IV techniques applied in a sequential fashion when initial insertion of a peripheral IV catheter fails (Fig. 62-1).

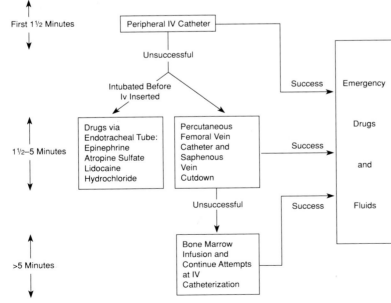

Figure 62-1.

2. Use an intraosseous infusion site for the least possible amount of time, but for no more than 2–3 days at one site.

3. All fluids infused through the intraosseous infusion site are filtered by a .22-μm in-line filter.

4. The intraosseous tubing is changed every 48 hours.

5. The dressing is changed every 24 hours.

Assessment

1. Assess pertinent history and physical findings to determine the need for rapid fluid or medication resuscitation.

2. Assess physical findings that would contraindicate the use of intraosseous infusion (for example, underlying infection, bony abnormality, or bone lesion).

3. Assess for allergies.

4. Assess the family's knowledge of the therapy and the reason for the intraosseous infusion.

Nursing Diagnoses

The following is a list of possible diagnoses and could apply, depending on the child's age, clinical situation, and physical condition:

High risk for injury

High risk for infection

Impaired skin integrity

Ineffective family coping, disabling

Impaired physical mobility

Pain

Planning

When preparing for an intraosseous infusion, the following equipment must be assembled:

Body or extremity restraints

Sterile barrier

2 2 × 2 split gauze dressing

Povidone-iodine ointment

4 Povidone-iodine swabs

1% lidocaine

1 3-mL syringe with 25-gauge needle for lidocaine

Sterile gloves

IV infusion set with tubing and filter

2-inch adhesive tape

1 10-mL syringe containing 5-mL of sterile normal saline

1 No. 11 scalpel blade

Needles to enter the bone marrow

    Standard bone marrow needles, trephine needles, 18- or 20-gauge short spinal needles, or 14-, 16-, or 18-gauge hypodermic needles may be used. Although trephine bone needles are preferred, they are rarely available during an emergency so the standard hypodermic needle is used most often. Since an open-channel needle may become obstructed with marrow or bone chips, a second smaller-gauge needle may have to be introduced through the lumen of the first needle to clear the obstruction.

Interventions

PROCEDURE	**RATIONALE/EXPECTED OUTCOME (EO)**

1. Gather equipment.

2. Bundle or "mummy" the child and further restrain the extremity with a limb holder. A small sandbag should be placed underneath the extremity immediately behind the operative site.

3. Wash hands.

EO: The child will have the infusion needle inserted in a safe, aseptic manner.

4. Open up sterile field.

5. Open povidone-iodine swabs and drop onto sterile field.

The insertion procedure is accomplished using sterile technique.

6. Drop scalpel blade onto sterile field.

7. Remove the protective sheaths from all needles connected to syringes and place needles and syringes on sterile field.

8. Open the package with marrow needle and drop onto sterile field.

9. Put on sterile gloves.

10. Cleanse area of intended insertion with povidone-iodine swabs, working in a circular motion from insertion site outward.

11. Assist the physician in the insertion of the needle. After the area has been cleaned and anesthetized, a small incision is made in the skin with a No. 11 blade.

The incision will facilitate insertion of the needle.

The needle is then inserted through the skin and into the bone until a sudden lack of resistance signals entry into the medullary cavity (Fig. 62-2).

EO: The child has the intraosseous needle inserted with minimal trauma.

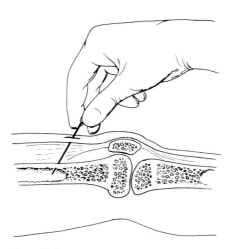

Figure 62-2.

PROCEDURE

The 10-mL syringe filled with saline is attached to the needle in the bone. Withdraw slightly through the needle and then infuse the saline.

12. Detach the syringe and connect the intraosseous tubing, infusing ordered fluids.
13. Apply a small dab of povidone-iodine ointment around the needle.
14. Place the split 2 × 2s around the needle in opposite directions.
15. Place tape over the 2 × 2s to hold the dressing in place.
16. Coil intraosseous tubing and secure it to the extremity (Fig. 62-3).

RATIONALE/EXPECTED OUTCOME (EO)

Marrow should be easily aspirated and saline easily administered without significant subcutaneous infiltration.

EO: The needle that has been inserted will irrigate without difficulty.

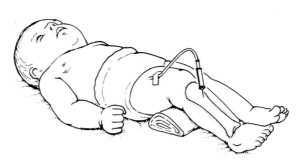

Figure 62-3.

17. Every hour, assess the restrained extremity for pulse, movement, sensation, temperature, and color.
18. Check for pressure areas every hour.
19. Every hour, touch site around the needle to check whether skin is soft or taut.

20. Check for symmetry of limbs. Complications may include:
    a. Local abscess or cellulitis
    b. Subcutaneous leakage from around the needle
    c. Osteomyelitis
    d. Sepsis.
21. If the infusion stops, the needle may be styletted and flushed with saline.
22. Document the procedure and the child's tolerance in the medical record.

Physical restraining devices are used to keep the child from moving and dislodging the needle.

EO: The child maintains patent intraosseous infusion.

EO: The child requires minimal restraint.

Taut skin indicates leakage of fluid under the skin or an infectious process around the needle.

EO: The child was strong, equal pulses, movement sensation, and temperature; the child has normal neurovascular checks in extremity.

Once a foreign body is introduced into the child's body, the risk of infection increases.

EO: The child is afebrile.

Marrow or bone chips may occlude the needle.

EO: The medical record will reflect the child's tolerance to the procedure.

Patient/Family Education: Home Care Considerations

1. Discuss with the family why the infusion is necessary. The child and parents need information and teaching in order to deal with intraosseous equipment, to cope with limitations of movement, and to help prevent complications.

2. Explain that the intraosseous needle is a short-term solution to circulatory access and that a more permanent line will need to be inserted via cutdown or central line insertion.

3. Teach the parents how to provide adequate stimulation for the child to meet his or her normal growth and development needs.

References

Berg, R.A. (1984). Emergency infusion of catecholamines into bone marrow. *American Journal of Diseases in Children,* 138, 810–811.

Fisher, D.H. (1990). Intraosseous infusion. *New England Journal of Medicine, 322*(22), 1579–1581.

Kanter, R.K., Zimmerman, J.J., Strauss, R.H., et al. (1986). Pediatric emergency intravenous access. *American Journal of Diseases in Children,* 140, 132–134.

LaFleche, F.R., Stepin, M.J., Vargas, J., et al (1989). Iatrogenic biolateral tibial fractures after intraosseous infusion attempts in a 3-month-old infant. *Annals of Emergency Medicine, 18*(10), 125–127.

Orlowski, J.P., Julius, C.J., Petras, R.E., et al (1989). The safety of intraosseous infusions: Risks of fat and bone marrow emboli to the lungs. *Annals of Emergency Medicine, 18*(10), 72–78.

Seigler, R.S., Tecklenburg, F.W., Shealy, R. et al (1989). Prehospital intraosseous infusion by emergency medical services personnel: A prospective study. *Pediatrics 84*(1), 173–177.

Spivey, W. (1987). Intraosseous infusions. *The Journal of pediatrics, 111*(5), 639–643.

Tidwell, B., & Parks, B. R. (1991). Intraosseous infusions. *Pediatric Nursing, 17*(1), 56–57.

Turkel, H. (1983). Intraosseous infusion. *American Journal of Diseases in Children,* 137, 706.

Hydration Assessment

63

Definition/Purpose

The kidney is the organ most responsible for maintenance of stable extracellular fluid volume and composition. During a variety of conditions, the kidney adjusts the amount and type of acids and ions that are secreted and absorbed from blood plasma.

Common Clinical Conditions

Dehydration: Hypernatremic (hypertonic)

Etiology

Hypernatremic dehydration results from a loss of both fluid and electrolytes. In this type of condition, however, the loss of free water exceeds the loss of sodium and other solutes. It can occur as a result of diarrhea, vomiting, burns, high fever, diabetes, insipidus, inappropriate parenteral alimentation, aggressive dialysis, increased respiratory insensible water loss, and administration of large amounts of sodium bicarbonate or mannitol. Diabetic ketoacidosis can also produce dehydration as a result of the osmotic diuresis produced by glucosuria. The administration of infant formula inappropriately mixed from concentrate can also produce hypernatremia.

Pathophysiology

The serum sodium concentration and serum osmolality will increase, even though total body sodium concentration is decreased. The increase in intravascular osmolality stimulates antidiuretic hormone (ADH) and aldosterone secretion. ADH secretion increases free water reabsorption, but aldosterone increases both water and sodium reabsorption. If the fluid loss is significant and reduces intravascular volume and compromises perfusion, aldosterone increases further, thus perpetuating hypernatremia. Fluid shifts from the cells into the vascular space as a result of osmosis; consequently, fluid lost in hypertonic dehydration is largely intracellular. The most important tissue damaged by these fluid shifts is the brain, resulting in cerebral damage, effusions, thrombosis, and hemorrhage.

Signs and Symptoms

Indications of hypernatremic dehydration include weight loss, depression of anterior fontanelle, doughy skin over the abdomen, gray skin color, dry mucous membranes, irritable, hyperactive reflexes, serum sodium over 150 m Eq/L, elevated CSF protein, and proteinuria.

Interventions

Management is geared to *gradual* correction of the fluid and electrolyte deficit and prevention of CNS complications (such as seizures). If the child is demonstrating signs of poor systemic perfusion (for example, tachycardia, vasoconstriction, poor capillary refill, oliguria, or hypotension), a single rapid infusion (10–20 mL/kg) may be ordered. Next, fluids and electrolytes can be replaced gradually over 48 hours so the serum sodium does not fall more than 10 m Eq/24 hrs.

Dehydration: Hypotonic

Etiology

Hypotonic dehydration occurs when the child's sodium losses exceed free water losses or when salt-poor solutions are infused. The most common causes of hypotonic dehydration include gastroenteritis and inappropriate intravenous therapy. Other causes include gastric suction, inappropriate ADH secretion, and water enemas.

Pathophysiology

Since sodium and chloride are distributed in the intravascular space, loss of salt can reduce intravascular osmolality. As a result, water moves from the intravascular to the intracellular space. The circulating blood volume is reduced.

Signs and Symptoms

Indications of hypotonic dehydration include sunken eyes, dry mucous membranes, depressed fontanel, tachycardia, tented skin turgor, irritability, cool and clammy skin, decreased peripheral pulses, decreased urine output, low cardiac output, decreased blood pressure, and serum sodium concentration of less than 130 m Eq/L.

Interventions

If signs of circulatory failure are evident, the immediate goal of therapy is restoration of adequate circulating blood volume. A rapid infusion of normal saline or lactated Ringer's solution (10–20 mL/kg) may be ordered. It may be repeated two or three times to ensure acceptable blood pressure and perfusion. Next, fluid replacement is calculated so that deficits are corrected within 24 hours, with the first half of the deficit corrected during the first 8 hours.

Dehydration: Isotonic

Etiology

Isotonic dehydration reflects a loss of total body water coupled with a loss of sodium in equal volumes. Children may lose fluid through the gastrointestinal tract, the kidneys, and the skin. Gastrointestinal losses account for most instances of isotonic dehydration.

Pathophysiology

The daily maintenance of fluid is directly related to caloric expenditure. Because skin surface area correlates best with caloric expenditure, this parameter often serves as a guide to fluid therapy. Alternately, weight alone can provide a basis for establishing requirements. The final sodium in the extracellular fluid (ECF) is a function of what is lost from the body and the composition of replacement fluids. The initial loss of fluid from the body depletes the ECF. Water shifts from the intracellular space to maintain the ECF, and this fluid is lost if dehydration persists.

Signs and Symptoms

Indications of isotonic dehydration include absence of tears, fewer wet diapers, dry skin and mucous membranes, tachycardia, hypotension, tachypnea, poor peripheral perfusion, urine specific gravity above 1.020, normal serum sodium, normal potassium, and elevated BUN.

Interventions

The child in shock demands fluid resuscitation and monitoring. An initial fluid bolus of 20 mL/kg of saline given in 30–60 minutes is the treatment of choice. Sufficient fluids are administered during the first 24 hours, with half the deficit replaced within the first 8 hours.

Standard of Care

Fluid Volume Deficit

Clinical Parameters	Mild	Moderate	Severe
1. Body weight loss			
Infant/Child	5% (50 mL/kg)	10% (100 mL/kg)	15% (150 mL/kg)
Adult	3% (30 mL/kg)	6% (60 mL/kg)	9% (90 mL/kg)
2. Skin turgor	Normal	Mild tenting	Severe, prolonged tenting
3. Fontanelle	Fat	Depressed/soft	Significantly depressed/sunken
4. Mucous membranes	Dry	Very Dry	Parched
5. Skin color/feel	Normal/moist	Gray/dry	Mottled/clammy
6. Urine output	1.0 mL/kg/hr	> .5 mL/kg/hr	Minimal to no urine output
7. Azotemia	Absent	Present	Present and severe
8. Pulse	Normal	Slightly elevated	Tachycardic
9. Blood pressure	Normal	Above normal	Reduced
10. Sensorium	Normal Consolable	Lethargic Irritable	Convulsions Lethargy
11. Eyeballs	Normal	Deep set	Sunken
12. Specific gravity of urine	1.015–1.020	1.020–1.030	< 1.030
13. Cardiovascular	CVP, BP normal	CVP, BP decreased	CVP, BP, capillary filling markedly decreased

Assessment

1. Assess the pertinent history and physical findings for:
   a. the course of the illness
   b. others sick at home
   c. home care regarding diet and fluids
   d. normal weight of the child
   e. normal bowel pattern
   f. vital signs
   g. level of consciousness
   h. level of hydration
   i. stool characteristics (amount, color, blood in stool, reducing substances)
   j. vomiting
   k. condition of skin
   l. indications of pain.

2. Assess the psychosocial and developmental factors in regard to coping mechanisms, habits, and the impact of isolation (if necessary).

3. Assess the family's knowledge of nutrition and diet, the communicability of the disease, and their readiness to learn.

Nursing Diagnoses

The following is a list of possible diagnoses and could apply, depending on the child's age, clinical situation, and physical condition:

Fluid volume deficit

Altered nutrition, less than body requirements

Impaired skin integrity

Diversional activity deficit

Pain

Planning

In planning to assess hydration, the following equipment must be assembled:

Thermometer

Stethoscope

Mechanical intravenous regulator

Blood pressure machine

Scale

Refractometer for specific gravity determination.

Interventions

PROCEDURE	**RATIONALE/EXPECTED OUTCOME (EO)**
1. Monitor vital signs every 4 hours or more often. Record and report abnormalities to the physician.	Continued loss of fluids by vomiting, diarrhea, burns, and GI suction causes imbalances in electrolytes and fluids. Excessive output without replacement leads to fluid deficits.
2. Monitor for signs of increasing dehydration as listed on accompanying Fluid Volume Deficit chart. (See Standard of Care.)	*EO: The child shows improving skin turgor and moist mucous membranes.*
3. Monitor IV every hour, regulating it with a mechanical device and microdrip chamber. Restrain the child to preserve patent IV.	
4. Record intake and output; weigh diapers if needed.	*EO: The child demonstrates urine output within acceptable limits (1 mL/kg/hr).*
5. Check specific gravity of urine every 4 hours.	*EO: The specific gravity of the child's urine will be 1.002–1.020.*
6. Weigh child daily at the same time and on the same scale; he or she may need to be weighed more often at the beginning of the treatment.	*EO: The child will return to pre-illness weight.*
7. Monitor laboratory reports and report abnormal values to the physician.	*EO: The child demonstrates normal laboratory values.*
8. Maintain NPO or diet as ordered by the physician. Resume diet slowly, progressing from clear liquids to half-strength and then full-strength formulas. Finally, reintroduce solid foods.	If the hydrational problem is due to vomiting or diarrhea, the body cannot absorb nutrients; thus, the child may lose weight and will fail to grow. *EO: The child will experience cessation of the cause of the hydrational problem and will maintain growth and development.*
9. Change previous diet if it has caused hydrational problems. Report tolerance for new diet to the physician.	
10. Lubricate the skin with lotion.	Diarrheal stools are alkaline and contain enzymes that excoriate the skin. *EO: The child will experience intact skin.*
11. Provide oral hygiene every 8 hours (or more often if needed.)	
12. Change position every 2 hours.	*EO: The child will be comfortable and experience relief from pain.*

PROCEDURE	**RATIONALE/EXPECTED OUTCOME (EO)**
13. Schedule time every hour for verbal and physical contact.	
14. Encourage parents to visit and interact with child.	*EO: The child will be free from boredom and emotional disturbances related to hospitalization and illness.*
15. Provide the infant and child with sucking stimulation.	The infant should be provided with security objects from home. Comfort measures (such as a pacifier) are especially important when the infant is denied food.
16. Use bright, washable toys, pictures, and mobiles to vary the environment.	

Patient/Family Education: Home Care Considerations

1. Instruct parents about the presumed cause of the illness and how to recognize and prevent it in the future.

2. Teach the danger signs related to dehydration (for example, loss of appetite, fever, vomiting, diarrhea, decreased urination, change in level of consciousness, absence of tears, and dry mucous membranes).

3. Explain the methods of treatment that parents may use at home to rehydrate their child (for example, a diet of clear liquids and the BRAT diet—bananas, rice, applesauce, and toast).

References

Barkin, B.M. (1990). Treatment of the dehydrated child. *Pediatric Annals, 19*(10), 597–603.

Hazinski, M.F. (1988). Understanding fluid balance in the seriously ill child. *Pediatric Nursing, 14*(3), 231–236.

Hinkle, A.J. (1989). Pediatric blood and fluid therapy. *Current Reviews of Nurse Anesthetics, 12*(6), 43–48.

Lybrand, M., Cooper, B.M., & Munro, B.H. (1990). Periodic comparison of specific gravity using urine from a diaper and collecting bag. *Journal of Maternal Child Nursing, 15*(4), 238–239.

Implantable Venous Port

64

Definition/Purpose

Vascular access problems develop most commonly in pediatric oncology patients receiving chemotherapy. Venous irritation from anticancer drugs and the need for repeated venipuncture for a period of months to years result in sclerosis, thrombosis, and destruction of surface veins. In children with poor peripheral veins, oncologists recommend placement of a central venous catheter for venous access to circumvent the high risk of extravasation from administration of vesicant chemotherapy. The use of the traditional Hickman and Broviac catheters has improved the quality of life and comfort of those undergoing therapy. The implantable catheter system potentially obviates three shortcomings of these traditional catheters: care of the catheter, altered body image, and the risk of infection.

Traditional catheters require dressing changes and frequent flushes when not in use, whereas the implantable system requires no dressings, and flushes are necessary only once every 4 weeks. Because the implantable system leaves little visible evidence of its presence, it is advantageous for adolescents who are concerned about their appearance. Most important, the risk of infection is theoretically less than that with traditional catheters. Recent studies implicate the catheter entrance site and catheter hub as entry portals for bacteria; with the implantable system, the skin acts as a contiguous barrier against the risk of infection.

The venous port is implanted under local or general anesthesia. The appropriate catheter tip is introduced into the superior vena cava. The catheter is then tunneled to a prepared subcutaneous pocket for the port. The port is held in place to the fascia with a nonabsorbable suture material. The port is positioned so the upper edge is palpable through the skin (Fig. 64–1).

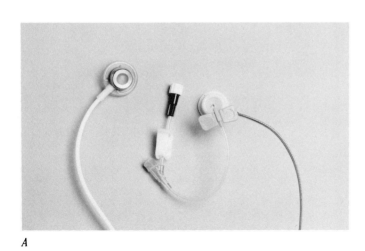

A

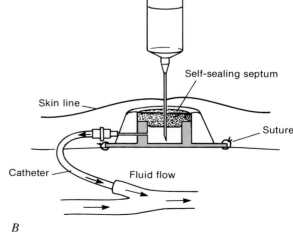

B

Figure 64-1.

Standard of Care

1. The injection site and the catheter tract must be inspected daily for signs of infection for example, redness, tenderness, and drainage at the port or tract site).
2. Following the injection of medication, the system must be flushed with 5 mL heparinized saline (100 U/mL).
3. Once every 3–4 weeks, the port must be flushed with 5 mL heparinized saline (100 U/mL).
4. The port can be entered only with a 22-gauge Huber needle.
5. Entering the port will be accomplished using sterile technique.
6. Change intravenous tubing every 24 hours.
7. Change needle every 7 days for a continuous infusion.
8. Change dressing every 3–5 days.

Assessment

1. Assess pertinent history for any previous experience with central catheters or venous ports.
2. Assess physical findings for location of previous central access sites.
3. Assess psychosocial and developmental factors for the child's coping mechanisms for painful procedures, age and developmental level, previous experience with central access ports, and habits or routines that would affect the success of a port.
4. Assess the family's knowledge and level of acceptance of the venous port.

Nursing Diagnoses

The following is a list of possible diagnoses and could apply, depending on the child's age, clinical situation, and physical condition:

Anxiety

Fear

High risk for infection

High risk for injury

Impaired skin integrity

Pain

Planning

In planning to care for a child with an implantable venous port the following equipment should be gathered:

Sterile barrier

Sterile gloves

3 povidone-iodine swabs

Sterile extension tubing

22-gauge Huber needle

2 6-mL syringes of saline

2 6-mL syringes of heparinized saline (100 U/mL)

Medication to be administered

Alcohol swabs

Adhesive bandage

Sterile 2 × 2 gauze pad
Tincture of benzoin
½-inch Steri-strips
Transparent dressing
IV tubing connected to infusion pump

Interventions

PROCEDURE

Inserting the Needle

1. Palpate the port to find the entry septum.
2. Put on sterile gloves.
3. Clean the injection site with povidone-iodine, starting at the center of the septum. Swab outward in a circular motion until an area 6 inches in diameter is cleaned.

4. Repeat procedure twice, using a new swab each time (Fig. 64-2).

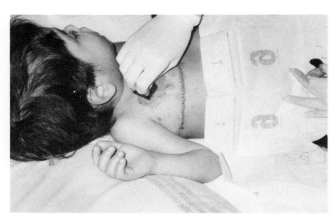

Figure 64-2.

RATIONALE/EXPECTED OUTCOME (EO)

EO: The child will have the port identified by palpation.

Once a foreign object has been introduced into the child's body, the risk of infection increases.

EO: The child will have the venous port entered using sterile technique.
The child will remain free from infection.

Regular needles   Huber needles

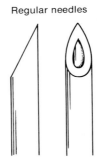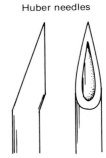

Figure 64-3.

5. Attach a 6-mL/syringe of heparin solution to the end of the extension tubing.
6. Attach the Huber needle to the other end of the extension tubing and prime the tubing and needle with the heparin solution (Fig. 64-3).

7. Palpate skin again to find the rim of the port. Insert needle through skin and septum at a 90° angle to the skin. Feel the needle go through the septum and reach a stopping point. Do not rock or rotate the needle once it is in place.
8. Aspirate a small amount of blood (Fig. 64-4).

This will expel all air from the needle and tubing. The Huber needle minimizes septum damage or coring.
EO: The Huber needle and tubing will be primed with heparinized solution.

EO: The child will experience quick resolution of the pain associated with entering the port.

This will damage the septum.

This will confirm the placement of the needle. It must be

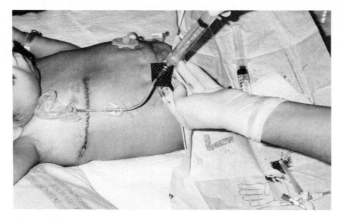

Figure 64-4.

PROCEDURE	**RATIONALE/EXPECTED OUTCOME (EO)**
	noted that at times you may not be able to aspirate blood but may still be able to infuse fluid.
	EO: The child will ideally have a good return prior to catheter irrigation.
Injecting a Bolus	
9. Using steady pressure, flush the port with 5 mL heparin solution.	If swelling occurs or the child complains of pain or burning as you inject the heparin, the needle is improperly positioned.
	EO: The child has the port irrigated without difficulty.
10. Disconnect syringe and discard.	Be sure to close slide-lock clamp whenever tubing end is disconnected from syringes.
11. Attach the 6-mL syringe of saline to extension tubing and flush.	
12. Close slide-lock clamp; disconnect the syringe and discard.	Flushing the system of the heparin solution prevents a reaction between the heparin and other medication to be infused.
13. Attach the syringe with the medication, open clamp, and inject slowly.	*EO: The child has medication infused through the port without difficulty.*
14. Close slide-lock clamp; disconnect syringe and discard.	
15. Attach 6-mL syringe of saline solution, open clamp, and flush the tubing, needle, and port.	Flushing the system of the infused medication assures that the total dose of the medication is injected into the blood and that the medication will not react with the heparin flush.
16. Close slidelock clamp and attach heparinized saline syringe; flush. Pull the needle straight out as the last $\frac{1}{2}$ mL is injected.	Heparin prevents clotting of the port.
	This prevents backflow of blood into the port.
17. Clean area on top of port with alcohol and apply adhesive bandage.	
18. Document medication given and any complaints voiced by the child. Note whether blood could be aspirated from the port.	*EO: The child and family will use appropriate coping strategies to promote adaptation of having a port in place.*
Continuous Infusion	
19. Prepare the site and insert the needle into the port as in steps 1–8 above, flushing the heparin solution	*EO: The child's skin will remain intact at the port site and along the catheter tract.*

PROCEDURE	**RATIONALE/EXPECTED OUTCOME (EO)**
out of the port and connecting the infusion line after the needle is in the port.	
20. Roll up the 2 × 2 gauze pad and place it under the needle hub.	This will support the needle.
21. Apply tincture of benzoin to the skin on both sides of the gauze pad.	This will help the Steri-strips adhere.
22. Secure the needle and tubing by applying Steri-strips across the needle hub using a chevron taping technique.	
23. Apply transparent dressing to cover injection site; pinch around junction of needle and extension tubing to make dressing occlusive.	The transparent dressing is an added barrier against infection. *EO: The child or the port will not be injured by dislodged needle.*
24. Begin the continuous infusion at the prescribed rate.	
25. When the infusion is complete, close slide-lock clamp and disconnect the IV line. Attach a 6-mL syringe of saline, open clamp, and flush the port. Close clamp and attach a 6-mL syringe of heparinized saline. Open clamp and flush, removing the needle as the last $\frac{1}{2}$ mL is injected.	
26. Clean area on top of port with alcohol and apply adhesive bandage.	
27. Document infusion (as before).	

Patient/Family Education: Home Care Considerations

1. The child and family will be educated about what a venous port is, what advantages it offers, and how the system works before and after the port is inserted.
2. Educate the family about what to watch for after the port is inserted:
   a. Examine skin around port daily to detect any changes.
   b. Notify the physician of fever or redness, tenderness, or swelling near the portal site.
   c. Notify the physician if the port has moved or if there is pain or a burning sensation at the site.
   d. Resist the urge to rub the skin over the port.
3. Stress to the family the importance of keeping appointments for heparinization of the port.
4. Encourage the child and family to carry an identification card so vital information is available when visiting the hospital, clinic, or emergency room.
5. Stress to the family the importance of the child's returning to school and participating in activities as able. Caution the family, however, against the child's participation in contact sports or other activities that could move or damage the port.

References

Kandt, K.A. (1991). An implantable venous access device for children. *Journal of Maternal Child Nursing, 16*(2), 88–91.

Lokich, J. (1985). Complications and management of implanted venous access catheters. *Journal of Clinical Oncology, 3* (5), 710–717.

Mirro, J. (1989). A Prospective study of Hickman/Broviac catheters and implantable ports in pediatric oncology patients. *Journal of Clinical Oncology, 7* (2), 214–222.

Raffensperger, J.G. (1990). *Swenson's pediatric surgery.* Norwalk, Connecticut: Appleton & Lange.

Shulman, R.J. (1987). A Totally implanted venous access system used in pediatric patients with cancer. *Journal of Clinical Oncology, 5* (1), 137–140.

Speciale, J.L., & Kaalaas, J. (1985). Infuse-A-Port: New path for IV chemotherapy. *Nursing '85, 15*(10), 40–43.

Strum, S. (1986). Improved methods for venous access: The Port-A-Cath, a totally implanted catheter system. *Journal of Clinical Oncology, 4* (4), 596–603.

Wallace, J., & Zeltzer, P. (1987). Benefits, complications and care of implantable infusion devices in 31 children with cancer. *Journal of Pediatric Surgery, 22,* 833.

Your child will soon be discharged from the hospital with a central line catheter. This teaching guide will introduce you to the skills you will be learning in order to care for your child with a central line catheter at home.

You will be practicing these skills with a nurse while your child is still in the hospital, so that by the time of discharge you will understand and feel comfortable caring for the catheter.

After reading this guide (it is yours to keep) please feel free to ask questions and express any concerns you may have. Remember that the nurse will demonstrate these skills to you first and that you will have many chances to practice and to ask questions.

A central line catheter can be inserted for many purposes. The catheter, generally located on the chest or abdomen, enters a vein and is advanced so that the end rests in a larger vein that enters the heart (Fig. 1)

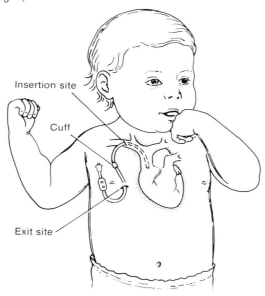

Insertion site

Cuff

Exit site

Figure 1.

The cuff you feel around the catheter at the exit site helps to hold the catheter in place. The area around the catheter heals within 2 to 3 weeks after insertion. After this, it is difficult to remove the catheter accidentally. Remember that the catheter is not painful to your child. This catheter can be used when a child has a limited number of veins and may have long-term needs for IV access. Blood samples can also be painlessly obtained from the catheter by your nurse or doctor.

The skills you will be learning include how to put on sterile gloves, how to flush the catheter with a heparinized saline solution, changing the dressing over the insertion site, and changing the injection cap.

How to Put on Sterile Gloves

1. Wash hands with hot soapy water for 1 full minute.
2. Peel open the package of the glove wrapper and place it on a clean workspace.
3. Pull the inside fold of the open wrapper in an outward direction, pulling it taut so it does not fold back.
4. Gloves are positioned inside the package so the right-hand glove is on the right and the left-hand glove is on the left. Both gloves have a cuff at the bottom.
5. With your left hand, pick up the lower *inside* edge of the cuff of the right-hand glove and insert your right hand.
6. With your gloved right hand, tuck your fingers *outside* the cuff of the left hand.
7. Pick up the left glove and insert your left hand, being careful not to let any part of your bare hand touch your gloved right hand.
8. Once both your hands are gloved, you may touch no body parts except your gloved hands to adjust your fingers in the gloves.

How to Flush the Catheter with a Heparinized Saline Solution

Purpose

The catheter requires flushing twice a day with a heparinized saline solution to prevent blood from clotting off the line. Flushings should be done approximately 12 hours apart. The concentration of heparinized saline solution you will be using is *10 units of heparin to every 1 mL of saline.*

1. Gather the following supplies:
   a. Package of sterile gloves
   b. Heparin saline solution (10 U/1 mL saline)
   c. 3-mL syringe with needle
   d. Povidone-iodine swabs
2. Select a quiet clean place in your home to flush the catheter. Keep work area clean and wipe down the surface with soap and water.
3. Wash hands with hot soapy water for 1 full minute.
4. If necessary, attach needle to syringe. DO NOT touch the tip of syringe or the end of the needle.
5. Wipe off the tip of the heparin bottle with a povidone-iodine swab.
6. Remove needle cover. Pull back plunger to 3-mL mark. Inject the 3 mL of air into the bottle; turn the bottle upside down.
7. Withdraw 3 mL of the heparin flush solution.
8. With the needle pointing up, tap the syringe to shift the air bubbles to the top of the syringe. Push out all of the air. *It is extremely important that no air bubbles ever enter the catheter!*
9. Carefully replace the needle cover.
10. Set up a sterile field by opening the package of sterile gloves on your clean flat surface, following the instructions at the beginning of this Teaching Guide.
11. Open a povidone-iodine swab and drop it onto the sterile field.
12. Carefully remove the protective cover from the prefilled syringe and place the syringe onto the sterile field.
13. Put on sterile gloves.
14. Wipe the injection cap with a povidone-iodine swab.
15. Holding the injection cap securely, take the syringe and insert the needle into the tip of the injection cap. (Again, be sure there are no air bubbles in the syringe.)
16. Before you begin injecting, you must open the clamp.
17. Slowly begin injecting the 3 mL of heparin solution into the cap. As you inject the last $\frac{1}{2}$ mL of solution, clamp the line shut (Fig. 2).

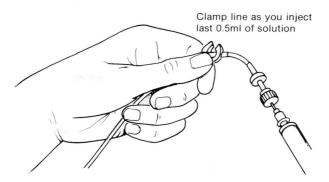

Clamp line as you inject
last 0.5ml of solution

Figure 2.

18. Close the clamp securely.

19. Pull out the syringe.

20. Carefully replace the needle cover and dispose of all supplies except the bottle of heparin solution. (An old coffee can may be used to dispose of used needles and syringes. Keep can out of reach of children.)

21. Double-check that you have securely closed the clamp on the catheter.

How to Change the Central Line Dressing

Purpose

To prevent infection and maintain skin integrity at the catheter insertion site. The dressing should be changed every 72 hours (every third day), or whenever the dressing becomes unsealed. Arrange for another person (other than the child) to act as a helper.

1. Gather the following supplies:
   a. Package of sterile gloves
   b. Alcohol swabs
   c. Transparent dressing
   d. Steri-strip
   e. Povidone-iodine swabs
   f. Povidone-iodine ointment.

2. Wash hands with hot soapy water for 1 full minute.

3. Set up sterile field by opening package of sterile gloves on a clean flat surface.

4. Open dressing and alcohol swabs and drop onto the sterile field. Tear the corner of povidone-iodine ointment package open.

5. Carefully remove the old dressing. Have helper restrain the child and hold catheter above the chest so the catheter does not touch the skin. Do *not* use scissors to cut the dressing away, as you may cut the catheter by mistake (Fig. 3).

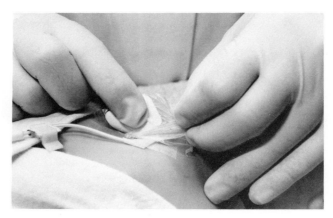

Figure 3.

6. Observe the insertion site for any signs of redness, swelling, pustules, or drainage.

7. Put on sterile gloves.

8. First, using an alcohol swab, cleanse the skin, starting at the catheter insertion site and moving outward from the insertion site in a circular manner. DO NOT TOUCH THE CATHETER WITH THE ALCOHOL SWAB, as it will damage the catheter. Let area dry thoroughly. (Do *not* blow on area to hasten the drying time).

9. Repeat Step No. 8, using a povidone-iodine swab (Fig. 4).

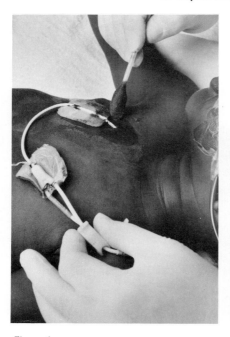

Figure 4.

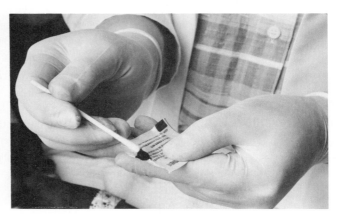

Figure 5.

10. Using another povidone-iodine swab, cleanse the length of the catheter that will be housed under the dressing, from the insertion site outward toward the hub.

11. If the child's skin is reactive to iodine, the iodine on the skin can be removed with alcohol, using a circular motion moving outward from the insertion site.

12. Place a small dab of iodine ointment at the insertion site (Fig. 5).

13. Smoothly apply the dressing over the insertion site and over the catheter. DO NOT COIL the catheter under the dressing. The edges of the dressing should seal over the skin (Fig. 6).

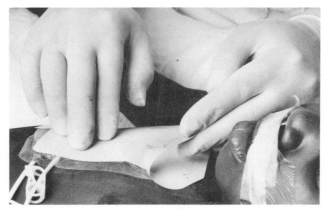

Figure 6.

14. Remove gloves.

15. Cut a notch in a Steri-strip.

16. Place this Steri-strip under the catheter as it exits the dressing, and overlapping the dressing. This will secure the dressing at the catheter exit site.

17. If necessary, you may secure the catheter with additional tape elsewhere on the chest or abdomen to prevent tension on the line.

How to Change the Injection Cap

Purpose

The Luer-lock injection cap must be changed once a week, using sterile technique, to prevent bleeding from the central line.

1. Gather the following supplies:
   a. Package of sterile gloves
   b. Standard heparin flush (you may need a little more than 3 mL) in a syringe with a needle attached
   c. New injection cap
   d. Several povidone-iodine swabs
   e. Mask
   f. Sterile field (or sterile glove package lining)

2. Wash hands with hot soapy water for 1 full minute.

3. Prepare the heparin flush solution as you would when just irrigating the catheter. (Draw up 10 mL of flush.)

4. Put on mask.

5. Open sterile field.

6. Open the new injection cap and drop it onto the sterile field. Also open the povidone-iodine swabs and drop them onto the sterile barrier.

7. Remove needle cap from prefilled syringe and place onto the sterile field.

8. Put on sterile gloves.

9. With a povidone-iodine swab in each hand, grasp the end of the catheter with one hand while unscrewing the cap with the other hand.

10. Pick up the new injection cap and screw it onto the end of the central line.

11. Take another povidone-iodine swab and wipe off the end of the injection cap.

12. Insert needle of flush into cap. Open clamp. Draw back on syringe enough to get air bubbles out of central line, yet not enough to draw blood into the syringe.

13. Irrigate with heparin flush as you normally do. *Remember to clamp the catheter closed before pulling the needle completely out.*

Instructions for Emergency Care

Your child has a _____ central line catheter in place.
           (type, size)

It was inserted on _____/_____/_____ at _____
                      (date)   (hospital)

by Dr. _____.
           (name)

When to Call your Doctor or Emergency Room

1. If your child has a fever.

2. If you see redness, drainage, or swelling around the catheter insertion site.

3. If the catheter is pulled out (totally or partially).

4. If the catheter cannot be flushed easily.

5. If the flush solution leaks from around the catheter when you irrigate.

6. If the catheter is damaged and is leaking from the tubing.

7. If your child complains of chest pain, shortness of breath, dizziness, or confusion.

When to Bring Your Child to the Emergency Room

1. If a break in the tubing occurs, quickly place the clamp on the catheter between the break and the child and bring him or her to the emergency room.

2. If you see blood backing up inside the catheter—even with the clamp in place—double the catheter back on itself and tightly secure it with tape or a rubber band. Bring your child to the Emergency Room.

Resources Available to You

Physician's Name: Dr. _____ Office Telephone: _____

Pediatric ER at _____ Telephone: _____
               (institution)

Social Worker's Name: _____ Telephone: _____

Outpatient Clinic Telephone: _____

Nurse Clinician Telephone: _____

Pharmacy Telephone: _____

Medical Supply Co. Telephone: _____

There is a national organization for patients with central line catheters and their families. It functions as a support group and resource center. For further information contact:

Lifeline Foundation, Inc.
30 East Chestnut St.
Sharon, MA 02067
(617) 784–3250

Tips

Generally, your child's activities do not need to be restricted because of the catheter. However, contact sports and swimming should be avoided. If you think the catheter or the chest wall may have been injured due to a fall or other accident, call your physician or emergency room.

When traveling away from home with your child, always be sure to carry extra supplies with you in case of an emergency. Depending on your child's age, you will also want to send extra supplies along to school so that the school nurse will have the needed equipment for care of the catheter. Do not assume that the school nurse knows how to care for your child's catheter. There are dozens of different catheters that require varied care, so make an appointment with the school nurse to go over the specific care needed for your child's catheter. Remember to order new supplies for your home use well before your present supplies run out.

At home and at school, a great deal of attention will be focused on the catheter. Keep in mind that your child may be nervous or frightened, and remember to explain exactly what you are doing during a procedure in order to decrease some of the fear. As your child grows and exhibits a sense of control, let him or her help with catheter care in an age-appropriate manner.

Your child (especially older children and teenagers) does not want to feel different from other kids their age. Other than providing some special care for the *catheter*, remember to treat your child as normally as possible. Do not smother or overprotect. Your child needs to participate in normal family activities. Do not isolate or restrict your child any more than is necessary to protect the catheter.

At first, this information may seem overwhelming. These instructions will make more sense once you have seen a demonstration. After a few practice sessions with the nurse, you will remember more and more steps and you will need to refer to the guide less frequently. We don't expect you to learn everything right away. Many parents have learned these skills and have done well caring for their child with a central line catheter at home. With time you can too!

Remember that the nursing staff is always available when questions or concerns arise.

Good Luck!

PATIENT TEACHING CHECKLIST

Skill	**Nurse Demonstration (Initials & Date)**	**Parent Return-Demonstration (Initials & Date)**
1. Putting on sterile gloves. (The parent should also have a basic understanding of sterile technique—what can and cannot be touched.)		
2. Drawing up 3 mL heparin saline flush for irrigation.		
3. Flushing the catheter.		
4. Completing a dressing change.		
5. Changing injection cap.		
6. Able to list signs and symptoms of infection at the insertion site.		
7. Knows when to call the physician.		
8. Knows what to do in an emergency if the catheter cracks or leaks.		

References

Children's Memorial Hospital. (1988). *Central Line Discharge Instructions.* Chicago: Children's Memorial Hospital.

Davol, Inc. (1988). *How to care for your Hickman or Broviac catheter.* RI: C.R. Bard, Inc.

Sanders, J.E. (1982). Experience with double lumen right atrial catheters. *Journal of Parenteral and Enteral Nutrition, 6*(2), 95–99.

Vane, D.W. (1990). Complications of central venous access in children. *Pediatric Surgery International 5*(3). 174–178.

Viall, C. (1990). Your complete guide to CV catheters. *Nursing '90, 20*(2), 34–41.

Gastrointestinal System Procedures

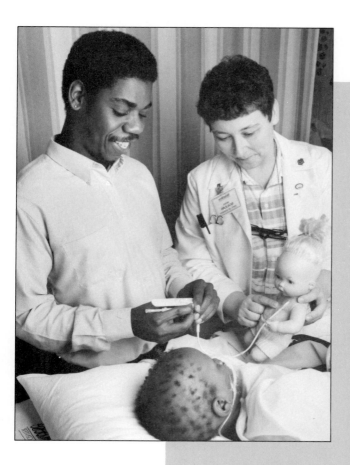

Unit X

Enema

65

Definition/Purpose

An enema is a rectal injection of a liquid for cleansing, therapeutic, or diagnostic purposes. Tap water and hypotonic solutions should be used with caution. Absorption of large amounts of fluid instilled into the bowel may produce hypotonicity of the extracellular fluid and hyponatremia. This, however, is more likely to occur in the infant rather than the older child.

Types of enemas:

1. Cleansing or Retention—These enemas may be used to empty the lower intestine. Isotonic saline or commercially prepared solutions (oil retention) may be used for this type of enema.

2. Therapeutic—Cool saline is used to reduce the body temperature of an infant with a high fever. Radiopaque solutions such as barium may also be used by a trained radiologist for the reduction of an intussusception.

3. Diagnostic—The most frequent use of diagnostic enemas is in the examination of the lower intestinal tract with liquid barium sulfate.

Standard of Care

1. The amount of fluid instilled varies with the age and size of the child and the reason for the enema (Table 65-1).

Table 65-1. Instillation Fluid

Age	Amount of Fluid
Infant (5–10 kg)	100–200 mL
Small child (11–30 kg)	200–300 mL
Large child (31–50 kg)	300–500 mL
Adolescent (over 50 kg)	500–700 mL

Table 65-2. Catheter Advancement

Age	Length of Advancement
Infant (5–10 kg)	1 inch
Small child (11–30 kg)	2 inches
Large child (31–50 kg)	3 inches
Adolescent (over 50 kg)	3–4 inches

2. Never force the catheter into the anal canal. If a well lubricated catheter does not advance easily, stop the enema (Table 65-2).

Assessment

1. Assess the pertinent history and physical findings for previous periods of immobility or illnesses requiring enemas.

2. Assess psychosocial concerns and developmental factors such as age, sex, usual coping mechanisms, available support, and habits.

3. Assess the child's and family's knowledge of the need for the enema and the procedure to be used.

Nursing Diagnoses

The following is a list of possible diagnoses and could apply, depending on the child's age, clinical situation, and physical condition:

Anxiety

Fear

Constipation/Diarrhea

High risk for injury

Pain

Planning

When planning to administer an enema, the following equipment must be gathered:

Container for the enema solution

Solution

Towels

Lubricant

Nonsterile gloves

Bedpan, diaper, or potty chair

Bath thermometer

Rectal catheter

Waterproof pad

Interventions

PROCEDURE	**RATIONALE/EXPECTED OUTCOME (EO)**
1. Explain the procedure to the child and the family.	The child and family will tend to cooperate with the procedure if they have had an explanation of what to expect. *EO: The child and family will be able to verbalize why the enema is being given.*
2. Fill the container with the enema solution warmed to body temperature (37.7°C or 100°F), unless the purpose is to reduce body temperature. In that case, a cool solution is used.	Cold fluid in a small child will cause hypothermia.
3. Provide for the child's privacy; close curtains around the bed. Drape the child, with the anus exposed.	The child's comfort and warmth will aid relaxation. *EO: The child will be afforded privacy during the procedure.*
4. Position waterproof pad under the child.	This protects bed linen.
5. Position the child: a. The child lies on the left side in the lateral recumbent position with knees drawn up to the chest (Fig. 65-1).	The knee–chest position helps distribute the solution throughout the lower intestinal tract; however, the exact position has not been found to alter the results.

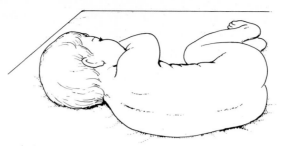

Figure 65-1.

PROCEDURE

b. The infant is placed on the back and the legs are lifted to expose the anal orifice (Fig. 65-2).
c. The Sims position is used for the older child, who lies on the left side, with the right thigh flexed about 45° to the body axis (Fig. 65-3).

RATIONALE/EXPECTED OUTCOME (EO)

EO: The child will be positioned in a comfortable manner.

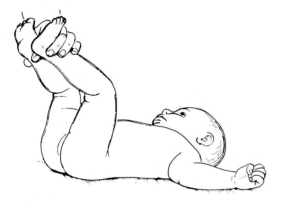

Figure 65-2.

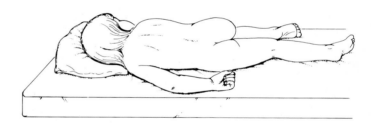

Figure 65-3.

d. The knee–chest position may be used for the older child. The child balances on the knees and chest, resting the head on the forearms (Fig. 65-4).

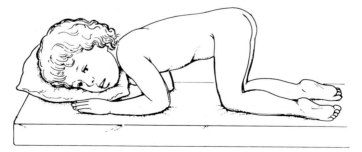

Figure 65-4.

6. Put on gloves.

This protects the nurse from microorganisms in the feces.

PROCEDURE	**RATIONALE/EXPECTED OUTCOME (EO)**
7. Lubricate the rectal catheter.	Lubrication will prevent irritation of the mucosal lining of the bowel.
	EO: The enema will be administered without injury to the bowel.
8. Introduce the catheter past the anal sphincter, into the anal canal and lower rectum.	
9. Once the tip of the catheter is in place, elevate the bag and instill the fluid slowly.	Water pressure increases with the height of the bag. The container should not be elevated more than 10 cm above the rectum. The rate of flow of fluid is influenced by the fluid's viscosity and the diameter of the instillation tube.
10. If the child shows symptoms of distress (for example, abdominal pain, shortness of breath, or chest pain), the flow of the fluid should be stopped.	
11. After the rectal catheter is removed, the child is urged to defecate and expel the contents of the enema. The buttocks may be held together to prolong retention of the fluid, especially in infants.	*EO: The child will defecate with the assistance of the enema.*
12. Place child on bedpan or potty chair or apply clean diaper.	
13. Wash hands and dispose of equipment.	
14. Document the enema procedure and how the child tolerated it. Also document the results of the enema.	The nurse needs to observe and record the results. Additional enemas may be necessary if the physician has ordered enemas until clear.

Patient/Family Education: Home Care Considerations

1. Instruct the family about the proper procedure for administering an enema.
2. Teach perineal hygiene, use of analgesic rectal ointment, or sitz baths for anal discomfort.
3. Instruct to plan for regular follow-up care.

References

Calandrino, C. (1989). Barium enema procedure for the pediatric patient. *Radiologic Technology, 60*(3), 209–214.

Taylor, C., Lillis, C., & Le Mone, P. (1989). *Fundamentals of nursing: The art and science of nursing care.* Philadelphia: J.B. Lippincott Co.

Caring for Children with Ostomies

66

Definition/Purpose

Many conditions necessitate diversion of fecal or urinary output in the pediatric population; these *ostomies* may be temporary or permanent. Among neonates, necrotizing enterocolitis, Eagle–Barrett syndrome ("prune belly") and imperforate anus are the conditions most frequently necessitating an ostomy. Infants born with spina bifida may also require fecal or urinary diversion, although this is far less common than in the past. In young children, Hirschsprung's disease (aganglionic sections of the intestine) may necessitate fecal ostomy formation. Regardless of the indication for surgery, the formation of stoma heralds the need for intensive parental support, guidance, and teaching from all members of the healthcare team. In institutions where Enterostomal Therapy Nurses are available, much of this responsibility is streamlined. In other situations, nurses in neonatal intensive care units and pediatric units must be equipped with skills necessary to provide care, and must be prepared to assist parents in assuming the responsibility for the care of their children upon discharge from the hospital. Following discharge, ongoing outpatient support is crucial to the success of parents in caring for their children as they adapt to care requirements that may change rapidly as developmental milestones are approached and achieved.

The anatomical location of the stoma depends on the pathology present; function of the stoma (such as the nature of the effluent, frequency of output, and pouching requirements) depends on its location. Ileostomies, openings into the small intestine, consistently produce highly corrosive, thin-to-mushy, greenish–brown or yellow effluent almost constantly (Fig. 66-1).

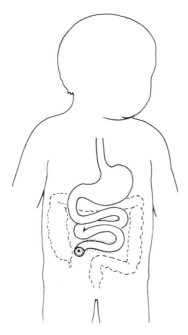

Figure 66-1.

Colostomies, openings into the large intestine, drain less frequently and produce stool that is less corrosive to the skin (Fig. 66-2). Urinary diversions (ureterostomies and nephrostomies) drain urine continuously (Fig. 66-3). Pouching a stoma is desirable from a

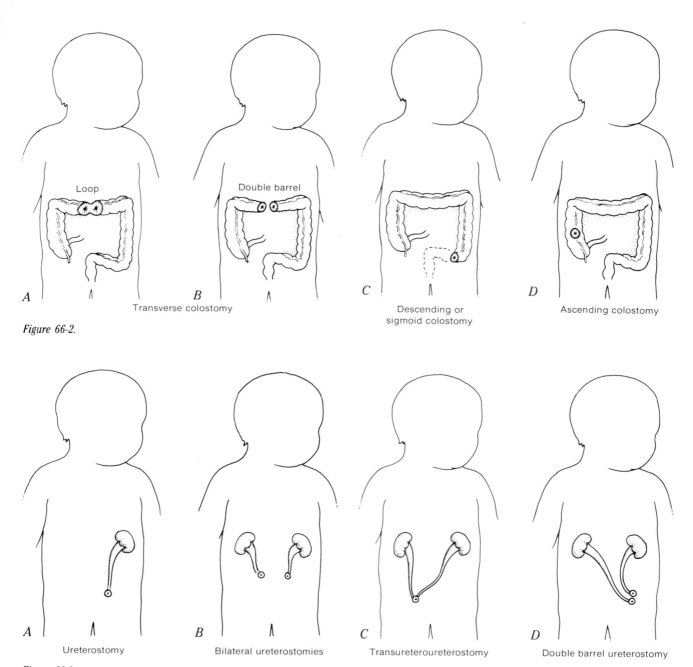

A *Transverse colostomy* B C *Descending or sigmoid colostomy* D *Ascending colostomy*

Figure 66-2.

A *Ureterostomy* B *Bilateral ureterostomies* C *Transureteroureterostomy* D *Double barrel ureterostomy*

Figure 66-3.

variety of viewpoints: skin protection is afforded by a properly fitted appliance, outputs can be measured accurately, and odor control and other phenomena of social importance are addressed. In a minority of cases, it may be appropriate to allow effluent to drain into a diaper; parents should be included in the decision of whether or not to pouch. The necessity to have control over elimination (i.e., ostomy management) becomes increasingly important as children become older and get involved in peer activities.

Standard of Care

1. Whenever possible, select the stoma site preoperatively. Consider the size and developmental stage of the child and his or her abdominal contour, including the presence of skin folds, scars, bony prominences, incisions, or umbilical cord.

2. Always consider pouching as a method for managing a diverted urinary or fecal stream. Although it is true that children under 3 years old are generally incontinent, it is unwise to expose the skin to corrosive enzymes or urine unnecessarily.

3. Select a pouch that affords maximum security, is easily applicable, is cost-effective, and is readily available.

4. Begin involving parents in stoma care and management as soon as possible.

5. Be prepared to reevaluate and make modifications in ostomy care frequently. Developmental changes such as activity and dietary progression will necessitate creative alternatives in management.

6. The pouch should be emptied as necessary; changing should be minimized.

Assessment

1. Determine age, weight, and developmental stage of the infant or child; assess the reason for surgery.

2. Determine the kind of ostomy—ileostomy, colostomy, (ascending, transverse, descending, sigmoid)—or urinary diversion (ureterostomy, nephrostomy). This information will be found on the operative documentation records.

3. Determine the type of stoma present. End stomas have one opening; loop stomas have two openings—a proximal (functional) lumen, and a distal (nonfunctional) lumen. Double-barrel stomas are two separate stomas—one functional and one nonfunctional.

4. Determine peristomal skin integrity. The skin around the stoma should look like the skin on the remainder of the abdomen, and should be free of redness, erosion, or irritation.

5. Decide the best method for managing output. Parents' preference and ability should be part of this decision. Ileostomies should always be pouched; colostomies and urinary diversions may be managed with diapers and absorbent dressing.

6. Assess parents' knowledge about the need for ostomy, any misconceptions they may have, and their general understanding of ostomy function and management.

7. Assess parents' readiness for learning and willingness to be responsible for emptying and changing pouch.

8. In children 3 years and older, assess readiness for involvement in ostomy self-care. Emptying can usually be achieved before changing; children will need reminders or cues for emptying.

Nursing Diagnoses

The following is a list of possible diagnoses and could apply, depending on the child's age, clinical situation, and physical condition:

Constipation/Diarrhea

High risk for impaired skin integrity

Body image disturbance

Knowledge deficit related to ostomy care

Planning

When planning to care for a child with an ostomy, the following equipment must be assembled:

For Pouch Change

Materials for cleaning (soft washcloth and towel, or paper towels; mild soap)

Pouching equipment:

Pouch with wafer-type skin barrier (Figure 66-4)

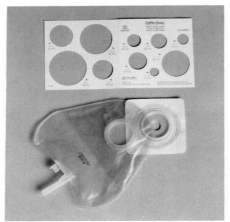 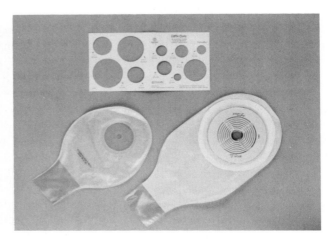

Figure 66-4.

Liquid skin barrier (may be eliminated in preterm infants)

Scissors

Pattern

Pouch closure (standard clamp or rubber band)

Disposable nonsterile gloves

For Emptying

Receptacle for effluent (graduated if output is measured)

Syringe (or bulb syringe) to aspirate contents of pouch of very small infants

Toilet tissue to clean end of pouch prior to closure

Water to rinse inside of pouch (optional)

Disposable nonsterile gloves

Interventions

PROCEDURE	**RATIONALE/EXPECTED OUTCOME (EO)**

Emptying Pouch

1. Explain procedure to child and parent, stressing that there will be no discomfort or pain related to the procedure. Ask for assistance with infants or with children who are unable to cooperate.

Older children will be able to assist with and cooperate in emptying if they understand the purpose, and realize that emptying the pouch is painless.

EO: The child and parent will understand that emptying the pouch before it is more than half full will prolong the wear time, and will make the pouch less visible under clothing.

PROCEDURE

2. Select an appropriate environment. The bathroom is ideal for children who can stand or kneel in front of the toilet.

3. Gather necessary equipment.

4. Put on gloves.

5. Open clamp or remove rubber band.

6. Empty contents of pouch into toilet or other receptacle; note the amount, color, consistency, and the presence of mucus or blood.

7. If desired, rinse the inside of the pouch with a small amount of lukewarm tap water. A small paper cup, a squirt bottle with a small nozzle, or a syringe may be used. Care should be taken to avoid the area directly around the stoma, because frequent washing can loosen the skin seal prematurely, causing leakage and the need for appliance replacement.

8. Wipe end of pouch clean with tissue; replace clamp or rubber band.

Changing Pouch

9. Explain procedure to child and parent explaining that there may be some discomfort or pain related to the procedure, especially during removal of the old pouch. Ask for assistance with infants or children who are unable to cooperate. Pouch changing should be planned, rather than waiting until the pouch leaks.

10. Long warm baths may help loosen the adhesive seal of an appliance.

RATIONALE/EXPECTED OUTCOME (EO)

Stool may carry hepatitis virus and contagious enterobacteria; stool contaminated with blood can also carry HIV (if child is HIV-positive).

Ileostomy effluent is thin to slightly mushy; its color can be green, greenish-yellow, or brown. The color and consistency of ileostomy effluent is affected by foods, fluids, and medications. Colostomy effluent gets thicker as the colostomy gets more distal, for example, a sigmoid colostomy may produce an almost-formed stool, while a transverse colostomy produces mushy stool. This is because a major function of the colon is water absorption; the longer the stool is in contact with the colonic mucosa, the more water is absorbed. In urinary diversions, output should be measured, the color and clarity of the urine noted, and the odor evaluated; urine will have a characteristic, but not unpleasant, odor. Foul-smelling, cloudy urine may indicate infection. Urine may also be assessed for pH; generally, acidic urine is less prone to infection than alkaline urine. The presence of mucus in urine from a urinary diversion is normal only when an ileal or colon conduit has been constructed; because a piece of intestine is used in both these procedures, the presence of mucous is expected.

EO: The child's effluent will be emptied from the pouch with attention paid to the amount, consistency, color, and presence of mucus or blood.

Older children will be able to assist with and cooperate in changing the pouch if they understand the purpose.

EO: The child and parent will feel more in control by changing the pouch before it leaks.

PROCEDURE

11. Once the appliance is off, wash the periostomal skin with an ostomy soap.

12. Rinse the skin well and pat dry. Examine skin for redness or breaks in the skin.

13. Place a Stomahesive wafer around the ostomy with the donut hole fitted close to the base of the stoma (Fig. 66-5).

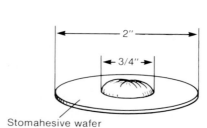

Stomahesive wafer

Figure 66-5.

14. Apply the collection pouch to the Stomahesive wafer. (If the child uses an Active-Life One Piece Drainable Custom pouch, remove the pouch (Step 10), wash skin (Steps 11 and 12) and place the pouch with backing attached and hole cut in the appropriate size to fit the child's skin around the stoma.)

15. If two stomas are present, cut an oval in the skin barrier to fit around both stomas.

16. Put a dab of Karaya paste between the stomas, making certain that there is no skin showing.

17. Let paste dry until shiny.

18. Apply bag, using circular motion around stoma.

19. Record the following observations in the medical record:
    a. Condition of skin
    b. Consistency of stools
    c. Amount and color of urine
    d. Appliance type applied.

20. Record child's and parents' response to the teaching of ostomy management.

RATIONALE/EXPECTED OUTCOME (EO)

Redness or breakdown is caused by leakage of effluent under the skin protector.

EO: The child's skin will remain intact.

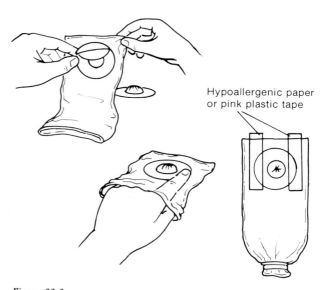

Hypoallergenic paper or pink plastic tape

Figure 66-6.

Use a circular motion with the index finger up inside the pouch, bonding it to the Stomahesive and minimizing the possibility of wrinkles that would permit leakage (Fig. 66-6).

Karaya paste will protect the skin between the stomas from the effluent.

Patient/Family Education: Home Care Considerations

1. Begin involving the family and the developmentally ready child in ostomy management as soon as possible following surgery.

2. Begin teaching by demonstrating care in a calm accepting manner.

3. Gradually begin to transfer tasks related to ostomy management (for example, emptying and changing pouch).

4. Encourage independent decision-making, and support parents' "gut feelings" about times for pouch change and anticipated wear time of the pouch.

5. Teach parents to trust their judgment regarding necessary alterations in pouching technique, but encourage them to check out ideas for different methods or equipment use with health care professionals first.

6. Arrange for follow-up visits; children and parents need to know that they are doing well.

7. Make arrangements for obtaining supplies through a reputable dealer who can answer questions and will refer parents to the healthcare worker.

8. Help parents explore financial aspects of reimbursement for ostomy supplies; most third party payers and some HMO/PPO arrangements will reimburse all or part of the cost of ostomy supplies.

9. Help parents contact other parents who have successfully managed a child or infant with a stoma.

10. Instruct parents to call a healthcare professional if any of the following occur:
    a. Significant changes in output (amount, color, and consistency)
    b. Failure of a child to grow and gain weight
    c. Skin irritation or excoriation around stoma
    d. Changes in the stoma itself
    e. Behavior changes in the older child that may be the result of body image and self-esteem disturbances.

11. Remind parents frequently that the stoma should not "rule" them, but rather that they should "rule" the stoma; encourage a normal daily schedule.

12. Offer to contact the child's school and teacher, as the parent desires, to discuss the child's ostomy management and any special needs for toileting.

References

Boarini, J.H. (1989). Principles of stoma care in infants. *Journal of Enterostomal Therapy, 16*(1), 21–25, 41.

Embon, C.M. (1990). Ostomy care for the infant with necrotizing enterocolitis: Nursing considerations. *Journal of Perinatal Neonatal Nursing, 4*(3), 56–63.

Jeter, K. (1982). The Pediatric patient: Ostomy surgery in growing children. In Broadwell, D, & Jackson, B. *Principles of ostomy care.* St. Louis: C.V. Mosby Co., 489–544.

Jeter, K. (1982). *These special children: The ostomy book for parents of children with colostomies, ileostomies, and urostomies.* Palo Alto, CA: Bull Publishing Co.

Madda, M.A. (1991). Helping ostomy patients manage medications. *Nursing 91, 21*(3), 47–49.

Motta, G. (1987). Life span changes: Implication for ostomy care. *Nursing Clinics of North America, 22*(2), 333–339.

Roback, S., & Boarini, J. (1988). Conditions requiring gastro-intestinal stomas in infants. *Journal of Enterostomal Therapy, 15*(4), 162–166.

Peritoneal Tap: Paracentesis

67

Definition/Purpose

A peritoneal tap (paracentesis) is a procedure by which the abdominal cavity is entered percutaneously to obtain information for the diagnosis of ascites, peritonitis, or intraperitoneal hemorrhage; and institute therapeutic measures such as dialysis and abdominal decompression to relieve respiratory compromise caused by a large collection of peritoneal fluid.

There are no absolute contraindications except bleeding disorders, disruption of the abdominal wall integrity due to burns or cutaneous lesions, or distention of the bowel that predisposes it to puncture.

Standard of Care

1. The procedure will be carried out using aseptic technique.
2. The area of the tap will be injected with local anesthetic to provide pain control.

Assessment

1. Assess the pertinent history and physical findings for a history of critical illness or trauma; abdominal surgery; current medications; respiratory, cardiac, renal, or liver disease; hypertension or a sudden gain in weight; and allergies (especially to iodine).
2. Assess psychosocial and developmental factors with regard to a fear of the unknown, changes in body appearance precipitating a disturbance in body image, habits, and what comforts the child during periods of stress.
3. Assess the child and family's knowledge of the proposed tap, along with their readiness and willingness to learn.
4. Assess the family's use of adaptive skills in dealing with the child's health problems.

Nursing Diagnoses

The following is a list of possible diagnoses and could apply, depending on the child's age, clinical situation, and physical condition:

Anxiety

Fear

High risk for infection

High risk for injury

Impaired skin integrity

Pain

Planning

In planning to assist the physician in performing a peritoneal tap, the following equipment must be gathered:

18-, 20-, or 22-gauge angiocatheter

Povidone-iodine

Sterile 4 × 4s

Sterile gloves

Sterile drape

1% lidocaine in 5 mL syringe with 22-gauge needle

20-mL syringe

50-mL syringe

Sedation (optional)

Interventions

PROCEDURE	RATIONALE/EXPECTED OUTCOME (EO)
1. Explain the procedure and the need for the tap to the child and family. Obtain written consent from the child's guardian.	*EO: The child and family will be given an opportunity to express their concerns and verbalize the reason for the procedure.*
2. Sedate the child as ordered.	The child undergoing a peritoneal tap may require sedation to permit safe access to the peritoneal cavity. If there is a large collection of fluid compromising respirations, the use of general anesthesia may be contraindicated.
	EO: The child will be medicated to provide comfort and a safe environment for the tap.
3. Place the child in either the sitting or lateral decubitis position with an adequate amount of restraint (Fig. 67-1).	Gravity is used to assist the drainage.
	EO: The child will be positioned to facilitate drainage of fluid from the peritoneal cavity.

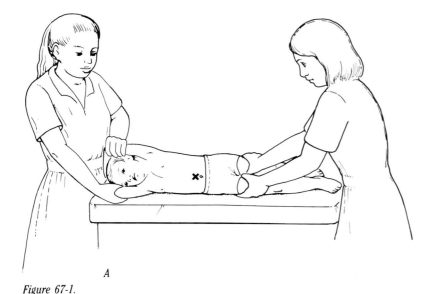

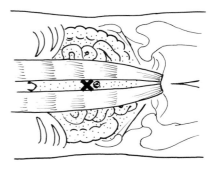

A *B*

Figure 67-1.

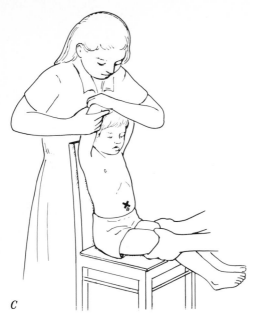

C

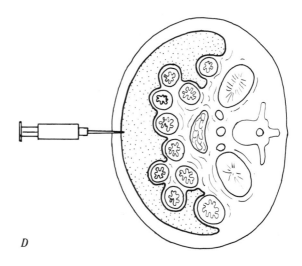

D

Figure 67-1. Continued

PROCEDURE

4. Put on sterile gloves and cleanse an area around the planned site with povidone–iodine-soaked 4 × 4s.

5. Drape the child with sterile towels.

6. The physician will inject the skin with 1% lidocaine.

7. The physician will direct the catheter or needle perpendicular to the abdominal wall, puncture the skin, and advance the catheter or needle until a popping sensation is felt. Verification of penetration into the peritoneum is accomplished by drawing fluid into the syringe.

8. The physician will slowly advance the catheter/needle while aspirating fluid. The needle will then be removed, leaving the catheter in place with fluid being withdrawn.

9. At the completion of the tap, the physician will pull the catheter straight out and apply a sterile gauze pad with pressure over the wound.

10. The abdominal sample will be sent for analysis (for example, culture, Gram stain, cell count, glucose, amylase, and RBCs). Label and bag the specimen.

11. The volume of fluid withdrawn should be measured and recorded.

12. The child will be monitored during and after the procedure for complications of the tap. The child's color, blood pressure, pulse, and respiratory rate will be observed every 5–15 minutes during the tap, and every 30 minutes for 2 hours after the tap.

RATIONALE/EXPECTED OUTCOME (EO)

The peritoneal cavity is sterile; thus surgical asepsis is observed.

EO: The child will be free from infection at the site of the tap.

Local sedation will make the procedure more comfortable.

The catheter tip can be repositioned once the needle is removed and the child can safely be turned to facilitate the drainage of fluid.

This will prevent bleeding or leakage of fluid from the tap site.

EO: The child's peritoneal fluid will be sent for analysis.

EO: The child's medical record will reflect the results of the tap.

EO: The child will not have injury to any internal structures.

PROCEDURE	**RATIONALE/EXPECTED OUTCOME (EO)**

a. Intraperitoneal

- Perforation of a hollow viscus — Usually seals off quickly, without leakage
- Perforation of a blood vessel — Usually seals off
- Introduction of contaminants — Minimized by strict aseptic technique

b. Extraperitoneal

- Hematoma formation secondary to trauma of the deep epigastric vessels
- Profound fluid shifts in the intravascular and extracellular fluid compartments, with resultant hypotension — *EO: The child will have fluid shifts identified and treated promptly.*

Patient/Family Education: Home Care Considerations

1. Develop a plan to teach the child and family about the current health problems and concerns.
2. Provide information and clarify any misconceptions regarding the procedure and the results of the fluid analysis.

References

Fleisher, G.R., & Ludwig, S. (1988). *Textbook of pediatric emergency medicine.* Baltimore: Williams & Wilkins.

Liu, P. et al. (1989). Percutaneous aspiration, drainage, and biopsy. *Journal of Pediatric Surgery,* *24*(9), 865–866.

Raffensperger, J.G. (1990). *Swenson's pediatric surgery.* Norwalk, CT: Appleton & Lange.

Nasogastric Tube Insertion

68

Definition/Purpose

Nasogastric intubation involves the insertion of a tube through the nasal passage into the stomach to assess gastrointestinal function, instill medications or feedings, or decompress the stomach.

Standard of Care

1. Change the nasogastric tube according to your hospital policy, keeping in mind that the softer tubes can remain in place as long as 3 weeks. When inserting the tube, alternate nares to decrease the chance of ulceration.
2. Provide mouth care every 4 hours.
3. Provide anesthetic spray or rinses for a sore throat.
4. Apply cream or ointment to nares and lips.
5. Monitor intake and output every 8 hours.
6. Monitor vital signs and symptoms of respiratory distress and gastrointestinal bleeding.
7. Provide physical and emotional support and age-appropriate stimulation to the child.

Assessment

1. Assess the medical history of the child, with emphasis on gastrointestinal disorders, congenital defects, and conditions affecting the nasal passages and the oropharynx.
2. Assess physical findings such as the child's weight, height, head circumference, nutritional intake, presence of bowel sounds, gastrointestinal bleeding, and level of consciousness.
3. Assess the child's developmental level, coping mechanisms, and previous experiences in a medical environment and with a nasogastric tube.

Nursing Diagnoses

The following is a list of possible diagnoses and could apply, depending on the child's age, clinical situation, and physical condition:

Altered nutrition, less than body requirements

High risk for injury

Ineffective airway clearance

Altered tissue perfusion

Body image disturbance

Pain

Planning

When inserting a nasogastric tube, assemble the following equipment:

Appropriate size nasogastric tube

½-inch tape

1 5-mL syringe or catheter tip syringe

Stethoscope

Lubricant

1 Transparent dressing

1 Hypoactive dressing

Non-sterile gloves

Interventions

PROCEDURE	**RATIONALE/EXPECTED OUTCOME (EO)**
1. Prepare child in a developmentally appropriate manner.	The child and parents will tend to cooperate with the procedure if they understand what to expect.
2. Gather necessary equipment. Select the correct size catheter, using the table below as a guide.	*EO: The child and parents will describe the tube insertion procedure correctly.* *The child will cooperate with the insertion as developmentally able.*

N/G Size	5F	8F	10F	12F	14F	16F
Child's Wt.	2 kg	3–9 kg	10–20 kg	20–30 kg	30–50 kg	50 kg+

3. Wash hands.	
4. Measure the length of tubing to be inserted by extending the tube from the tip of the child's nose to the earlobe, and then to the lower end of the xyphoid process (Fig. 68-1).	This measurement is the approximate length of the tube needed to reach the stomach.

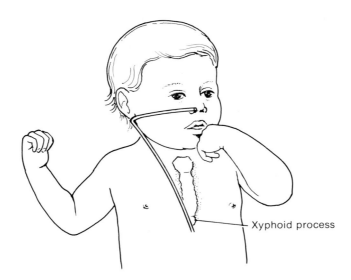

Xyphoid process

Figure 68-1.

PROCEDURE

5. Mark the tube with a piece of tape at this spot.

6. Put on gloves.

7. Lubricate the tube with water or a water soluble gel. Have the child sit up at a 45° angle, if possible. Insert the tube into the selected nostril, and advance it to the posterior pharyngeal wall, using gentle pressure. Direct the tube along the floor of the nostril and toward the ear on that side. As the tube is advanced and rotated, ask the child to swallow (have an infant suck on a pacifier).

8. Continue to insert tube until tape mark is at the nostril. If the tube meets resistance, withdraw it, relubricate it, and insert it in the other nostril. Also withdraw the tube immediately if any vomiting or any change in respiratory status is noted (for example, cyanosis, tachypnea, tachycardia, nasal flaring, retractions, expiratory grunting, wheezing, or prolonged coughing or choking).

9. Remove guide wire (if applicable).

10. Verify correct placement of the tube using the following methods (Table 68-1).

RATIONALE/EXPECTED OUTCOME (EO)

This serves as a measurement landmark.

Lubrication and swallowing or sucking facilitates passage of the tube.
This avoids injuring the turbinates along the lateral wall.

EO: The child will experience minimal discomfort.

The tube should never be forced because of the danger of injury.
Respiratory distress may indicate placement in the bronchus.

EO: The child will have no respiratory compromise from the tube.

Table 68-1. Methods of Determining Placement

Action	Tube in Stomach	Tube in Lungs
Attach distal end of tube to syringe and aspirate.	Gastric contents will fill the tube.	No fluid will be in the tube.
Introduce 1–5 mL of air into tube with a syringe while simultaneously listening over the gastric region with a stethoscope.	A distant popping, swooshing, or gurgling should be heard.	There will be no sound.
Place end of tube in a glass of water while the child exhales.	Few bubbles will appear.	A steady stream of bubbles will appear.

11. Secure the tube by first placing a small hypoactive dressing on the child's cheek and then securing the tube to the dressing with a transparent tape. Avoid pressure on the turbinates (Fig. 68-2).

12. Label the tube with insertion date.

13. Attach the tube to a feeding bag and pump apparatus (Fig. 68-3).

14. Document the insertion procedure, size of tube, patency, and the child's response.

Securing the tube in this manner will prevent skin breakdown and will prevent bleeding and ulceration of the nares.

EO: The child will maintain the tube in the correct position and will be free from side effects.

The tube needs to be changed according to hospital policy and the type of tube being used.

EO: The procedure will be documented in the medical record for future reference.

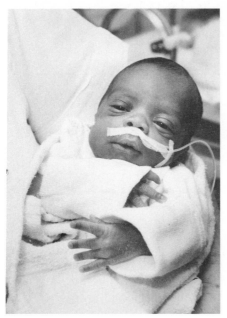

Figure 68-2.

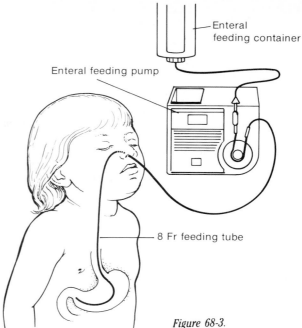

Enteral feeding container

Enteral feeding pump

8 Fr feeding tube

Figure 68-3.

Patient/Family Education: Home Care Considerations

1. Instruct the child and parents how to insert a nasogastric tube and how to check for placement.

2. Review signs and symptoms of respiratory distress (for example, cyanosis, tachycardia, tachypnea, nasal flaring, retractions, expiratory grunting, wheezing, and prolonged coughing or choking).

3. Instruct the child and parents about the irrigation of the tube.

4. If the tube is going to be used for medication administration or feeding, instruct the child and parents about technique for preparing medications and feedings.

5. Instruct the family about comfort measures:
   a. Inspect the nostril for discharge and irritation.
   b. Clean nostril and tube with a moist cotton-tipped applicator.
   c. Apply a water soluble lubricant to the nostril if it is dry.
   d. Change tape as required.
   e. Give frequent mouth care.

6. Identify potential body image disturbances that may develop (especially with the older child), and guide the family in coping with these issues.

References

Camp, D., & Otten, N. (1990). How to insert and remove nasogastric tubes quickly and easily. *Nursing '90, 20*(9), 59–64.

Lynn, M.R. (1991). Gastric tube insertion length: Routine or researchable? *Journal of Pediatric Nursing, 6*(2), 127–128.

Metheny, N., Dettenmeier, P., Hampton, K., et al. (1990). Detection of inadvertent respiratory placement of small-bore feeding tubes: A report of 10 cases. *Heart and Lung, 19*(6), 631–638.

Metheny, N.A., Spies, M.A., & Eisenberg, P. (1988, August). Measures to test placement of nasoenteral feeding tubes. *Western Journal of Nursing Research,* 367–379.

Walsh, S.M., & Banks, L.A. (1990). How to insert a small bore feeding tube safely. *Nursing '90, 20*(3), 55–59.

Yoldmen, C., Grindle, J., & Carl, D. (1980). Taking the trauma out of nasogastric intubation. *Nursing '80, 10*(9), 64–67.

Nasojejunal Tube Insertion

69

Definition/Purpose

The two major sites for delivery of tube feedings are the stomach and small bowel. The child with delayed gastric emptying or a tendency toward pulmonary aspiration may benefit from transpyloric feeding. Also because the small bowel recovers normal peristalsis very rapidly after surgery, access to the jejunum permits earlier infusion of enteral feedings than would otherwise be possible by the oral–gastric route.

Despite its potential benefits, transpyloric feeding has drawbacks. The feeding bypasses the stomach's antinfective mechanisms and appears to result in less mixing of the formula with pancreatic enzymes. In preterm infants, fat malabsorption may thus be greater during jejunal feedings than during intragastric ones. Also, the position of nasojejunal tubes must be ascertained frequently, as they are likely to become malpositioned proximal to the pylorus.

Standard of Care

1. Change the nasojejunal tube according to manufacturer's specifications.
2. Provide mouth care every 4 hours.
3. Provide anesthetic spray or rinse for a sore throat.
4. Offer infant a pacifier to enhance nutritive sucking.
5. Monitor intake and output every 8 hours.
6. Monitor vital signs every 4 hours, with attention to the signs and symptoms of respiratory distress and gastrointestinal bleeding.
7. Provide physical and emotional support and age-appropriate stimulation to the child.

Assessment

1. Assess the medical history, with emphasis on gastrointestinal disorders, congenital defects, and conditions affecting the nasal passages and oropharynx.
2. Assess physical findings such as weight, height, head circumference, nutritional intake, presence or absence of bowel sounds, level of consciousness, and gastrointestinal abnormalities.
3. Assess the child's developmental level, coping mechanisms, and previous experience in a medical environment.

Nursing Diagnoses

The following is a list of possible diagnoses and could apply, depending on the child's age, clinical situation, and physical condition:

High risk for injury

Airway clearance, ineffective

Body image disturbance

Pain

Planning

In planning for the insertion of a nasojejunal tube, the following equipment must be obtained:

Feeding tube (5F, 6F, 8F)

$\frac{1}{2}$-inch tape

5- or 10-mL syringe

Stethoscope

Lubricant

Non-sterile gloves

pH paper

Interventions

PROCEDURE	**RATIONALE/EXPECTED OUTCOME (EO)**
1. Explain the insertion procedure to the child and parents.	The child and parents will tend to cooperate if they understand what to expect. *EO: The child and parents will describe the insertion procedure correctly.*
2. Assemble the necessary equipment.	
3. Determine the required insertion length of the tube by measuring the distance from the bridge of the nose to the ear, then to the ankle; or from the nose to the ear and then 10 cm below the umbilicus.	This measurement is the approximate length of the tube needed to reach the jejunum. *EO: The child will cooperate with the insertion as developmentally able.*
4. Mark the tube with tape or a red marker.	This serves as a measurement landmark.
5. Lubricate the tube with a water soluble lubricant.	Lubrication and swallowing or sucking, as well as positioning the child on the right side, facilitate passage of the tube.
6. Position the child on his or her right side.	
7. Gently thread the tube through the nostril to $\frac{1}{2}$ the measured length. Encourage the infant to suck on a pacifier to facilitate passage. Observe the child for bradycardia, apnea, or color changes.	Respiratory distress may indicate placement in the bronchus. *EO: The child will have no respiratory compromise from the tube.*
8. Using pH paper, test the position of the tube. If it is in the stomach, the pH should be 3–5.	
9. If the tube is in the stomach, continue to insert the tube to the predetermined point.	
10. Tape the tube in place.	
11. Test the position of the tube in the following manner:	*EO: The child's tube will be in the jejunum.*
a. Attach a 10-mL (or smaller) syringe to the feeding tube and gently aspirate.	Aspirated jejunal contents should be golden yellow in color with a pH of 6 or above.
b. Inject 2–5 mL of air into the tube, while holding a stethoscope over the right lower quadrant.	If the tube is in position as air is injected, a crackling or swishing sound will be heard.
c. If there is no aspirate, leave the tube open and subject to gravity for 1–2 hours. Test again with pH paper. If there is still no aspirate, remove the tube and insert again.	

PROCEDURE	**RATIONALE/EXPECTED OUTCOME (EO)**
12. When the pH becomes 6 or above, obtain an x-ray for certain placement.	
13. Document the insertion date, tube size, and tolerance of the child.	*EO: The procedure will be documented in the medical record for future reference.*
14. Follow the recommendation of the manufacturer regarding tubing changes.	

Patient/Family Education: Home Care Considerations

1. Instruct the child and parents how to insert a nasojejunal tube and how to check for placement.

2. Review signs and symptoms of respiratory distress (for example, cyanosis, tachycardia, tachypnea, nasal flaring, retractions, expiratory grunting, wheezing, and prolonged coughing or choking).

3. Instruct the child and parents about irrigation of the tube.

4. If the tube is going to be used for medication administration or feeding, instruct the child and family on the technique for preparing medications and feedings.

5. Instruct the family on comfort measures:
   a. Inspect the nostril for discharge and irrigation.
   b. Cleanse the nostril and the tube with a moist cotton-tipped applicator.
   c. Apply a water soluble lubricant to the nostril if it is dry.
   d. Change tape as required.
   e. Provide frequent mouth care.

6. Identify potential body image disturbances that may develop (especially with the older child), and guide the family in coping with these issues.

References

Moore, M.C., & Greene, H.L. (1985). Tube feeding of infants and children. *Pediatric Clinics of North America, 32*(2), 401–415.

Sporing, E., Walton, M., & Cody, C. (1984). *Pediatric nursing policies, procedures and personnel.* Oradell, NJ: Medical Economics Books.

Wesley, J.R. (1988). Special access to the intestinal tract. *Enteral feeding: Scientific basis and clinical applications.* Columbus, OH: Ross Laboratories.

Gastrostomy Tube Insertion

70

Definition/Purpose

A gastrostomy is an opening made in the stomach and abdominal wall for the purpose of external gastric drainage or feeding. Usually there is an indwelling rubber or Silastic tube, although a tubeless gastrostomy can be constructed.

A gastrostomy is performed in children who cannot be fed adequately by mouth, and as an adjunct in the management of some surgical diseases.

Feeding problems requiring a gastrostomy include:

1. Swallowing incoordination as a result of neurologic disorders
2. Motility disorders of the esophagus
3. Recurrent aspiration of feedings
4. Respiratory-dependent children
5. Difficult or time-consuming feedings in brain-damaged children.

Surgical problems requiring a gastrostomy include:

1. Postoperative care of neonates with intestinal obstructions, short bowel syndrome, or other disorders in which feeding may be delayed
2. Esophageal atresia requiring staged or delayed repair
3. Pyloroplasty, in which gastric emptying may be delayed
4. Esophageal stricture, either from reflux esophagitis or caustic injury.

Standard of Care

1. The initial Pezzer or mushroom catheter will be changed by the physician. Only balloon-type catheters should be removed by the nursing staff.
2. After the initial tube is removed by the physician, the gastrostomy tube should be changed every 4 weeks.
3. If the Pezzer or mushroom catheter is dislodged, call the physician immediately.

Assessment

1. Assess the pertinent history for the condition necessitating a gastrostomy, including congenital disorders, injuries, oral–motor dysfunction, gastroesophageal reflux, anorexia, and malnutrition.
2. Assess the physical findings such as nutritional status and vital sign measurements (height and weight). Plot values on growth charts.
3. Assess the psychosocial and developmental concerns related to coping mechanisms, support systems, and body image (in the older child).
4. Assess the child and family's knowledge of the care of the gastrostomy tube, feeding techniques, and skin care.

Nursing Diagnoses

The following is a list of possible diagnoses and could apply, depending on the child's age, clinical situation, and physical condition:

Anxiety

Fear

Impaired skin integrity

High risk for infection

Body image disturbance

High risk for injury

Pain

Planning

In planning to change a gastrostomy tube, the following equipment is needed:

Balloon catheter

Towel

Water soluble lubricant

6-mL empty syringe

6-mL syringe filled with tap water

Sterile gloves

Interventions

PROCEDURE	**RATIONALE/EXPECTED OUTCOME (EO)**
1. Explain to the child and family the procedure that will be used to change the tube. Allow the child to hold the equipment and participate in the process.	A well-informed child and family will tend to cooperate with the tube change. *EO: The child and family will express concerns to the healthcare workers, thus helping to alleviate their anxiety and fear.* *EO: The child and family will have a chance to discuss the actual or perceived change in body image due to the gastrostomy tube.*
2. Remove the new catheter from the package and attach the 6-mL syringe filled with water to the inflation port.	
3. Inflate the balloon with 3–5 mL water (Fig. 70-1).	The balloon should be checked for leakage prior to insertion.

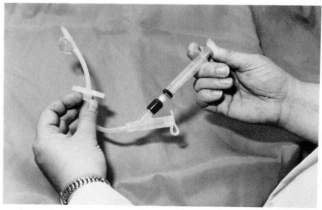

Figure 70-1.

PROCEDURE

4. Deflate the balloon, leaving the syringe attached to the catheter.

5. Lubricate the catheter end with water soluble gel and set aside (Fig. 70-2).

RATIONALE/EXPECTED OUTCOME (EO)

The lubricant will facilitate insertion into the stoma.

EO: The child will have the catheter changed with minimal discomfort.

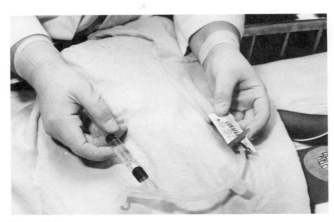

Figure 70-2.

6. Put on sterile gloves.

7. If a dressing is used around the catheter, remove the old dressing.

8. Attach an empty 6-mL syringe to the inflation port of the catheter in place and deflate the balloon (Fig. 70-3).

The balloon must be deflated fully before the old tube is removed. If not fully deflated when removed, the balloon will be traumatized.

EO: The child will have the old catheter removed without injuring the stoma.

9. With a towel over the catheter, pull out the old catheter and cover the stoma with the towel (Fig. 70-4).

The abdominal contents may spill out of the stoma, especially if the child cries or if the procedure is carried out too soon after feedings.

10. Holding the new catheter about 3 inches from the balloon end, insert the catheter into the stoma.

11. Inflate the balloon with 3–5 mL of water.

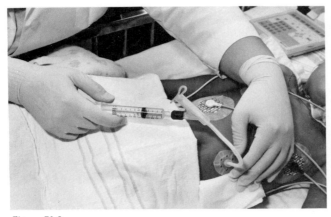

Figure 70-3.

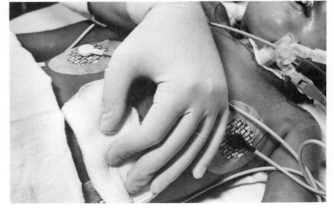

Figure 70-4.

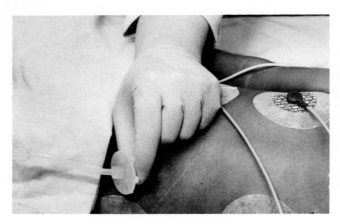

Figure 70-5.

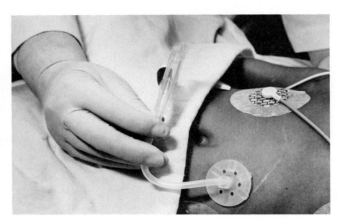

Figure 70-6.

PROCEDURE	**RATIONALE/EXPECTED OUTCOME (EO)**
12. Grasp the body of the tube and withdraw it until tension is felt from the balloon against the stomach wall (Fig. 70-5).	This will prevent leakage of stomach contents and migration of the balloon into the intestines.
13. If the catheter being used has a retention ring, position the ring to ensure tube placement. No dressing is necessary (Fig. 70-6).	*EO: The child's skin will remain intact around the stoma. The child will not experience an infection at the stoma site.*
If the catheter being used has no ring, secure tube with tape so that it does not migrate inward. Place a 2 × 2 slit dressing around the tube and tape.	If a dressing is used, change it immediately if it becomes wet. A dressing will promote skin maceration, breakdown, and infection.
14. Document the catheter change and the condition of the skin. Document the type and size of the catheter and the amount of water used to inflate the balloon.	This provides accurate documentation of the procedure and a point of reference for other caregivers.
	EO: The child's medical record will reflect the child's tolerance to the tube change, the condition of the skin, and the size and type of catheter used.

Patient/Family Education: Home Care Considerations

1. Teach the family how to change the gastrostomy tube.
2. Emphasize to the family the importance of maintaining excellent skin integrity.
3. Instruct the family in food preparation technique and the correct method of giving feedings.
4. Review symptoms requiring immediate medical attention with the family:
   a. Infection and skin breakdown around tube
   b. Leakage of fluid around opening
   c. Nausea, vomiting, or diarrhea
   d. Tube dislodgment or occlusion and inability to replace the tube
5. Emphasize to the family the need for follow-up medical care.
6. Refer the family to community resources for care and support once the child is discharged.

References

Huddleston, K., Vitarelli, R., Goodmundson, J., et al. (1989). MIC or Foley: Comparing gastrostomy tubes. *Journal of Maternal Child Nursing, 14*(1), 20–23.

Irwin, M. (1988). Managing leaking gastrostomy sites. *American Journal of Nursing, 88*(3), 359–360.

McGee, L. (1987). Feeding gastrostomy: Indications and complications—part 1. *Journal of Enterostomal Therapy, 14*(2), 73–78.

McGee, L. (1987). Feeding gastrostomy: Nursing care—part II. *Journal of Enterostomal Therapy, 14*(5), 201–211.

Medical Innovations Corporation. (1987). *Patient information: MIC gastrostomy tube.* Milpitas, CA: Medical Innovations Corportion.

Motta, G. (1989). Catheters as gastrostomy tubes? A cost saving alternative. *Continuing Care, (6),* 11–12.

Nelson, C.L.A., & Hallgren, R.A. (1989). Gastrostomies: Indications, management and weaning. *Infants and Young Children, 2*(1), 66–74.

Ross Laboratories. (1987). *General guidelines for gastrostomy care.* Columbus, OH: Ross Laboratories.

Gastrostomy Feeding Button

71

Definition/Purpose

The reasons for a gastrostomy tube are varied, ranging from asphyxia to gastrointestinal disorders and irreparable burns of the esophagus. The recently developed *gastrostomy feeding button* answers questions and concerns about the cosmetic appearance of conventional gastrostomy tubes. The major indication for insertion of a feeding button is the need for long-term enteral feedings. Pediatric patients who need this type of feeding include:

1. Children with poor oral–motor function as a result of central nervous system damage
2. Children with esophageal atresia
3. Children with oral or esophageal burns.

Children requiring short-term gastrostomy tubes are not suitable candidates for the button, since insertion requires a well-established gastrostomy site.

The button is a small flexible silicone device that has a mushroom-like dome at one end and two small wings at the other end. There is a one-way valve inside the device to prevent reflux of stomach contents (Fig. 71-1).

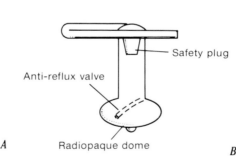

Safety plug

Anti-reflux valve

A   Radiopaque dome   *B*

Figure 71-1.

Advantages

1. Cosmetically pleasing
2. Simple care
3. Decreased incidence of skin irritation
4. Increased comfort and mobility
5. Decreased risk of dislodgment
6. Decreased risk of migration and intestinal obstruction
7. Ease in replacement
8. Minimal leakage
9. Immersible in water
10. Absence of reflux of gastric contents through the tube.

Limitations

1. Requires a well-established site
2. Limited number of sizes (18–20 French)
3. Valve may become clogged
4. Requires specialized feeding tubes
5. More costly than conventional tubes
6. Feeding tube disconnects easily with activity
7. Pressure necrosis may occur if button size is too small.

Standard of Care

1. Site care should be performed once or twice daily.
2. Rinse equipment with water after every feeding.

Assessment

1. Assess the pertinent history and physical findings for conditions necessitating a gastrostomy, nutritional status, and vital measurements (such as height and weight).
2. Assess developmental factors such as age, coping mechanisms, support systems, habits, and routines.
3. Assess the child and family's knowledge of the surgical procedure, its complications, the use of a traditional gastrostomy tube before a button can be inserted, and their readiness and willingness to learn.

Nursing Diagnoses

The following is a list of possible diagnoses and could apply, depending on the child's age, clinical situation, and physical condition:

Anxiety

Fear

Impaired skin integrity

High risk for injury

Body image disturbance

High risk for infection

Pain

Planning

When planning to care for a child with a feeding button, the following equipment must be gathered:

Insertion
Stoma measuring device

Obturator

Gastrostomy button

Lubricant (water soluble)

Soap and water or povidone-iodine scrubs

Feeding
Adaptor and feeding catheter

Syringe (60-mL)

Feeding bag

Feeding solution

Water

Routine Care
Soap and water

Peroxide

Cotton-tipped applicator

Baby bottle brush

Interventions

PROCEDURE	**RATIONALE/EXPECTED OUTCOME (EO)**
1. Explain the insertion procedure to the child and family.	Adequate preparation is important to ensure understanding and cooperation.
	EO: The child and family will ask questions of the healthcare worker and will have decreased anxiety or fear when they receive information.
2. Remove existing gastrostomy tube.	
3. Clean skin around the stoma with soap and water or povidone-iodine scrubs.	Clean skin is important to prevent skin infection or irritation.
4. The physician will determine the appropriate shaft length by following these steps:	Shaft length must be determined to minimize complications related to leakage of gastric contents and excessive pressure on the skin or gastric mucosa.
a. Insert the measuring device into the stoma.	*EO: The child will have the proper size button inserted to prevent injury to the abdomen.*
b. Pull up on the device until the balloon or tip is seated against the stomach wall (Fig. 71-2).	
c. Note the number of circumferential marks visible above the skin. Allow for slight in-and-out play.	
d. Withdraw the measuring device.	

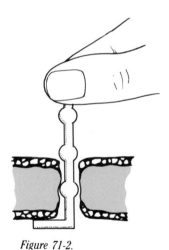

Figure 71-2.

5. Insert the obturator into the button and distend the button several times before insertion.	This will ensure patency of the antireflux valve.
6. Lubricate the dome of the button and the stoma with a water soluble lubricant.	Lubricant eases the insertion.
	EO: The child will not experience any undue discomfort during the insertion.
7. With the obturator in place, grasp the button with your second and third fingers beneath the skin disk. Place thumb on base of obturator and stretch the button until it reaches maximum length (Fig. 71-3).	The obturator lengthens the button and provides stiffness for ease of insertion into the stoma.
8. Use downward and to-and-fro rotary motion to advance the button into the stoma. When skin disc is at skin level, remove the obturator (Fig. 71-4).	Gentle insertion will prevent trauma to tissues.

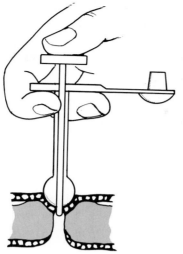

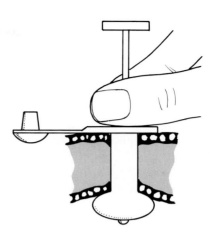

Figure 71-3.

Figure 71-4.

PROCEDURE

9. Check that the antireflux valve is in the closed position. If it is not closed, either push the obturator gently back into the button until the valve goes back, or insert an 8F or 10F suction catheter into the button until the valve goes back.
10. Insert plug into button (Fig. 71-5).

RATIONALE/EXPECTED OUTCOME (EO)

If the valve is not properly seated, leakage of gastric contents will occur.

EO: The child will have an improved self-concept after the insertion of the button.

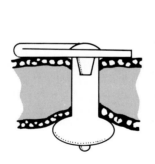

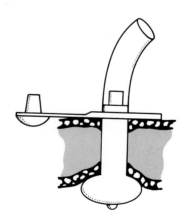

Figure 71-5.

Figure 71-6.

Feeding

11. Attach the adapter and feeding catheter to a syringe or bag.
12. Fill the syringe or bag and catheter with the feeding.
13. Open the safety plug and attach the catheter to the button (Fig. 71-6). Position the child on either side, with head elevated.
14. Elevate the feeding container and, using gravity, let the feeding flow in for at least 30 minutes.

EO: The child will be safely fed through the button.

Filling the catheter prevents large amounts of air from entering the stomach and causing abdominal distention.

A pump may be used for a child on continuous feedings.

PROCEDURE	**RATIONALE/EXPECTED OUTCOME (EO)**
15. When the feeding is complete, flush the button with at least 10 mL of water.	
16. Close the safety plug.	

Medications

17. Open the safety plug and attach the catheter to the button.	
18. Thick medications may need to be diluted with water; medications in tablet form should be crushed and mixed with water, milk, or juice before instilling them in the button.	
19. Give medicines before or after the feeding; do not mix medicine into the total amount of feeding to be given.	
20. Rinse the button with 10 mL of water after administering the medicine.	
21. Rotate the button when performing site care.	This will prevent skin breakdown because the device is flush with the skin and irritation can occur from leakage of stomach contents. *EO: The child's skin will remain intact at the site of the stoma.*
22. Wash around the stoma with mild soap and water.	The button can be immersed in water; thus site care can be accomplished during a bath. *EO: The child will not develop an infection at the stoma site.*
23. If the skin becomes red, irritated or excoriated, clean site with half-strength peroxide.	
24. Let the site dry thoroughly before covering the area with clothes.	

25. Document the following in the medical record:
  a. Size of the button inserted and shaft length
  b. Skin condition
  c. Feeding tolerance
  d. Any problems encountered.	

Patient/Family Education: Home Care Considerations

1. The nurse will demonstrate the correct method of giving the feeding and the parent will return the demonstration.

2. The nurse will demonstrate the proper position for feeding and the parent will return the demonstration.

3. The nurse will provide the parent with information regarding equipment cleaning and storage, and food preparation.

4. The nurse will instruct the parent on the importance of skin care (for example, rotating the button and cleaning around the stoma).

5. The nurse will review the symptoms requiring medical attention with the parents:
   a. Tube dislodgment
   b. Diarrhea
   c. Vomiting
   d. Bleeding at stoma
   e. Infection or breakdown of the skin.

6. The nurse will instruct the parents on the importance of medical follow-up.

References

Gauderer, M.W., Picha, G.J., & Izant, R.J. (1984). The gastrostomy button—A simple skin level nonrefluxing device for long-term enteral feedings. *Journal of Pediatric Surgery, 19*(6), 803–805.

Huddleston, K.C., & Palmer, K.L. (1990). A button for gastrostomy feedings. *Maternal/Child Nursing, 15*(5), 315–319.

Huth, M., & O'Brien, M. (1987). The gastrostomy feeding button. *Pediatric Nursing, 13*(4), 241–245.

Reynolds, E., & Kirkland, S. (1989). Alternatives in gastrostomy management: The button. *Journal of Enterostomal Therapy, 16*(3), 134–136.

Enteral Feeding (Tube Feeding)

72

Definition/Purpose

Nutritional support of children includes prevention, recognition, and therapy of secondary protein–calorie malnutrition. The steps involved in patient care include nutritional assessment, estimation of nutritional requirements, implementation of therapy, and monitoring of therapy for efficacy and complications.

To identify children in need of nutritional support, screening is performed when children are admitted to the hospital, including the diagnosis, history of recent weight loss, and weight-for-height. When nutritional depletion is determined, the clinician must determine the most effective means of resolving the problem (Table 72-1).

Table 72-1. Conditions for Which Tube Feeding May Be Useful

Gastrointestinal

Short bowel syndrome
Inflammatory bowel disease
Chronic liver disease
Glycogen storage disease type 1
Chronic nonspecific diarrhea
Surgery of the GI tract

Neurologic

Long-term coma
Severe mental retardation (making it difficult or impossible for child to suck or
    swallow without aspiration)

Metabolic—Hypermetabolic Status

Burns
Sepsis
Multiple trauma
Cardiac disease
Respiratory disease

Congenital Anomalies

Cleft lip
Esophageal atresia
Tracheoesophageal fistula

Other

Anorexia or weight loss
Growth failure
Malnutrition—Acute or chronic: hypoproteinemia
Cancer with associated surgery, radiation, and chemotherapy

The role of tube feedings ranges from supportive therapy to primary management of the disease state. The two major sites for delivery of tube feeding are the stomach and the small bowel. The decision whether to use a nasogastric, gastrostomy, or nasoduodenal/jejunostomy tube is based on two major factors—length of use and physiologic concerns.

In general, children who have functional GI tracts but who are unable or unwilling to eat may be tube-fed by the nasogastric or orogastric route when they require night feedings, when they require continuous drip feedings after severe diarrhea, or when they are in hypermetabolic states from major burns, sepsis, or trauma. Usually these children will require tube feeding for a maximum of 10 weeks.

Feeding by transpyloric jejunal tube reduces the risk of gastroesophageal reflux and aspiration as long as the tube delivering the formula is in place. Indications for this type of tube may include short-term coma, congenital GI anomalies, impaired gastric motility, upper GI surgery, and history of GE reflux or aspiration pneumonia.

When children are to be managed by enteral tube feedings for longer than 8 to 10 weeks, a gastrostomy or jejunostomy should be considered. Figure 72-1 provides an algorithm for selection of a feeding route.

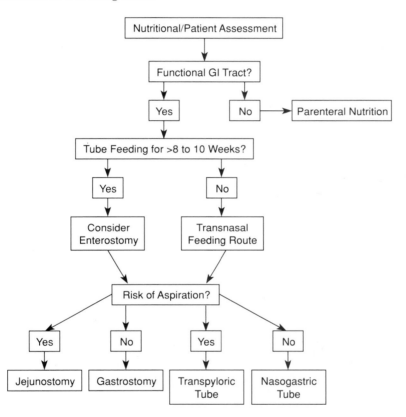

Adapted from Rombeau, I.L., Jacobs, D.O.. (1984). Nasoenteric tube feeding. In Rombeau J.L., Coldwell M.D. (eds): Clinical Nutrition, Vol. 1. Enteral and Tube Feeding. Philadelphia: W. B. Saunders, pp. 261–274.

Figure 72-1.

Standard of Care

Guidelines for Storage and Administration of Feedings

Storage	Recommendation
Sterile* canned/bottled liquid products	Store at temperatures <30.5°C (85°F). Cover and refrigerate opened, unused product labeled with date and time opened.
	Use/discard within 24 to 48 hours or in accordance with manufacturer's recommendations and/or hospital policy.
Powdered products	Store in cool, dry area. Cover opened, unused product labeled with date and time opened.
	Use/discard in accordance with manufacturer's recommendation and/or hospital policy.

Guidelines for Storage and Administration of Feedings (*continued*)

Storage	Recommendation
Nonsterile liquid products†	Store in refrigerator from time of preparation to time of use, labeled with date, time, and nature of preparation.
	Use/discard according to hospital policy.

Administration	Recommendation
Container and pump set	Change every 24 hours in accordance with gavage or pump-set manufacturer's recommendations and/or hospital policy. Consider more frequent changes when nonsterile feedings are given.
	Rinse with water between feedings.
Hang time	Sterile feedings* may be hung for 8 to 12 hours or in accordance with manufacturer's recommendations and/or hospital policy.
	Nonsterile feedings' should not remain in feeding container for >6 to 8 hours (or for >2 to 4 hours, if blenderized).
Feeding-tube irrigation	Rinse with water (e.g., 20 to 30 mL) before and after each intermittent feeding or every 3 to 4 hours during continuous feeding.

* Sterile feedings include industrially produced or pre-packed liquid formulas that are "commercially sterile."
† Nonsterile feedings are those that may contain live bacteria and include hospital- or home-prepared (blenderized) formulas, reconstituted powdered feedings, and commercial liquid formulas to which nutrients and/or other supplements have been added in the kitchen, pharmacy, home, or ward. (From Moore, M.C. (1988). Enteral feeding: Scientific basis and clinical applications. Columbus, OH: Ross Laboratories.)

Assessment

1. Assess the pertinent history and physical findings for a condition or disease necessitating enteral feedings.
2. Assess psychosocial concerns and developmental factors, including age, coping mechanisms, support systems, routines, habits, and body image.
3. Assess the family's knowledge of the procedure and their readiness and willingness to learn.

Nursing Diagnoses

The following is a list of possible diagnoses and could apply, depending on the child's age, clinical situation, and physical condition:

Anxiety

Fear

Nutrition: less than body requirements, altered

Fluid volume deficit

Self-concept disturbance

Pain

Planning

In planning to care for a child with enteral feedings, the following equipment is needed:

Weight scale

Urine measuring device

Formula

Enteral administration set and container

10–60 mL syringe (catheter tip)

Water for irrigation

Enteral pump for continuous feedings (Fig. 72-2)

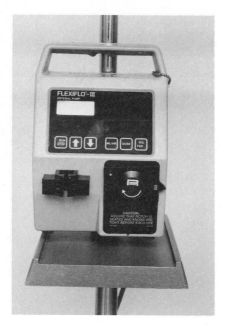

Figure 72-2.

Interventions

PROCEDURE

1. Provide an opportunity for the child and parent to express their fears and concerns. If surgery is required, review postoperative routine with all involved. Let the child handle the tube that will be inserted.

2. Monitor vital signs every 4 hours.

3. Record intake and output with specific gravity.

4. Weigh child daily, on the same scale, in the same clothes at the same time each day.

5. Monitor for signs of dehydration, as well as the effectiveness of intravenous fluids and enteral feeds.

6. Measure abdominal girth every 4–6 hours and record.

7. Provide oral hygiene frequently to keep mucous membranes moist and prevent discomfort.

8. Maintain placement and patency of the tube. Irrigate with normal saline before and after each intermittent feeding (or every 3–4 hours if feeding continues).

9. Note the color and amount of drainage return.

RATIONALE/EXPECTED OUTCOME (EO)

Adequate preparation helps to decrease fear and anxiety while increasing ability to cope.

EO: The child and parents will have adequate knowledge of the tube feeding process and surgical intervention (when appropriate).

Fluid loss can occur through feeding tubes. Dehydration and osmolar overload can occur in children who receive too high a concentration of formula in too short a period of time.

EO: The child will have adequate urine output (1 mL/kg/hr).

EO: The child stabilizes and demonstrates consistent weight gain.

Dehydration may be the result of diarrhea, fever, or excess fluid loss due to sweating.

EO: The child has normal skin turgor and moist mucous membranes.

Feeding administered too rapidly or in high volume may cause abdominal distention, which may cause aspiration.

EO: The child will experience minimal discomfort from the feedings and tube.

PROCEDURE	**RATIONALE/EXPECTED OUTCOME (EO)**
10. Monitor bowel sounds every 8 hours.	*EO: The child has active bowel sounds.*
11. Vent stomach before and after feedings, and any time the abdomen becomes distended.	
12. Position the child on his or her side with the head elevated, if possible.	
13. For feedings, unclamp the tube, attach a syringe, and aspirate gastric residual. Measure and record the residual. If it is less than half of previous feeding, return gastric aspirate to the stomach and proceed with the feeding. If residual is more than half of the previous feeding, notify the physician and stop the feeding until new orders are obtained.	Beginning a feeding when there is a large residual may cause vomiting and aspiration. *EO: The child will have his or her stomach aspirated to check residual.*
14. Administer the first feeding of clear liquids in small amounts; then increase the strength of formula feedings from ¼- to ½-strength noting the child's tolerance. Add the formula to a syringe or feeding bag, and, using gravity, allow the formula to flow in. A complete feeding should take 30–60 minutes. Use a pump for continuous feedings, preparing and hanging up 4 hours' worth of formula at a time.	Begin with a dilute-to-hypotonic concentration. The volume is advanced over a period of several hours to several days until fluid maintenance is achieved. Once the volume has been stabilized, the caloric density is increased.
15. Stop continuous feedings for at least 30 minutes before and during treatments such as physical or pulmonary therapy.	This will prevent aspiration of stomach contents.
16. Monitor urine and blood glucose 2–4 times a day; monitor serum electrolytes to ensure that the formula is appropriate for the child's metabolic requirements.	*EO: The child has normal electrolytes and blood sugars.*
17. Provide a pacifier for an infant to associate sucking with a feeling of fullness. Hold, cuddle, and talk to the child during the feeding.	*EO: The child and parents will adapt to an altered body image, and will cope with the loss of normal eating patterns.*
18. Encourage the child to sit at the table during mealtimes to promote normal behavior.	*EO: The child achieves expected developmental milestones.*

Patient/Family Education: Home Care Considerations

1. Instruct the child and parents about the principles of tube feeding as described above.
2. Teach the child and parents about potential complications and side effects and the appropriate action to take for each.
3. Teach parents to administer medications by tube; reinforce the administration of medications using a syringe to inject the medication into the tube rather than adding them to the feeding bag.
4. Have parents demonstrate feeding technique, preparation of the formula, anchoring techniques, and verification of tube placement.
5. Instruct child and parent in comfort measures and the care of mucous membranes.
6. Provide parents with a list of resources and references to a home health agency if appropriate.
7. Stress the need for medical follow-up.
8. Stress the importance of excellent skin care.

9. Review the symptoms requiring immediate medical attention: tube dislodgment, occlusion, bleeding, infection, vomiting, excessive diarrhea, polyuria, or skin breakdown.

Table 72-2. Summary of Potential Complications of Tube Feeding

	Signs and Symptoms	**Cause**
Physical	Nausea	Poor gastric emptying
	Diarrhea	Receiving medication that causes the above symptoms, including delayed gastric emptying
	Abdominal distention	Being fed too quickly or with formula that is too cold
	Abdominal discomfort	Ingesting contaminated formula
	Reflux—Aspiration	Intolerance to hypertonic formula
		Low serum albumin—(It has been demonstrated that colloid-osmotic pressure, to which serum albumin is a major contributor, is associated with tolerance to enteral tube feeding. Children with low serum albumin (>3 g/dL) have increased GI intolerance to enteral feeding.)
		Fecal impaction
Mechanical	Occlusion	Tube too small for the viscosity of the formula or medication
	Nasopharyngeal erosion	Lack of irrigation of the tube
	Otitis media	Inappropriate skin care or taping of the tube
	Sinusitis	Gastric obstruction due to migration of a ballooned tube through the pylorus
	Esophagitis	Long-term use of a nasal or oral tube instead of a gastrostomy
	Infection	
	Leakage around tube	
	Gastric obstruction	
Metabolic	Electrolyte imbalance	Inadequate administration of free water
	Dehydration	Hyperglycemia resulting in osmotic diuresis
		Other underlying medical conditions (such as renal or endocrine)

References

Belknap, M.D., Davidson, L. J., & Flournoy, D.J. (1990). Contamination of enteral feedings and diarrhea in patients in intensive care units. *Heart and Lung, 19*(4), 362–370.

Garvin, G., & Franck, L.S. (1989). Preventing delivery of enteral formula via parenteral route. *Pediatric Nursing, 15*(1), 17–18.

Moore, M.C. (1985). Tube feeding of infants and children *Pediatric Clinic of North America, 32*(2), April, 401–415.

Moore, M.C. (1988). *Enteral feeding: Scientific basis and clinical applications.* Columbus, OH: Ross Laboratories.

Moore, M.C. (1988). *Enteral nutrition support of children.* Columbus, OH: Ross Laboratories.

Sands, J.A. (1991). Incidence of pulmonary aspiration in intubated patients receiving enteral nutrition through wide- and narrow-bore nasogastric feeding tubes. *Heart and Lung 20*(1), 75–80.

Breast Milk Collection and Storage

73

Definition/Purpose

The Committees on Nutrition of the American Academy of Pediatrics and the Canadian Paediatric Society have recommended breast-feeding for infants. The success of lactation will depend on the attitude of the professional staff, a hospital climate that is conducive to breast-feeding, and the realization that mothers need instruction and support.

Human milk is the best source of nutrition for infants during the first months of life. The collection, processing, and storage of human milk may be initiated to meet the needs of the preterm infant, of the full-term newborn infant who temporarily cannot breast-feed, or of sick infants with intractable diarrhea, short gut syndrome, or intolerance to cow's milk or soy proteins.

An important property of breast-feeding is human milk's relative freedom from bacterial contamination. However, contamination can be a major problem with banked human milk. The precautions that are necessary to make human milk microbiologically safe require careful attention when the milk is collected and stored prior to feeding.

Standard of Care

1. Mothers may use mechanical or manual units for providing breast milk for their infants.
2. Breast milk will be used in the same order as it is pumped.

Assessment

1. Assess the mother's level of understanding of the methods of collecting breast milk and of the quantity of milk to be placed in each container.
2. Assess the infant for changes in vital signs, laboratory findings, physical changes, behavioral changes, and the response to therapeutic modalities.
3. Assess the anxieties and fears of the mother and provide explanations and support. Assess the mother's coping mechanisms and her support systems.

Nursing Diagnoses

The following is a list of possible diagnoses and could apply, depending on the child's age, clinical situation, and physical condition:

Anxiety

Fear

High risk for infection

Impaired skin integrity

Planning

In planning to collect and store breast milk, the following equipment is needed:
Sterile culture bottle

Breast pump
Sterile gauze wipes
Sterile water
Soap

Interventions

PROCEDURE

1. Explain to the mother the methods of obtaining and storing breast milk for the use of her hospitalized infant.
2. *Breast milk sampling for infection control*
   a. Before the initial use of breast milk, a sample of the milk will be sent for culture analysis.
   b. After the initial assessment, milk should be cultured every 2 weeks.
3. *Care of the Breast Pump*
   a. All parts of the breast pump must be washed in warm soapy water and rinsed well before each use.
   b. The pump parts must be sterilized every 12 hours.
4. *Collection and Storage of Milk*
   a. Mothers are to wash their hands thoroughly with soap immediately before touching their breasts.
   b. Assemble the sterile pump equipment beside the pump (Fig. 73-1). Instruct the mother to avoid touching the inside of the plastic parts or contaminating them by coughing or sneezing on them.

RATIONALE/EXPECTED OUTCOME (EO)

EO: The infant's mother will have her questions answered and have a thorough explanation of the breast-feeding and breast milk storage technique.

Salmonella and group B streptococcal infections have occurred from infected breast milk. Also, other bacteria and viruses (for example, CMV, rubella, and hepatitis B) have been identified.

EO: The mother's milk will be cultured before administration.

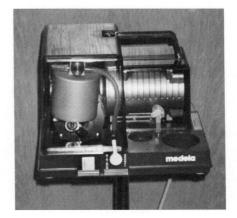

Figure 73-1.

c. Instruct the mother to express and discard the first several drops of milk from her breast.
d. Instruct the mother to wash her nipple in the following manner:
   • Wet sterile gauze wipes with sterile water.

This clears the milk ducts of residual milk, which contains the highest concentration of bacteria.
EO: The mother's nipples will remain intact with minimal discomfort.

PROCEDURE

    • Apply Phisoderm soap to one wipe and cleanse area concentrically from nipple to outer areola.
    • Wet another sterile gauze wipe with sterile water and rinse concentrically as above.
    • Dry nipple with a dry, sterile gauze wipe.
  e. Begin use of breast pump.
  f. After the breast is empty, pour the milk into a sterile specimen container (such as the ones used for cultured urine specimens). Do not fill the container more than $\frac{3}{4}$ full.
  g. Label the container with the infant's name, the date, and the time of collection. *Freeze the milk immediately.* Milk should not remain in a refrigerator-freezer longer than 2 weeks before it is transferred to a deep freeze. Milk should be placed on ice or in a cooler to remain frozen enroute to the hospital.
  h. Fresh milk can be brought to the hospital if the infant is feeding and the milk will be used within 24 hours.

5. *Thawing and Feeding*
  a. Frozen milk is thawed at room temperature before use.
  b. Milk is then labeled with the date and time thawed and placed in the refrigerator. The unused portion is discarded after 24 hours.
  c. Acceptable culture results for initiation of continuous feedings are <103 cfu/mL of skin flora bacteria.
  d. Acceptable culture results for initiation of bolus feedings are <104 cfu/mL of skin flora bacteria.
  e. In the event of unacceptable cultures, previously collected milk should be discarded and a new culture obtained.

RATIONALE/EXPECTED OUTCOME (EO)

Storage of milk in bottles with a nipple cap permits contamination because of the hole in the nipple.

EO: Breast milk will be stored for the infant in an appropriate and safe manner.

These organisms are *Sepidermidis*, alphastreptococci, and *Corynebacterium*. The presence of other bacteria is not acceptable for continuous feedings.
These organisms are *Sepidermidis*, alphastreptococci, and *Corynebacterium*. The presence of other bacteria should be brought to the attention of the neonatologist.
EO: The infant will be free from any infection transmitted by the breast milk.

Patient/Family Education: Home Care Considerations

1. Instruct the mother on how to sterilize the breast pump. Either of these methods is acceptable:
  a. Sterilize by washing in a dishwasher equipped with sanicycle.
  b. Sterilize by boiling for 20 minutes:
    • Place a clean washcloth in bottom of 4–5 quart saucepan.
    • Place all disassembled parts in pan.
    • Fill the pan to within 1 inch of the rim with cold water. Bring water to a rapid boil for 20 minutes.
    • Drain off the water and let the parts cool in the saucepan.

2. Instruct the mother to rest when at home. Fatigue is a common contributor to problems in breast-feeding.

3. The mother should be cautioned to avoid excessive caffeine and drug intake while breast-feeding.

4. Refer the family to a support group or a lactation specialist.

References

American Academy of Pediatrics. (1989). Transfer of drugs and other chemicals into human milk. *Pediatrics, 84*(5), 924–936.

Forbes, G.B. (1985). *Pediatric nutrition handbook*. Elk Grove Village, IL: American Academy of Pediatrics.

Meier, P., & Wilks, S. (1987). The bacteria in expressed mother's milk. *Maternal/Child Nursing, 12*(6), 420–423.

Wilks, S., & Meier, P. (1988). Helping mothers express milk suitable for preterm and high-risk infant feeding. *Maternal/Child Nursing, 13*(2), 121–123.

Obtaining a Stool Specimen

74

Definition/Purpose

Stool may need to be collected when a child exhibits any form of gastrointestinal dysfunction. The most frequent problem in childhood is acute diarrheal disturbances.

Stool can be collected for the following purposes:

1. To check for the presence of blood, ova, parasites, bacteria, fat, or sugar
2. To determine the status of the child and the effectiveness of therapy.

The demonstration of fecal leukocytes in diarrheal stool is well-correlated with inflammatory (usually bacterial) disease. Erythrocytes suggest amebic colitis. Stool should be examined as soon as possible after passage, and before barium or cathartics are given. Helminth ova and protozoal cysts can be identified in older specimens, but the identification of free-living motile forms requires the examination of fresh warm stool.

Standard of Care

1. Isolate child if an acute infectious gastroenteritis is suspected.

Assessment

1. Assess the pertinent history and physical findings for clues to the length of the illness; others that may be ill at home; diet, and normal and current bowel patterns (for example, frequency, amount, color, presence of blood, sugar, or proteins, and abdominal cramping).
2. Assess the child's developmental level, habits, and coping mechanisms.
3. Assess the family's knowledge of reasons for the test, the procedure for collecting the stool, the probable outcome, and the discharge regimen.

Nursing Diagnoses

The following is a list of possible diagnoses and could apply, depending on the child's age, clinical situation, and physical condition:

Anxiety

Impaired skin integrity

Diarrhea

Planning

When planning to obtain a stool specimen, the following equipment must be gathered:

Tongue blade

Plastic liner for diaper (when stool is watery)

Specimen container

Nonsterile gloves

Interventions

PROCEDURE	**RATIONALE/EXPECTED OUTCOME (EO)**
1. Explain the stool collection procedure to the child and family.	The family will help with the collection procedure if they appreciate the importance of the specimen. *EO: The family will voice their questions and will assist in the collection.*
2. If a stool specimen is needed from a child whose stools are loose or watery enough to absorb into the diaper, line the diaper with a piece of plastic. Place the liner between the diaper and the skin. If stools are soft, use diaper only.	The liner will allow the loose, watery stool specimen to be collected from the liner and not be absorbed into the diaper. *EO: The child will have the stool specimen collected in a timely manner.*
3. Check the diapered child frequently to see if defecation has occurred. Stool may be obtained from the bedpan of a toilet-trained child.	A fresh specimen should be obtained so test results will not be distorted by time lapse.
4. Put on gloves.	
5. Remove the soiled diaper and clean perineal area before applying a clean diaper.	Cleaning the perineal area will prevent skin irritation from the stool. Diarrheal stool is alkaline and contains enzymes that cause excoriation when in contact with the skin. *EO: The child will experience no diaper rash or impaired perianal skin integrity.*
6. Remove a small amount of stool from the diaper or bedpan with the tongue blade and place it in the specimen container.	
7. Send labeled specimen to the laboratory.	
8. Accurately describe and document the following: a. Time the specimen was collected b. Color, amount, consistency, and smell of stool c. Test collected for d. Condition of the skin	The medical record will demonstrate the collection of the specimen.

Patient/Family Education: Home Care Considerations

1. Reinforce with the family the information given by the physician regarding the results of this test. Correct any misinformation and fill in gaps of needed information.

2. Explain the need for continuous monitoring of the child once treatment has begun. Help the family coordinate follow-up appointments and repeat tests.

3. If the child has impaired perianal skin integrity, the following instructions may be helpful to the family:
   a. Clean diaper area with water and mild soap after each bowel movement.
   b. The infant or small child may sit in a pan of warm water for 5 minutes.
   c. Use a heat lamp on perineal area for 5–10 minutes every 2–4 hours during naptime, and before ointment is applied. (Use a 60 watt bulb and keep the lamp 18–20 inches from the child.)
   d. Apply medicated ointment, powder, or corn starch to the area.
   e. Cloth diapers may be less irritating to the skin than disposable ones.

References

Krom, F.A., & Frank, C.G. (1989). Clinitesting neonatal stools. *Neonatal Network, 8*(2), 37–40.

Levine, M. (1985). Infant diarrhea: Etiologies and newer treatment. *Pediatric Annals, 14*(1), 15–18.

Patient Education Aid. Diaper rash. (1984). *Patient Care, 18*(18), 93–94.

Suddarth, D. (1991). *The Lippincott manual of nursing practice.* (5th ed.). Philadelphia: JB Lippincott Company.

Yannelli, B., et al. (1988). Yield of stool cultures, ova and parasite tests and *Clostridium difficile* determinations in nosocomial diarrheas. *American Journal of Infection Control, 12,* 246–249.

Nutritional Assessment

75

Definition/Purpose

The purpose of a nutritional assessment is to collect data for estimating a child's nutritional requirements. This process involves evaluating the adequacy of nutrient intake, assimilation, and utilization. The effect of these factors on the child's body size and composition can then be identified and effective interventions planned to maintain or replenish the child's nutritional status at or near normal levels.

With the development of nutritional support services in pediatrics, strides have been made in developing nutritional therapies for children, as well as understanding the nutritional requirements of low–birth-weight infants. Improvements in the ability to replenish the nutritional reserves of pediatric patients with cancer, enteritis, and cystic fibrosis make accurate assessment of nutritional status more important for monitoring changes during therapy.

Primary protein–calorie malnutrition (PCM) is rare in the United States; however, PCM can be secondary to many chronic diseases and has been documented in 30% to 60% of pediatric inpatients. Unrecognized PCM may contribute to growth failure, medical complications, impaired immunocompetence, increased surgical morbidity and mortality, and reduced intellectual development.

An assessment begins with making a presumptive diagnosis of unrecognized diseases or defects. The "at risk" concept should be used as a first step in any nutritional assessment. This term represents the presence of biological or environmental factors that predispose to disease and of easily recognizable warning signs that malnutrition is impending.

Each child carries a set of risks for malnutrition which, if identified, establishes the nature of appropriate assessment. Below is a table of risk factors for malnutrition in childhood (Table 75-1).

Table 75-1. Risk Factors for Malnutrition

Family history of obesity
Low socioeconomic status
Malabsorption or gastrointestinal disease
Cancer
AIDS
Chronic pulmonary disease
Chronic renal disease
Drug effects
Cystic fibrosis
Fad diets or eating disorders
Burns
Trauma
Adolescent pregnancy

Awareness of the risks in a child, family, and community is the first step in any nutritional assessment.

Standard of Care

1. Techniques of nutritional assessment are traditionally divided into history, physical examination (anthropometric measurements and an estimation of body composition), and laboratory measurements.

2. All children, especially those who are hospitalized and fall into the "at risk" category, deserve a nutritional assessment and intervention.

Assessment

1. Admission screening procedures must identify those children at high nutritional risk. The following assessment criteria determine those children at risk:

Growth

    a. > 5% body weight loss in the past month
    b. Length and height for age < 5th percentile
    c. Weight for height < 5th percentile; < 80% of standard

Condition or Disease

    a. Any diagnosis associated with PCM

Laboratory

1. a. Serum albumin < 3.0 g/dL
    b. Lymphocyte count < 1000
    c. Creatinine–height index < 80% of standard
    d. Hemoglobin/Hematocrit
2. Assess historic data for information related to nutrition:
    a. Previous measurements of growth which provide a comparison to current data
    b. Social and family history, which affect a child's eating habits and nutritional status
    c. Previous illness or present diagnosis which may limit food intake, while increasing metabolic needs
    d. Current medications that may compromise nutrient absorption and utilization.
3. Assess nutritional data for information related to deficiencies:
    a. Quantity, quality, and frequency of food or formula
    b. Family eating patterns
    c. Cooking and storage facilities
    d. Socioeconomic status (for example, use of WIC, food stamps, and food pantries)
    e. Cultural habits (such as vegetarianism)
    f. Feeding history
    g. Dentition
    h. Food allergies and intolerances
    i. Method of preparing formula
    j. Stool pattern
    k. History of vomiting or diarrhea
    l. History of formula changes
    m. Transition from breast milk to formula
    n. Introduction of solid food
    o. Oral–muscular development
    p. Feeding environment (for example, is the child fed alone, in a group, or in front of the TV?).
4. Assess the physical findings related to nutritional status, such as changes in hair, skin, and oral mucosa, as well as behavioral abnormalities, such as psychomotor retardation and failure to interact with others.
5. Assess the family's interactional patterns and how these affect feeding; also assess their willingness to change and to accept support from outside the family, their level of knowledge, and their readiness and willingness to learn.

Nursing Diagnoses

The following is a list of possible diagnoses and could apply, depending on the child's age, clinical situation, and physical condition:

Altered growth and development

Altered nutrition: less or more than body requirements

Impaired skin integrity

Planning

In planning a child's nutrition assessment, the following equipment will be needed:

Scale

Non-stretch tape measure

Growth chart

Interventions

PROCEDURE	RATIONALE/EXPECTED OUTCOME (EO)
1. During the initial physical examination, the areas most likely to show effects of malnutrition are:	
a. Hair	a. Hair lacks normal pigmentation and luster and becomes easily pluckable.
b. Skin	b. Skin is dry and rough, with petechiae or ecchymoses.
c. Eyes	c. Eyes are pale, dull, and dry.
d. Lips, tongue, and gums	d. Lips are cracked, fissured, or pale. Tongue is swollen, with loss of normal papillae.
e. Subcutaneous fat (musculoskeletal)	e. There is wasting or obesity, bowed legs, and epiphyseal enlargement.
f. Behavior	f. Child becomes apathetic and irritable.
Examine the child thoroughly and record findings.	
2. Recumbent length/height, weight, and head circumference are routine measurements for the anthropometric component of a nutritional assessment.	
a. Record length weekly for children under 2 years old.	The best interpretation of a child's growth is made from serial observations rather than a single measurement. In general, stunted height is indicative of chronic malnutrition and low weight is indicative of acute malnutrition.
b. Record height weekly for children over 2 years old.	*EO: The child will gain weight within recommended ranges.*
c. Record weight daily (Table 75-2).	
d. Record head circumference daily of children under 36 months old.	
Plot all of the above on age-appropriate graphs at logical intervals.	The growth chart is an important part of the nutritional assessment.
	EO: The child resumes a normal growth pattern for his or her developmental level.

Table 75-2. Normal Weight Gain for Children

Age	g/day
0–3 months	25–35
3–6 months	15–21
6–12 months	10–13
1–6 years	5–8
7–10 years	5–11

PROCEDURE

Plot values on a longitudinal basis at birth: also at 1, 2, 4, 6, 9, 12, 18, and 24 months and every 6–12 months thereafter. All measurements must be corrected for gestational age. To correct for gestational age, the number of weeks of prematurity (using 40 as full-term) are subtracted from the child's current age. That age is then used to plot on the growth chart.

3. Routine laboratory tests represent the most objective assessment of nutritional status, particularly for early detection of marginal deficiencies before clinical signs are apparent.

　　a. Albumin

　　b. Hemoglobin or hematocrit
　　c. Total lymphocyte count (TLC)

　　d. Urine creatinine

Note the results of these tests.

4. Record a 3-day intake for assessment of energy and protein. (Table 75-3).

RATIONALE/EXPECTED OUTCOME (EO)

For the most part, premature infants will catch up to normal weight by 24 months, normal length by 36 months, and normal head circumference by 18 months, at which time correction is no longer needed.

EO: The child will have measurements plotted on growth charts, taking into account corrections for prematurity.

EO: The child's laboratory test results will be analyzed with respect to nutritional deficits.

　　a. Albumin is an indicator of visceral protein status. However, because of its large body pool and long half-life (20 days) it responds slowly to changes in nutritional status.
　　b. These are useful in screening for iron deficiency.
　　c. This is an index of visceral protein status. A depressed TLC places the child at risk.
　　d. This is used to calculate the creatinine–height index, which is an indirect measure of skeletal muscle mass.

Table 75-3. Nutritional Requirements for Infants and Children

Age	Cal/kg/24 hr
0–6 months	120
6–12 months	100
12–36 months	90–95
4–10 years	80
> 10 years (male)	45
> 10 years (female)	38

Nutrient	% of Total Calories
Carbohydrates	40–45%
Fat	40%
Protein	20%

Patient/Family Education: Home Care Considerations

1. Refer child and family to a dietitian to ensure continuous attention to nutritional interventions.

2. Guide the family through questions about breast- versus bottle-feeding, and when and how to introduce solid food.

3. Guide parents who follow special dietary practices, such as vegetarianism or religious proscription of foods, to supplement the child's diet with nonanimal protein substitutes, iron, etc.

References

——. (1988). *Nutritional Assessment: What Is It? How Is It Used?* Columbus, OH: Ross Laboratories.

Deen, D. (1990). Nutritional assessment for the primary care pediatrician. *Pediatric Annals, 4,* 244–260.

Howard, R.B., & Winter, H.S. (1984). *Nutrition and feeding of infants and toddlers.* Boston: Little Brown & Company.

Pipes, P.L. (1989). *Nutrition in infancy and childhood.* St. Louis: C.V. Mosby Company.

Queen, P. M., Boatright, S.L., & McNamara, M.N. (1983). Nutritional assessment of pediatric patients. *Nutritional Support Services. 3*(3) 23–31.

Snow, L.S., & Fry, M.E. (1990). Formula feeding in the first year of life. *Pediatric Nursing. 16*(5) 442–446.

Suitor, C.J.W. (1984). *Nutrition: Principles and application in health promotion.* Philadelphia: J.B. Lippincott Co.

Colon Irrigation

76

Definition/Purpose

Colon irrigation is a method of expelling feces from the intestines. Irrigations are performed to evacuate a hypoactive bowel (as seen in Hirschsprung's disease), and in preparation for abdominal or bowel surgery. The complete emptying of the bowel before surgery reduces the risk for peritonitis due to spilling of bowel content. Ordinary enemas or suppositories are of little value for this purpose.

Hirschsprung's disease, or congenital aganglionic megacolon, results from a congenital absence of the parasympathetic ganglion cells within the muscular wall of the distal colon and rectum. The parasympathetic nerves normally regulate autonomic peristalsis in the bowel; however, in Hirschsprung's disease, there is no peristalsis; thus the infant or child fails to pass stool or has a chief complaint of constipation. Colon irrigations are a daily requirement for these children.

Since the colon in Hirschsprung's disease is abnormally distended, the absorptive surface is increased. The absorption of enema fluids can dilute the extracellular fluids of the body, resulting in water intoxication. This is avoided by using a technique that avoids the buildup of a large volume of fluid in the bowel.

Standard of Care

1. Irrigations must be done at the same time each day.
2. Irrigations should be done with a warm saline solution unless stated otherwise.

Assessment

1. Assess the child's pertinent history, with reference to the course of the illness, medical or surgical history, family history of gastrointestinal problems, nutritional status, and eating patterns.
2. Assess the physical findings for discomfort, pain, nausea, vomiting, bowel sounds, abdominal distention, presence of blood or mucus in the stool, excoriation of perineal skin from diarrhea, nutritional status, and eating patterns.
3. Assess the psychosocial and developmental factors related to the child's developmental level, the family's ability to learn about the disease process, the need for irrigations, and the follow-up care required.

Nursing Diagnoses

The following is a list of possible diagnoses and could apply, depending on the child's age, clinical situation, and physical condition:

Anxiety

Constipation

Diarrhea

High risk for injury

Impaired skin integrity

Pain

Planning

In planning to perform a colon irrigation, the following equipment should be gathered:

Asepto syringe

Rectal tube (14–18 F for infants; 24–30 F for toddlers and older children)

Water-soluble lubricant

Extra diapers, washcloths, and towels

Saline solution

Non-sterile gloves

Interventions

PROCEDURE	RATIONALE/EXPECTED OUTCOME (EO)
1. Assemble all necessary equipment.	
2. Saline solution should be at room temperature.	Cold saline can cause hypothermia.
3. If the patient is old enough to understand, explain the procedure; also explain the procedure to all family members.	Prepared, well-informed child and parent will tend to cooperate with the procedure. *EO: The child will maintain current level of functioning and family members will verbalize an understanding of the child's specific needs.*
4. Place the infant or young child on the back or abdomen; place the older child on the left side.	
5. Place diapers or towels under the child.	
6. Put on gloves.	
7. Draw up prescribed amount of saline in asepto syringe.	
8. Put a small amount of lubricant along the length of the rectal tube. Insert the tip of the tube into the rectum and allow any gas or stool to escape.	If the tube is difficult to insert, lubricate it with more gel. *EO: The child will not have unnecessary discomfort from the insertion of the tube.*
9. Thread the tube into the rectum, using a twirling motion, to a depth of 3–4 inches.	The twirling motion and the fluid injection while advancing the catheter prevents perforation of the bowel. *EO: The child will have irrigations performed without injury to the bowel.*
10. Using the asepto syringe, inject a small amount of the saline solution as the catheter is advanced further.	
11. With the rectal tube completely inserted in the rectum, begin to instill the saline solution. Instill ¼ of the total amount; then disconnect the syringe from the tube, allowing the saline and feces to drain out through the tube. Allow the fluid and feces to drain into a cup, basin, or a diaper that can be weighed afterwards to determine exact output.	If unable to instill the solution: a. Check the tube to be sure that nothing is clogging the opening. b. Withdraw the tube to make sure that it is not kinked. *EO: The child will defecate during the procedure.*
12. Continue to instill ¼ of the total amount of solution and allow for drainage, while slowly withdrawing the rectal tube 1–2 inches with each irrigation until the entire length of the tube is removed.	Stop the irrigation if: a. The return is bloody b. Resistance is felt when irrigating c. The child complains of severe pain d. There is no fluid return after several irrigations. *EO: The child will have the irrigations stopped if complications develop.*

PROCEDURE	**RATIONALE/EXPECTED OUTCOME (EO)**
13. To facilitate drainage, gentle palpation of the abdomen or change of position may be attempted.	
14. Clean the perineal area after completing the irrigation.	*EO: The child's skin will remain intact.*

15. Document in the medical record:
    a. The total amount of irrigation solution instilled
    b. The total amount of irrigation solution and feces expelled
    c. The nature of the feces (color, presence of blood, etc.)
    d. How the child tolerated the procedure
    e. Condition of the skin.	

Patient/Family Education: Home Care Considerations

1. Educate the family as to the reason for the irrigations, the procedure itself, and when to notify the physician of complications.
2. Assist the family in obtaining the necessary equipment.
3. Teach them perineal hygiene and the use of sitz baths for anal discomfort.
4. Assist the family in planning for regular follow-up care.

References

Dehner, L. (1987). *Pediatric surgical pathology.* Baltimore: Williams & Wilkins.

Raffensperger, J.G. (1990). *Swenson's pediatric surgery.* Norwalk, CT: Appleton & Lange.

What is an Ostomy?

An ostomy is a surgically created opening. The location of the ostomy is specified by the prefix: *colo* means the opening is in the colon; *ileo* means the opening is in the ileum or small intestine; *nephro* means the opening is in the kidney; *uretero* means the opening is in the ureter; *jejuno* means the opening in the jejunum.

It is important to remember that an ostomy is not a disease or illness and is not contagious. The ostomy does not restrict play, school success, or social interaction.

What is a Stoma?

The word stoma means mouth. It refers to the nipple of exposed intestines or urinary tract. Most stomas are red because they are actually mucous membranes. They bleed easily because there is no skin covering, but the bleeding stops as quickly as it starts. Stomas also have no feeling because there are no nerve endings. As fragile as stomas appear, they can be slept on or rolled on without undue concern.

Types of Colostomies

1. Ascending colostomy
   This type of colostomy is located on the child's right side. Since the stool has not gone very far in the intestines, water and minerals have not had time to be absorbed. There are plenty of digestive juices left in the stool. These can digest normal skin and tissue if they come in contact with skin. It is therefore important to contain this stool in a bag that fits properly. The stool will usually be the consistency of toothpaste but may be only thick liquid if solid food is restricted.

   When there is no reason to remove the colon farther along the digestive tract, the surgeon will make a mucous fistula (opening between the colon and the abdominal wall) in the ascending colon, which will be at rest. This resting portion of the colon is alive and will secrete mucous, thus requiring the fistula for the mucous to escape.

2. Transverse colostomy
   This type of colostomy is located in the middle of the child's body and is usually created to rest or protect the colon below it. It may be required for only a short time. The stool is rarely formed, but it may be thicker than the stool from a right-sided colostomy because it has passed over more absorptive bowel surface.

3. Descending/Sigmoid Colostomy
   This type of colostomy is located on the left side of the body. Since most of the colon is functioning, the stool is formed as it would be if it came out of the rectum.

How to Manage Colostomies

Single Stoma

1. Wash hands. Wash around stoma with a mild soap and water.
2. Pat skin dry.
*3. Place a protective wafer around the stoma.
*4. Apply the adhesive disk of the bag to the wafer. Using a circular motion inside the bag with your fingers, bond the bag adhesive to the wafer.
5. Fold the bottom of the bag twice, pleat it across, and wrap it with a rubber band. Wash hand.

* You may use a bag and wafer that comes as a one-piece unit.

Stoma plus Mucous Fistula

1. Wash hands. Wash around stoma and fistula with mild soap and water.
2. Pat skin dry.
*3. Place a protective wafer around the two stomas.
4. Place a dab of protective paste in the space between the stomas, making sure that no skin is left showing.
5. Give the paste time to dry until shiny.
6. Apply the bag and bond it to the protective wafer as before.
7. Close the bottom of the bag with a rubber band. Wash hands.

* You may use a bag and wafer that comes as a one-piece unit.

Types of Ileostomies

1. *Conventional ileostomy*
   When the colon is sacrificed, water and minerals will not be absorbed. Pasty fecal material is passed through the stoma frequently during the day, with most of the activity occurring after meals. Fecal material usually does not have an offensive odor as it leaves the small intestines. Odor mounts as stool collects in the bag.

2. *Continent ileostomy*
   This operation creates an internal sac or reservoir made from the end of the small intestines. The pouch is made with a valve created from the intestine that prohibits the passage of stool and gas. It is emptied regularly, every 4 to 6 hours, by inserting a catheter into the pouch and draining the contents. There is a stoma, but no appliance is required.

How to Manage Ileostomies

1. Wash hands. Wash around stoma with a mild soap and water.
2. Pat skin dry.
3. Place a protective wafer around the stoma. The general rule for fitting the wafer is to allow $\frac{1}{8}$ inch extra for the stoma to expand. (For example, if the stoma is 1 inch, the wafer should be $1\frac{1}{8}$ inch).
4. Place karaya powder around the base of the stoma.
5. Snap on the pouch or apply the pouch as in the colostomy. Close the bottom of the bag. Wash hands.

There are dozens of variations in colostomy and ileostomy care. The system doesn't matter as long as your child is comfortable, the skin remains in excellent condition, and the procedure is affordable.

Diet

Colostomies

Infants usually do not have a problem with stool odor as long as they are on formula or a bland diet. In older children, odor-producing intestinal gas is caused by certain foods. To control odor, eliminate gassy foods and make sure your child eats applesauce, yogurt, or buttermilk each day. Do not give any medication to control gas.

If your child's stools change in consistency (become looser or harder), discuss this with your child's doctor or nurse. Excessive loss of fluid can cause dehydration quickly. If the stool is foul-smelling, this usually indicates that your child is ill. If the stool is dry or sticky, have your child drink more fluids. Both constipation and diarrhea can be caused by diet, illness, or medication.

Ileostomies

Your child's diet should include foods and liquids necessary to replace water and salts lost through the constant discharge of stool. All food should be chewed well because the stoma cannot stretch to pass a large piece of undigested food. Medications may change the color and consistency of the stool. Also, infants and small children may produce stools the same color as the food they eat.

Guide to Foods for Children with Ostomies

Easily Digested Foods

Rice

Potatoes

Noodles

Cream Soups

Potassium-Rich Foods

Banana	Tea
Cocoa	Tomatoes
Colas	Rye crackers
Oranges	Grapefruit

Sodium-Rich Foods

Bacon	Tuna
Butter	Mustard
Salt	Crackers

Gas-Producing Foods

Cabbage	Eggs	Cauliflower
Asparagus	Fish	Green peppers
Broccoli	Onions	Sauerkraut
Cucumbers	Radishes	

Hard-to-Digest Foods

Celery	Pineapple
Coconut	Olives
Corn	Whole grain cereal
Nuts	Pickles
Popcorn	Mushrooms
Grapes	Fried foods

Skin Care Considerations

1. Redness around the stoma
   If the skin is intact (not blistered or bleeding), this is usually due to pressure from the skin barrier and requires no treatment.

2. Redness, blistering, or weepy skin
   This is usually caused by leakage of discharge onto the skin. Remove the skin barrier, wash the area well and put on a clean appliance, making sure that the seal between the skin and barrier is tight. If there are irregularities in the skin around the stoma, paste may be used to fill the crevices and help maintain a tight seal.

3. Red skin with a pinpoint rash
   This may indicate a yeast infection. Your doctor needs to see the rash and prescribe something to clear it up. Do not apply any ointment or cream, as this will prevent the skin barrier from adhering properly. Never use a heat lamp to dry a rash, because it can burn the stoma.

Daily Living Tips

1. *Bathing.* A child may be bathed in a tub or shower with or without an appliance in place. Bath water will not enter the stoma. Avoid soaps that contain cold cream, oil, or lanolin.

2. *Clothing.* Your child will not require any special clothing. For infants, it is desirable to cover the bag completely to prevent the child from pulling at the appliance.

3. *School.* Most parents find school officials very cooperative. As a rule, you will want the school nurse, principal, and teachers (especially physical education or home room) to be aware of your child's condition. Emphasize that you want your child to be treated no differently than the other children in the school; however, your child does have special needs. These may include the need for privacy in showering after gym, the need for frequent fluid intake, and the need for access to the bathroom to service the appliance. The ostomy is emptied as frequently as necessary to prevent the weight of the stool or urine from pulling the protective wafer away from the skin.

   The school nurse should have detailed instructions on the care of the ostomy and should have extra supplies and a change of clothing in case of leakage.

4. *Travel.* Always take enough supplies to last the entire trip. Carry at least half of your supplies with you in case baggage is lost. At a minimum you will want to carry with you a complete appliance, accessories, water in a plastic bottle, and a zip-lock bag in which to empty the pouch in an emergency.

Where to Get Help

The United Ostomy Association
2001 W. Beverly Boulevard
Los Angeles, California 90057
(213) 413-45510

National Foundation for Ileitis and Colitis
295 Madison Avenue
New York, New York 10017
(212) 685-3440

References

Hancock, L.A. (1988). Ostomy Care and Puppets Too. *Journal of Pediatric Health Care, November/December*, 167–170.

Jeter, K.F. (1982). *These Special Children: The Ostomy Book For Parents of Children with Colostomies, Ileostomies and Urostomies.* Palo Alto, CA: Bull Publishing Company.

_____. (1984). *Ostomy and Your Child—A Parents' Guide.* Princeton, NJ: Convatec, A Squibb Company.

A gastrostomy tube has been inserted into your child's stomach through the abdominal wall. This tube permits the intake of the food, water and medications that the body requires. The following information needs to be retained by you for future reference:

_____ Date of gastrostomy insertion

_____ Balloon volume

_____ Size of gastrostomy tube

_____ Doctor's name

_____ Doctor's telephone

_____ Nurse's name

_____ Nurse's telephone

Insertion of Gastrostomy Tube

Do not attempt to replace the gastrostomy tube unless you have been given instructions on the correct placement by the surgical team.

Steps

1. Wash your hands before beginning the insertion procedure.
2. Check the new tube prior to placement.
   a. If the tube has a ring used for positioning, make sure that it will slide up and down along the tube.
   b. Inflate the balloon by filling it with water to make sure it will not leak. Then deflate the balloon.
3. Moisten the tip of the tube with water or water-based lubricant. Do not use oil or a petroleum-based jelly, because these may cause balloon damage.
4. Gently guide the tube through the opening and into the stomach, about 1–1½ inches on infants and children, and 2–4 inches on adolescents. The entire balloon should pass through the tract (Fig. 1).

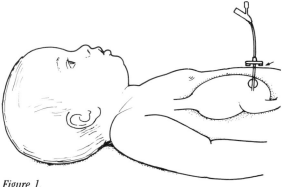

Figure 1.

5. Attach a 5 mL syringe filled with water to the inflation valve and inflate the balloon with 3–4 mL of water. Do not use air, and do not exceed 5 mL of water in the balloon.

6. Grasp the body of the tube and withdraw it until tension is felt from the balloon against the stomach wall.

7. Position the ring to ensure secure placement of the tube. Allow 1–2 mm of space between the skin and the ring.

8. The ring holds the tube in place; therefore, there is no need for gauze or tape at the insertion site.

9. Close or clamp the newly inserted tube.

Removal of Gastrostomy Tube

Steps

1. Wash your hands before beginning the removal procedure.

2. Using an empty 5-mL syringe, attach the syringe to the inflation/deflation valve and withdraw the water from the balloon.

3. Gently pull on the tube until it comes out.

4. Cover the stoma with a gauze or towel to prevent drainage of stomach contents until a new tube is inserted.

Maintenance of the Gastrostomy Tube

Daily Care of the Gastrostomy Site

1. Inspect the skin for redness, tenderness, swelling, irritation, and presence of purulent drainage or gastric leakage.

2. Inspect the tube for inward or outward migration. At the time of insertion, you may either mark the tube at the skin entry point or measure and record the length of the tube from skin level to the end.

3. Cleanse the skin with soap and water. Use a spiral pattern, beginning next to the site and moving outward. Dry the area thoroughly. You may need to use cotton-tipped swabs to clean and dry under the ring.

4. Avoid a dressing around the tube. A dressing will promote skin maceration, breakdown, and infection. If a dressing is used, change it immediately if it becomes wet.

Problem Solving

1. Leakage around the tube

Causes:
a. Improper positioning of the child
b. Too rapid feeding rate
c. Balloon decreased in size due to leakage of water from balloon
d. Blocked tube
e. Increased size of gastrostomy tract
f. Decreased GI function
g. Tube migration inward
h. Tube migration outward.

Actions:
a. Keep the child in an upright position during the feeding and for 30–60 minutes after. This may be accomplished by using a pillow or infant seat.
b. Slow the rate of infusing the feeding.
c. Check for balloon leakage by using a syringe to withdraw the water from the balloon. If less than originally instilled, either add more water or change the tube.
d. Flush the tube with water.
e. Keep the tube well-stabilized with the ring. Avoid excess tension, which could result in damage to the gastric mucosa. Prevent your child from pulling on the tube.
f. If your child vomits or has abdominal distention, suspend the feedings and notify a member of the surgical team.

g. Check length of the tube or look for the mark you made when you inserted the tube and readjust as needed.

2. Skin redness or irritation around tube

Causes:
a. Gastric leakage around tube
b. Allergic reaction to soap
c. Reaction to tube material.

Actions:
a. Assess the cause of leakage and correct the problem. Keep skin dry, clean, and free from drainage. If a dressing is used, change it when it becomes soiled or wet. Use a waterproof barrier (such as an ointment or wafer) around the site to protect the skin from gastric drainage.
b. Try plain water for cleansing, or switch to a different soap.
c. Use tube made of biocompatible material.

3. Tube blockage

Causes:
a. Inadequate flushing of tube
b. Curdling of formula
c. Medication administration.

Actions:
a. Flush feeding tube with warm water before and after each feeding, before and after the administration of medications, and every 3–4 hours if your child is on continuous feeding.
b. Flush the tube with warm water after checking the residual.
c. Do not mix medications with formula. Medication should be in liquid form or crushed finely and diluted in water. Multiple medications should be given one at a time with the tube rinsed in between with 5–10 mL of water.

4. Feeding bag disconnects

Causes:
a. Buildup of oily deposits
b. Feeding bag connector does not fit snugly in gastrostomy tube.

Actions:
a. Keep the feeding port and the bag connector clean. Remove oily buildup with a diet soft drink, using a tiny amount of soda on a cotton-tipped swab and cleansing the top 2 inches around the inside of the tube.
b. Ask the surgical team or medical supplier for an adaptor to fit both the feeding bag and gastrostomy tube.

5. Balloon fails to deflate

Causes:
a. Valve is clogged.

Actions:
a. Cut off the feeding port adaptor above the ring. This will allow the balloon to drain.

Feeding Through the Gastrostomy

Equipment Needed:

Feeding bag

Formula

Water.

Steps:

1. Place your child on the right side and prone with head elevated, or in a sitting position in a chair. These positions enhance the emptying of the stomach.

2. If the feeding is refrigerated, warm it to room temperature.

3. Pour the prescribed amount of feeding into the feeding bag. Allow the feeding to flow into the tubing by opening the regulator clamp on the bag.

4. Attach the feeding bag tubing to the gastrostomy tube.

5. Using gravity, let the prescribed feeding flow in over the the course of 30–45 minutes. After all the feeding has infused, pour the prescribed amount of water into the bag and let the water flow in using gravity for 5 minutes.

6. After the flush of water has infused, open the regulator clamp on the bag completely and allow the empty feeding bag to remain attached to the gastrostomy. This will vent the stomach, allowing built-up gas to escape. Vent the stomach for 15 minutes; then disconnect the feeding bag, rinse the bag with water, and clamp or close the gastrostomy. (If you suspect your child has a buildup of gas in the stomach, you may at any time connect an empty feeding bag to the gastrostomy tube, open the regulator clamp, and vent the stomach.)

Administering Medications Through the Gastrostomy

Do's

1. Use the liquid form of the medication whenever possible.

2. Check your pharmacy if in doubt about the availability of medication in liquid form and whether or not tablets are crushable.

3. If a tablet must be crushed, be sure it is crushed finely and dispersed well in warm water.

4. Use a 30–60-mL syringe with 10–30 mL of warm water to rinse feeding tube before and after giving the medication.

5. If more than one medication is to be given, administer each separately, rinsing the tube with 5 mL of water between medications.

6. Administer medication at the appropriate time in relation to the feeding. Some medications should be given with food, whereas others should be given on an empty stomach. Check with your pharmacy when in doubt.

Don'ts

1. Do not mix medication with the feeding formula.

2. Do not crush enteric-coated or time-release capsules or tablets.

3. Do not mix medications together.

When to Call Your Doctor or Nurse

1. If the gastrostomy tube comes out and you are unable to replace it within 1 hour.

2. If your are unable to flush the gastrostomy tube with water.

3. If there is bleeding through or around the tube.

4. If there is purulent drainage, redness, or skin breakdown around the tube.

5. If your child's stomach looks distended even after you have vented the tube.

6. If your child has excessive diarrhea or constipation.

7. If your child demonstrates a painful response either during or after feedings, or when the tube is manipulated.

8. If your child has a temperature of 38.3°C (101°F) or higher.

References

Medical Innovations Corporation. (1987). *Patient information: MIC gastrostomy tube.* Milpitas, CA.

Ross Laboratories. *Instructions for use: 18 Fr replacement gastrostomy tube.* Columbus, OH.

Ross Laboratories. (1986). *Administering oral medications through an enteral feeding tube.* Columbus, OH.

Ross Laboratories. (1987). *General Guidelines for gastrostomy care.* Columbus, OH.

PATIENT TEACHING CHECKLIST

All of the following skills must be learned before discharge. The nursing categories must be dated and signed by the nurse who has assumed responsibility for teaching. Parents are to sign and date each task as mastery is achieved. (See skills as outlined in "Gastrostomy Home Instructions".)

Child and/or Parent Should Be Able to:	Nurse Demonstration (Initials & Date)	Parent Return-Demonstration (Initials & Date)
1. Verbalize an understanding of the purpose of the gastrostomy.		
2. Insert a new gastrostomy tube.		
3. Remove the old gastrostomy tube.		
4. Verbalize daily maintenance of the tube.		
5. Verbalize problems that could appear and what corrective actions should be taken.		
6. Demonstrate a safe feeding technique.		
7. Demonstrate a safe method of administering medications through the gastrostomy tube.		
8. Verbalize an understanding of when to call the doctor or nurse.		

Purpose

Rectal irrigations are performed to soften and remove stool from the bowel tract. The irrigation should be done at a convenient time for your family, but it must be done at the same time every day.

Procedure

1. Assemble the following equipment:
   - Rectal tube (size specified by physician)
   - Asepto syringe
   - Water-soluble lubricant
   - Extra diapers, washcloth, and towel
   - Saline (salt) solution (The amount will be specified by physician.)

   To prepare the saline solution, mix 2 teaspoons of table salt with 1 quart (32 ounces) of water. Leave at room temperature.

2. Prepare your child for the procedure by placing the child on his or her back or abdomen with diapers or a towel underneath. Place the older child on his or her left side.

3. Put a small amount of lubricant along the length of the rectal tube. Insert the tip of the tube into the rectum, and allow any gas or stool to escape.

4. Next, thread the tube into the rectum, using a twirling motion, to a depth of 3–4 inches. The twirling motion helps to pass any tight spots.

5. Using the asepto syringe, put in the saline solution continuously as the tube is advanced further into the rectum.

6. With the rectal tube all the way inside the rectum, begin instilling the saline solution. Instill $\frac{1}{4}$ of the total amount and then disconnect the syringe from the tube, allowing the saline to drain out. Continue to instill $\frac{1}{4}$ of the total amount of solution and allow for drainage, while slowly withdrawing the rectal tube 1–2 inches with each irrigation until the entire length of the tube is removed.

7. Cleanse the area after completing the irrigation.

Helpful Hints:

1. If the tube is difficult to insert:
   a. Make sure it is well-lubricated.
   b. Gently and slowly twist the rectal tube while putting in the saline.

2. If unable to instill solution:
   a. Check tube to make sure nothing is clogging openings at the end of the tube.
   b. Withdraw and reinsert the tube.

3. Stop irrigation if any of the following occur:
   a. Resistance to the irrigation is felt.
   b. The returns are blood-tinged.
   c. The child complains of severe abdominal pain. The irrigation procedure may feel uncomfortable or "funny," but it should not cause severe pain.
   d. There is no fluid return after several irrigations.

PATIENT TEACHING CHECKLIST

Child and/or Parent Should Be Able to:	Nurse Demonstration (Initials & Date)	Parent Return-Demonstration (Initials & Date)
1. Verbalize an understanding of the purpose of colon irrigations.		
2. Verbalize how to prepare the saline solution.		
3. Verbalize how to position the child.		
4. Perform the irrigation.		
5. Anticipate problems and complications of the irrigations.		

Genitourinary System Procedures

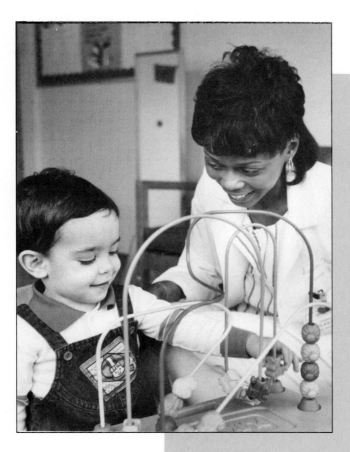

Unit XI

Obtaining a Urine Specimen from the Infant and Young Child

77

Definition/Purpose

The relatively high frequency of urinary tract infections and anomalies in infants and children makes examination of the urine a necessary task. Because the frequency of voiding is unpredictable in infants and young children, attaching a container to the genitalia is most successful for obtaining single specimens. Disposable, sterile, thin plastic bags with nonirritating adhesive flaps are commonly used. These bags have a flap valve to prevent voided urine from refluxing out of the bag.

Urine can be collected for the following purposes:

1. To check for the presence of sugar, acetone, bacteria, blood, ketones, cells, casts, bacteria, or crystals.
2. To aid in diagnosis of renal abnormalities and screening for the adequacy of renal function.
3. To determine the effectiveness of therapy by measuring pH and specific gravity.

Standard of Care

1. A thorough preparation of the perineum is necessary before collecting urine for any purpose.

Assessment

1. Assess the pertinent history and physical findings for signs of infection (for example, cloudy or foul-smelling urine, fever, irritability, failure to thrive, urgency, or dysuria); renal failure (for example, abnormal blood test results, fluid imbalance, pulmonary edema, or congestive heart failure); diabetes (for example, abdominal pain, blurred vision, polydipsia, polyphagia, or polyuria), or other diseases that could be detected by analysis of the urine. Assess for a past family history of kidney disease, diabetes, urinary tract infection, or enuresis.
2. Assess the age, developmental level, and coping strategies of the child and family. Assess the present history for toilet training, if age-appropriate.
3. Assess the family's knowledge of the reasons for the urine test, the procedure for collecting the urine, the outcomes, and the discharge regimen.

Nursing Diagnoses

The following is a list of possible diagnoses and could apply, depending on the child's age, clinical situation, and physical condition:

Anxiety

High risk for infection

High risk for injury

Impaired skin integrity

Pain

Planning

When planning to apply a urine collection bag, the following equipment is needed:

Sterile water

Antiseptic solution or soap

Sterile cotton balls or 4 × 4s

Urine collector

Specimen container

Non-sterile gloves

Interventions

PROCEDURE	**RATIONALE/EXPECTED OUTCOME (EO)**
1. Explain the urine collection procedure to the child and family.	The family will cooperate with the collection if they understand the procedure. *EO: The family will exhibit decreased anxiety.*
2. Position the child so that the genitalia are exposed by placing the child on the back with legs in frog-like position (Fig. 77-1).	Proper positioning will facilitate cleansing and allow for proper placement of the collection bag. *EO: The child will be positioned to provide optimal cleaning and placement of the bag.*

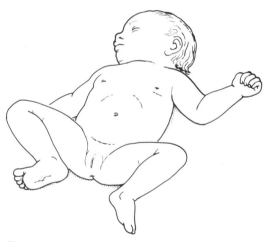

Figure 77-1.

3. Cleanse the genital area. Wash hands and put on gloves.	During the cleansing, be gentle to avoid any injury to the skin. *EO: The child will exhibit minimal discomfort.*
Male—Wipe tip of penis with cotton ball and soap solution in circular motion down towards the scrotum. Repeat the procedure with sterile cotton ball saturated with sterile water to rinse soap from the area. Let the area air-dry and replace the foreskin.	
Female—Wash hands and put on gloves. Wipe labia majora with cotton ball and soap solution from top to bottom (clitoris to anus) once only with each cotton ball. Then spread the labia apart with one hand, while wiping labia minora in the same manner with the other hand. Repeat procedure with ster-	This method of cleansing will prevent contamination of the genitalia from the anus and will prevent contamination of the urine specimen.

PROCEDURE	RATIONALE/EXPECTED OUTCOME (EO)

ile cotton ball saturated with sterile water to rinse the area of the soap. Let air-dry.

4. Remove the paper backing, exposing the adhesive surface of the collection bag.

5. For the male, insert the penis through the opening in the bag. For the female, apply the round opening over the vulva and beneath the urethral orifice.

6. Press the adhesive surface firmly against the skin (Fig. 77-2).

The procedure will not have to be repeated, if the collecting bag is properly placed.

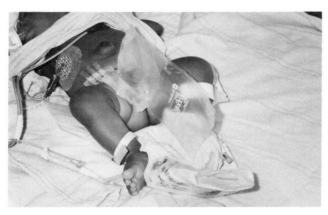

Figure 77-2.

7. Diaper the child and make him or her comfortable. Remove gloves and wash hands.

8. Check the child every 30–60 minutes for the appearance of urine in the bag.

9. When the child has voided, remove the bag gently and pour the specimen into a collecting container.

10. Clean and dry the area, and rediaper.

11. Send specimen to laboratory.

Prompt delivery of specimens to the laboratory will prevent growth of organisms.

EO: The child will have the urine collected and analyzed.

12. Accurately chart and describe the following:
    • Time specimen was collected
    • Amount of urine voided
    • Color of urine
    • Type of test to be performed
    • Condition of the skin of perineal area.

The medical record will document the collection of the specimen.

Severe diaper rash may limit the use of urine bags. Not only can the adhesive exacerbate an existing rash, but an active dermatitis increases the chances of contaminating the urine specimen, even with adequate skin preparation. The child may need to be catheterized for a urine specimen.

EO: The child's skin will remain intact.

13. Follow up on the test results.

If a culture from a bag is sterile, it is acceptable. If bacterial growth is demonstrated, another specimen must be obtained by a more reliable method before treatment is begun. (See Chap. 78, Suprapubic Bladder Aspiration.)

Patient/Family Education: Home Care Considerations

1. Reinforce the information given by the physician to the family regarding the results of the test. Correct any misinformation and fill in gaps of needed information.

2. Explain the need for continuous monitoring of the child once treatment has begun. Help the family coordinate follow-up appointments and repeat tests.

3. If an infection is detected, the following instructions may be helpful:
   a. Increase fluid intake with regular and frequent voidings to promote bladder washout of bacteria.
   b. Avoiding constipation helps to ensure better bladder emptying.
   c. Good perineal hygiene, including wiping from front to back after a bowel movement, is important.
   d. Eliminating pinworms prevents inflammation, excoriation, and secondary increase in skin flora.
   e. Bubble bath, by producing inflammation at the meatus, may produce increased bacteria and should therefore be avoided.

References

Fleisher, G., & Ludwig, S. (1988). *Textbook of pediatric emergency medicine.* Baltimore: Williams & Wilkins.

Suddarth, D. (1991). *The Lippincott manual of nursing practice.* (5th ed.). Philadelphia: J.B. Lippincott Co.

Suri, S. (1988). Simplifying urine collection from infants and children without losing accuracy. *Maternal/Child Nursing; 13*(6); 438–441.

Suprapubic Bladder Aspiration

78

Definition/Purpose

Needle aspiration of the bladder to obtain a sterile urine specimen for culture analysis has become a common method of urine collection in infants and children under 2 years old. Above the age of two, sterile urine should be collected by urethral catheterization.

This technique is applicable to young children because their distended bladders are intra-abdominal. As the individual becomes older, the bladder becomes positioned more in the intrapelvic area. Also, the bladder of infants and children is more spindle-shaped than adults' and lies closely opposed to the lower anterior abdominal wall.

Standard of Care

1. The entire procedure will be carried out under strict aseptic technique.
2. An assistant is always needed to position the child.

Assessment

1. Assess the pertinent history for congenital defects, bladder distention, operative sites, previous urinary tract infection, and the condition now requiring the aspiration.
2. Assess the physical findings of possible neurogenic bladder, bladder obstruction, fever, and hydrational status.
3. Assess developmental factors, the family's knowledge of the purpose of the aspiration, and the necessary follow-up treatment.

Nursing Diagnoses

The following is a list of possible diagnoses and could apply, depending on the child's age, clinical situation, and physical condition:

Pain

High risk for infection

High risk for injury

Impaired skin integrity

Planning

To assist in the preparation for suprapubic bladder aspiration, the following equipment must be assembled:

Sterile gloves

3 povidone-iodine swabs

23-gauge straight 2–3 cm needle

3- or 5-mL syringe

Sterile urine container

Adhesive bandage

Interventions

PROCEDURE

1. Explain the bladder aspiration procedure to the family.

2. For the procedure to be successful, the infant's bladder must be full.

3. Position the infant supine, holding the legs in the frog-leg position (Fig. 78-1).

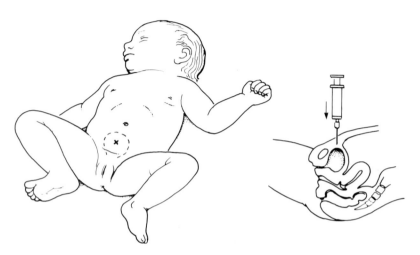

Figure 78-1.

(Steps 4–10 will be performed by the physician.)

4. Prepare the skin by cleansing it with povidone-iodine solution.

5. Put on sterile gloves.

6. Palpate the pubic symphysis in the midline as a landmark, and locate the aspiration site 1–2 cm above the pubic symphysis, in the midline.

7. Position the needle perpendicular to the plane of the abdominal wall.

8. Pierce the skin in a single steady movement.

9. After the needle enters the skin, gently aspirate the syringe as the needle is advanced. Entry into the bladder is signaled by the appearance of urine in the syringe.

10. After the specimen is obtained, withdraw the needle and apply an adhesive bandage.

    To prevent the infant from spontaneously voiding before the aspiration:
    • Handle the infant gently before and during the aspiration.

RATIONALE/EXPECTED OUTCOME (EO)

EO: The family will understand the need for the aspiration and express appropriate concerns to the staff.

This can be confirmed by a documented period of a dry diaper for longer than 30–45 minutes, gentle abdominal palpation, or by low abdominal transillumination.

EO: The child will be positioned to provide optimal alignment for the procedure to be completed safely.

EO: The child will not acquire a focus of infection at the aspiration site.

If urine is not obtained, do not remove the needle from below the surface of the abdomen. Instead, change the angle of the needle and reinsert (20° caudad or 20° cephalad to the perpendicular).

EO: The child will have a urine sample collected and evaluated.

EO: The child will experience minimal side effects from the procedure.

PROCEDURE	RATIONALE/EXPECTED OUTCOME (EO)

- Compress the male urethra gently before the aspiration.
- Place little finger into the female's rectum and apply pressure anteriorly, obstructing the female urine outflow.

11. Observe the child for complications of the procedure:
    a. Gross hematuria
    b. Anterior abdominal wall abscess
    c. Bowel puncture
    d. Peritonitis
    e. Anaerobic bacteremia.

Microscopic hematuria virtually *always* occurs. Gross hematuria is uncommon.

EO: The child remains free from injury.

Patient/Family Education: Home Care Considerations

1. Reinforce with the family the information regarding the results of the bladder aspiration given by the physician. Correct any misinformation and fill in gaps of needed information.

2. Explain to the family the need for repeat urine tests and for continuing medication administration.

Reference

Fleisher, G., & Ludwig, S. (1988). *Textbook of pediatric emergency medicine.* Baltimore: Williams & Wilkins.

Indwelling Urethral Catheter

79

Definition/Purpose

A catheter is introduced through the urethra into the bladder. Two categories of urinary catheters are straight catheters and retention catheters. The straight catheter is a single lumen tube with a small eye about $\frac{1}{2}$ inch from the insertion tip. The retention or Foley catheter contains a second smaller tube throughout its length on the inside. This tube is connected to a balloon near the insertion tip. After catheter insertion, the balloon is inflated to hold the catheter in place within the bladder. The outside end of the retention catheter is bifurcated, one opening to drain the urine, and one end to inflate the balloon (Fig. 79-1).

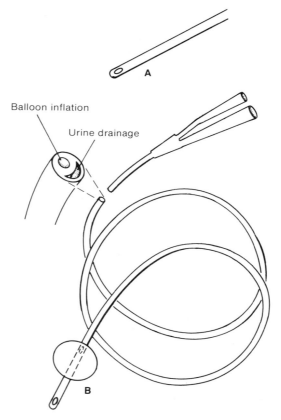

Figure 79-1. Two types of catheters commonly used. **(A)** Straight (Robinson) catheter. **(B)** Retention (Foley) catheter with balloon inflated.

Catheters are sized by the diameter of the lumen and are graded on a French scale of numbers; the larger the number, the larger the lumen (for example, 8F, 10F, 12F, etc). The balloons of retention catheters are sized by the volume of fluid used to inflate them. The most common size for children is a 5-mL balloon.

Indwelling catheters may be used after surgical procedures on the urinary tract or in any critically ill child who needs constant monitoring of fluid status.

Standard of Care

1. This entire procedure will be carried out under strict aseptic technique.

Assessment

1. Assess the history and physical findings for congenital defects, incontinence, bladder distention, or conditions requiring constant monitoring of urinary output, specific gravity, occult blood, glucose, acetone, pH, protein, and electrolytes.
2. Assess developmental factors related to body image, dependency, embarrassment about urine collection devices in view of visitors, and normal habits and routines.
3. Assess the child's and family's knowledge of the purpose and care of the catheter.

Nursing Diagnoses

The following is a list of possible diagnoses and could apply, depending on the child's age, clinical situation, and physical condition:

High risk for infection

Urinary retention

Functional incontinence

Anxiety

Planning

In preparation for inserting an indwelling urinary catheter, the following equipment must be gathered:

A sterile catheterization kit containing:

Gloves (sterile and nonsterile)

Drapes

Antiseptic solution (povidone-iodine)

Cotton balls

Forceps to apply the antiseptic solution

Water soluble lubricant

Specimen container

Catheter (of the appropriate size)

Drainage bag

Syringe (prefilled with sterile water) to inflate the balloon

Tape

Safety pin

Interventions

PROCEDURE	RATIONALE/EXPECTED OUTCOME (EO)
Insertion	
1. Explain the reason for inserting the retention catheter, how long it will be in place, and the way in which the urinary drainage equipment needs to be	Relieving the child's tension can facilitate insertion of the catheter because the sphincters will be more relaxed.

PROCEDURE

handled to maintain the drainage of urine. Reassure the child and family that the procedure may be uncomfortable, but not painful.

2. Provide privacy.

3. Assist the child to a supine position with knees flexed and thighs externally rotated. An assistant is needed to hold the child in the position.

4. Drape the child.

5. Pour the povidone-iodine solution over the cotton balls.

6. Put on sterile gloves.

7. Lubricate the insertion tip of the catheter with the water soluble gel.

8. *Female:* Separate the labia majora with the thumb and index finger and clean the labia minora on each

RATIONALE/EXPECTED OUTCOME (EO)

EO: The child and parent will express concerns and ask questions regarding the catheterization.

Raising the pelvis gives the nurse a better view of the urinary meatus.

Water soluble gel facilitates insertion by reducing friction.

The hand that touches the child becomes contaminated while the other hand remains sterile.

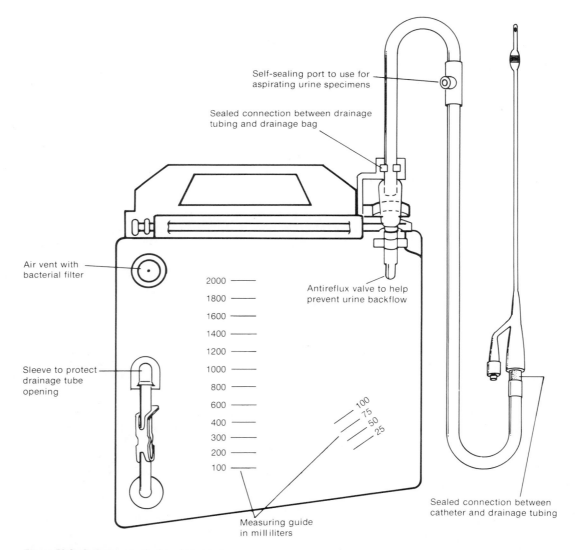

Self-sealing port to use for aspirating urine specimens

Sealed connection between drainage tubing and drainage bag

Air vent with bacterial filter

Sleeve to protect drainage tube opening

Antireflux valve to help prevent urine backflow

2000
1800
1600
1400
1200
1000
800
600
400
300
200
100

100
75
50
25

Measuring guide in milliliters

Sealed connection between catheter and drainage tubing

Figure 79-2. Catheter attached to drainage bag.

PROCEDURE

side, using forceps and soaked cotton balls. Use a new swab for each stroke, moving downward from the pubic area to the anus. Then separate the labia minora with two fingers, using the same hand. Expose the urinary meatus. Clean from the meatus downward and then on either side, using a new swab for each stroke.
Keep the labia apart.

Insert the catheter approximately 2.5 cm into the urinary meatus or until urine flows.

Male: Grasp the penis firmly behind the glans, and spread the meatus between the thumb and forefinger. Retract the foreskin of an uncircumcised male. The hand holding the penis is now contaminated. Clean the meatus with the soaked cotton balls and forceps in a circular motion. Discard each swab after one wipe. To insert the catheter, lift the penis to a position perpendicular to the body and exert slight traction. Insert the catheter 2.5 cm until urine flows.

9. Attach the catheter to the drainage bag (Fig. 79-2).

10. Inflate the balloon of the catheter to the size specified on the catheter. Apply slight tension on the catheter until resistance is felt (Fig. 79-3).

RATIONALE/EXPECTED OUTCOME (EO)

Cleaning from anterior to posterior cleans from the point of least contamination to that of greatest contamination.

Keeping the labia apart prevents the risk of contamination.
EO: The child will have a urinary catheter inserted in an aseptic atraumatic manner.

To avoid an erection, firm pressure rather than light pressure is used to grasp the penis.

To bypass resistance at the sphincters, twist the catheter or wait until the sphincter relaxes. Lifting the penis straightens the curvature of the urethra.

Resistance indicates that the catheter balloon is inflated and the catheter is anchored in the bladder.

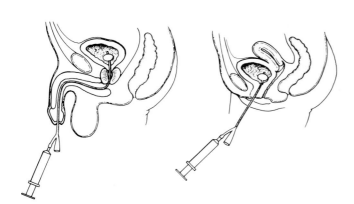

Figure 79-3.

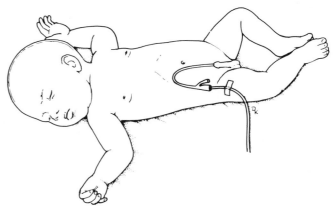

Figure 79-4.

11. Dry the perineum and replace the foreskin for males. Anchor the catheter to the inside of the female's thigh and the outside of the male's thigh (Fig. 79-4).

12. Coil the drainage tube beside the child on the bed and fasten it to the bedclothes with a clamp or safety pin. Hang the drainage bag on the side of the bed. Record the insertion time and the size of the catheter.

Maintenance

13. Observe and record the color, odor, amount, and appearance of urine each time the collection unit is emptied. Wear gloves to empty the bag.

Taping restricts the movement of the catheter, reducing irritation in the urethra. In the male, taping the catheter to the inside of the thigh with the penis bent over the catheter could cause internal tissue erosion.

The drainage tubing should not loop below its entry into the drainage bag, because this impedes the flow of urine by gravity.

EO: The child will maintain a properly functioning urinary drainage system.

PROCEDURE

14. Check the patency of the drainage system every 2 hours.
15. Determine specific gravity and pH of urine.
16. Record total intake and output at least every 8 hours.
17. Be alert for signs of renal calculi (flank pain and low abdominal pressure); pyelonephritis (fever, chills, and vomiting); or urinary tract infection.

    Infants: Poor sucking, poor feeding, vomiting, lethargy, fever, jaundice, and failure to thrive

    Toddlers: Abdominal pain, dysuria, fever, anorexia, urinary frequency, urinary urgency, and bedwetting

    Older child: Frequency, urgency, abdominal pain, dysuria, and fever.

18. Cleanse perineum daily with mild soap and water; rinse and dry thoroughly. Assess the area around the urinary meatus for:
    - Odor
    - Inflammation and swelling
    - Discharge (Note color, amount, and consistency).

19. Obtain urine specimens with a sterile 25-gauge needle and 5-mL syringe. After cleaning rubber port with antiseptic swab, insert needle and withdraw the specimen.

20. Clamp tubing whenever the drainage bag is lifted to the height of the mattress.

21. Never disconnect catheter from drainage bag unless absolutely necessary.

Removal

22. Reassure the child and parent that the removal of the catheter will not be painful, although it may feel "funny."

23. Put on nonsterile gloves.

24. Insert an empty syringe into the balloon inflation tube of the catheter and draw out all of the fluid.

25. Gently withdraw the catheter from the urethra.

26. Dry the genital area with cotton balls.

27. Dispose of the catheter and drainage system according to hospital policy.

28. Record the time the catheter was removed and the amount, color, and consistency of the urine in the bag.

29. Encourage the child to drink fluids if medically indicated.

30. Monitor the child's intake and output. Record time of first void after catheter removed, as well as the amount and color of the urine.

RATIONALE/EXPECTED OUTCOME (EO)

Stasis of urine in the bladder predisposes the child to bladder infection.

EO: The child will maintain normal urine composition.

Hourly output should average 1 mL/kg/hr.
A catheter left in place for more than a few hours increases the risk of bacteriuria.
Organisms frequently found: *E coli, Klebsiella, Proteus pseudomonas,* and *Aerobacter*

EO: The child will be free from bacterial growth and nosocomial infection.

This will prevent reflux of urine back into the bladder from tubing.

EO: The child will maintain gravity flow drainage without backflow into the bladder.

EO: The child will have the urinary catheter removed without trauma.

The balloon needs to be deflated to prevent trauma to the urethra when the catheter is withdrawn.

PROCEDURE	**RATIONALE/EXPECTED OUTCOME (EO)**
31. Assess the frequency of voiding or any unusual symptoms related to voiding.	Prolonged drainage of urine through a catheter causes loss of bladder tone. The child may have frequency or dysuria with the first few voids after the catheter is removed. *EO: The child regains normal bladder function after catheter removal.*

Patient/Family Education: Home Care Considerations

1. If the child is to be discharged with an indwelling catheter or needing intermittent catheterization, the child and parents will require instruction to ensure adequate catheter care.

2. The child or parent must demonstrate intermittent catheterization and routine catheter care.

3. The parent must be given a list of signs and symptoms of urinary tract infections and renal calculi.

4. Initiate referrals for home health care.

5. Provide written instructions for bladder training if it is to be done at home.

Reference

Joseph, D.B., Bauer, S.B., Colodney, A.H., et al. (1989). Clean, intermittent catheterization of infants with neurogenic bladder. *Pediatrics, 84*(1), 78–82.

Pearson-Shaver, A., et al. (1990). Urethral catheter knots. *Pediatrics, 87*(5), 852–854.

Peritoneal Dialysis

80

Definition/Purpose

Peritoneal dialysis is indicated for the child with acute renal failure when other management has failed to control hypervolemia, hypertension, bleeding, electrolyte imbalance, or acid–base imbalance. Indications for dialysis include the following:

1. Hypervolemia with congestive heart failure, hypertension, or hypertensive encephalopathy
2. Deterioration in neurologic status
3. Bleeding unresponsive to blood component therapy
4. Serum potassium concentration above 6.5–7.0 m Eq/L
5. BUN greater than 125–150 mg/dL
6. Serum calcium concentration above 12 mg/dL
7. Serum sodium concentration above 160 m Eq/L
8. Metabolic acidosis or alkalosis
9. Ingestion of any of the following substances:
   a. Salicylates
   b. Phenytoin
   c. Heavy metals
   d. Barbiturates.

Fluids cross the peritoneal membrane through diffusion and osmosis. Diffusion is the random movement of particles in solution toward a uniform concentration throughout the available volume. Osmosis is the movement of a solvent through a semipermeable membrane from an area of higher concentration to an area of lower concentration of solutes, equalizing the concentration.

Peritoneal dialysis is the diffusion of a solute through a semipermeable membrane (the peritoneum) from the child's blood to the dialysate. Fluids pass through the membrane by means of osmosis. The purpose is to remove toxic substances, body wastes, and fluid, and to maintain life until kidney function is restored.

The dialysate is removed and replaced repeatedly. The rate and amount of water removed from the child depends on the osmotic pressure generated by the dextrose in the dialysate. The solutions are available in 1.5%, 2.5%, and 4.25% dextrose solution and 500 mL, 1000 mL, and 2000 mL bags (Table 80-1).

Table 80-1. Peritoneal Dialysis Solutions (2-liter volumes)

Components	1.5% Dextrose	2.5% Dextrose	4.25% Dextrose
Dextrose in water	15 mg/L	25 mg/L	42.5 mg/L
Sodium	132 mEq/L	132 mEq/L	132 mEq/L
Calcium	3.5 mEq/L	3.5 mEq/L	3.5 mEq/L
Magnesium	1.5 mEq/L	1.5 mEq/L	1.5 mEq/L
Chloride	102 mEq/L	102 mEq/L	102 mEq/L
Lactate	35 mEq/L	35 mEq/L	35 mEq/L
Osmolality	347 mOsm/L	398 mOsm/L	486 mOsm/L
pH	5.5	5.5	5.5

(Courtesy of Diamed, Travenol Laboratories, Inc.)

Before dialysis, a catheter is inserted into the peritoneal cavity. A Teflon catheter is usually used in the acute situation and is removed following that episode. A Silastic catheter with a Dacron cuff (a bacterial barrier) is inserted when chronic dialysis is anticipated. This catheter can be left in for years if cared for properly.

The dialysis exchange consists of a 3-phase cycle. Each cycle includes:

1. Inflow—The time it takes for the dialysate to flow into the peritoneal cavity (5–10 minutes).

2. Dwell—The time the dialysate is in contact with the peritoneal cavity. (The length of time is determined by the amount of fluid and waste products that needs to be removed.)

3. Outflow—The time it takes the dialysate to drain from the peritoneal cavity (5–10 min).

There are three methods used to dialyze a child. They are:

1. *Manual method.* The catheter is attached to tubing and the prescribed fluid (10–50 mL/kg), warmed to body temperature, flows in by gravity. The tubing is clamped when the prescribed amount of fluid has infused. The fluid remains in the peritoneal cavity for a prescribed length of time and is then drained into a bag secured below the child.

2. *Continuous ambulatory peritoneal dialysis (CAPD).* The permanent catheter is attached to tubing and the prescribed amount and type of fluid is allowed to flow into the abdomen. The catheter is then clamped and the dialysate allowed to dwell 2–4 hours. (During the night, the fluid is allowed to dwell 7–8 hours.) During this time, the empty dialysate bag is folded and kept on the child. At the end of the dwell time, the bag is lowered to a clean surface and unclamped, and the fluid is allowed to flow out by gravity. The process is repeated 3–5 times a day, 7 days a week.

3. *Continuous cycling peritoneal dialysis (CCPD).* This method cycles fluid through the night with a cycling machine and has a long dwell time during the day, which affords the child more freedom for daily activity (Fig. 80-1).

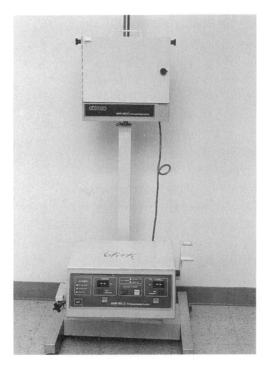

Figure 80-1.

Peritoneal dialysis differs from hemodialysis in that it requires a simple technique with no sophisticated equipment. However, it does take longer than hemodialysis and has increased risks for peritoneal and pulmonary infection and large albumin or protein loss. Peritoneal dialysis can be performed at home, depending on the child and parent's motivation to learn the required information. Advantages of home dialysis are economic, relative convenience, fewer medical complications, and a greater degree of independence. The major disadvantage is the disruption of the family schedule and the fact that success or failure depends a great deal on the abilities of the child and the family.

Standard of Care

1. Maintain strict aseptic technique at all times, including dressing changes, catheter care, and skin care.

Assessment

1. Assess the pertinent history and physical findings to determine if the child is in congestive heart failure or pulmonary edema due to fluid overload; if the child has rales, dyspnea, edema, headache, mental confusion or convulsions; if the child has an increased BUN, creatinine, serum–ammonia, uric acid, potassium, phosphorus or magnesium, and if the child is anemic or has delayed wound healing, joint pain, or loss of muscle mass. Also assess if the child is anuric, oliguric, proteinuric, or has an increased urine specific gravity and osmolality. Assess for allergies, especially to iodine.
2. Assess the psychosocial and developmental concerns related to denial, anxiety, depression, irritability, changes in memory and personality (associated with electrolyte imbalances), and adaptation to body image changes.
3. Assess the child's and family's knowledge of the disease process, prognosis, treatment options, complications, home maintenance, and readiness and willingness to learn.

Nursing Diagnoses

The following is a list of possible diagnoses and could apply, depending on the child's age, clinical situation, and physical condition:

Anxiety

Constipation

Pain

High risk for injury

Fluid volume excess or deficit

High risk for infection

Altered nutrition: more than, less than body requirements

Ineffective breathing pattern

Ineffective family coping compromised

Diarrhea

Planning

When planning to initiate or discontinue dialysis, the following equipment must be assembled:

Initiation
Sterile gloves
Mask
3-way tubing
Povidone-iodine solution
Appropriate bag of dialysate
Drainage bag
4 × 4s (6)
Povidone-iodine ointment
IV pole
Tape
Appropriate medication (if any) to be
 added to dialysate (such as antibiotics
 or heparin)
Cotton-tipped applicator

Discontinuation
Catheter cap
Sterile gloves
Mask
4 × 4s (3)
Tape
Povidone-iodine solution

Interventions

PROCEDURE	RATIONALE/EXPECTED OUTCOME (EO)
Initiation of Dialysis	
1. Explain each step of the procedure. Audiovisual materials, handouts, and the use of a teaching doll will assist in the explanation.	Lack of knowledge about the procedure leads to increased anxiety. Question-and-answer sessions about the dialysis and lifestyle changes are a sign of adaptation. *EO: The child and family will demonstrate behaviors reflective of decreased anxiety.*
2. Plan the child's care with as much involvement of the child and family as possible.	
3. Assemble all equipment needed.	
4. Wash hands.	
5. Record baseline assessment of weight, blood pressure, pulse, temperature, and respiratory rate.	
6. Put on mask.	The mask minimizes airborne bacterial contamination. *EO: The child will have dialysis initiated in a safe manner.*
7. Inject medication ordered into the injection port on the bag after cleaning the port with a povidone-iodine swab. Shake the bag to mix the solution.	This will evenly distribute the medication in the fluid.
8. Close all clamps on the tubing.	
9. Spike the dialysate bag with the tubing.	The tip must remain sterile.
10. Spike the drainage bag's outflow with the tubing.	
11. Hang bags on the IV pole.	
12. Prime the tubing by opening clamps 1, 3, and 4, allowing the fluid to flow from one end of the tubing to the other. Then close the clamps (Fig. 80-2).	This eliminates air bubbles.
13. Remove the dressing from the child's abdomen.	
14. Check the catheter insertion site for redness, swelling, or other signs of infection and irritation.	Exit site infection is a complication of having a catheter in place. *EO: The child's skin around the catheter will remain intact and will not become infected.*

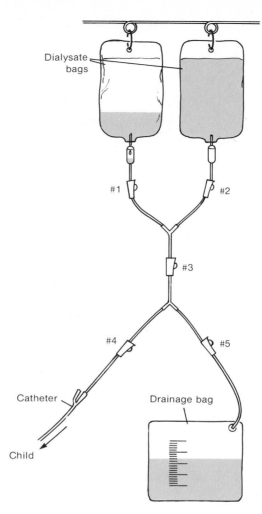

Dialysate bags

#1

#2

#3

#4

#5

Catheter

Drainage bag

Child

Figure 80-2.

PROCEDURE	**RATIONALE/EXPECTED OUTCOME (EO)**
15. Pour povidone-iodine solution over 3 sterile 4 × 4s.	
16. Put on sterile gloves.	
17. Using a soaked 4 × 4, begin cleaning the skin around the catheter insertion site, moving outward in a circular motion. Using a second 4 × 4, once again clean the skin.	
18. With the third soaked 4 × 4, clean the catheter, moving in one direction, from the insertion site out.	
19. Use a cotton-tipped applicator to apply povidone-iodine ointment to the insertion site.	
20. Apply a dressing around the catheter by laying a slit 4 × 4 around the catheter one way, and a second 4 × 4 in the opposite direction.	
21. Remove the cap from the child's catheter and connect the tubing to the catheter.	The system is now closed (sterile).
22. Remove gloves and securely tape the catheter and dressing to the child's abdomen.	Tension on the catheter may cause exit site irritation or trauma which may lead to infection.

PROCEDURE

23. Infuse the prescribed amount of dialysate into the patient by opening clamps 2, 3, and 4.

24. Close all the clamps and allow the fluid to dwell in the child's peritoneum for the prescribed time.

25. When the prescribed time is up, open clamps 4 and 5 and drain the fluid out of the peritoneum for 5–10 minutes or as ordered.

26. Close clamp 5 and restart the infusion process. Put on gloves. Empty the drainage bag and record the amount. Keep an accurate record of the fluid exchange balance.

27. Record dialysate color and clarity. Report a cloudy or bloody outflow to the physician.

28. If the outflow is slow, ask the child to change position, or apply firm pressure to the lower abdomen.

29. Monitor the child for signs of infection (for example, increased temperature, abdominal pain, increased WBC count, and cloudy dialysate).

30. Obtain cultures of dialysate and catheter exit site as necessary.

31. Assess for bowel sounds, bowel movements, abdominal distention, and increased nasogastric drainage, if nasogastric tube is present.

32. Assess for discomfort during the infusion or dwell phases. Look for nonverbal behavior that indicates discomfort in the younger child.

33. Change the child's position, offer frequent back rubs, provide age-appropriate diversions, administer analgesics when indicated, and make sure that all the solution is draining out.

34. Warm dialysate to core temperature before infusion.

35. Monitor serum albumin level, serum electrolytes, BUN, and creatinine.

36. Reinforce plans for dietary teaching; review foods permitted in diet.

37. Allow 2 hours after eating for digestion of food before dialysate infuses.

38. Auscultate breath sounds with vital signs.

39. Turn and deep breathe the child every 2 hours.

RATIONALE/EXPECTED OUTCOME (EO)

Solute(s) diffuse through the peritoneum from the child's blood to the dialysate.

The dialysate with the toxic substances, wastes, or excess fluid is drained from the body.

Dialysate solutions are hypertonic, causing shifts in fluid, and may cause too rapid removal of fluid.

EO: The child will maintain fluid balance by exhibiting normal vital signs, good skin turgor, and moist membranes.

Cloudy fluid = infection
Red fluid = bleeding

Mechanical problems with catheter drainage may cause fluid overload. Outflow or inflow may be impeded by fibrin clots. Call physician if position changes do not assist the flow.

Peritonitis is the major complication of peritoneal dialysis.

EO: The child will remain free from infection.

The catheter and fluid may cause irritation of the peritoneal cavity, thus decreasing bowel activity.

EO: The child will have normal bowel activity.

The amount of dialysate may cause abdominal distention and create a feeling of pressure on the abdominal organs.

EO: The child will demonstrate behaviors that indicate comfort during the procedure.

Ambulation is acceptable if the child is physically able.

Due to the dialysis, children have large amounts of protein loss.

EO: The child has maintained adequate nutrition.

The presence of dialysate causes a feeling of fullness with decreased appetite and, in some cases, vomiting.

An abdomen with dialysate fluid causes a decrease in inspiratory effort, which leads to pneumonia or atelectasis.

EO: The child will be free of respiratory complications.

Hypoventilation is accentuated in the lower lobes when the child is in the supine position. Atelectasis may be noted.

PROCEDURE	**RATIONALE/EXPECTED OUTCOME (EO)**

40. Administer oxygen, if needed.

41. Note amount and color of respiratory secretions.

Discontinuation of Dialysis

42. Assemble equipment.

43. Wash hands.

44. Put on sterile gloves and mask.

45. With one hand, pick up a sterile 4 × 4 and grasp the end of the tubing.

EO: The child will have dialysis discontinued in a safe manner.

46. With the other hand, grasp the catheter and gently disconnect the tubing from it.

47. Put the injection cap on the catheter.

48. Wipe the junction point between the catheter and the injection cap with a povidone–iodine-soaked gauze.

49. Place a 4 × 4 over the catheter and tape in place.

50. Record the child's vital signs and weight. Compare pre- and postdialysis values.

51. Discuss usual family routines, the need for the dialysis, and the change in lifestyle required by the treatment.

Try to adjust the dialysis schedule to accommodate normal routines.

EO: The family identifies aspects of daily life and schedules treatments to allow the child to participate.

52. Explain home dialysis and the fact that its success depends on the people involved and their ability to deal with stress and long-term illness.

53. Suggest that the child and family participate in a support group with other dialysis patients where common feelings can be shared.

EO: The family indicates awareness of community resources.

Patient/Family Education: Home Care Considerations

1. Instruct the child and family in all potential complications (for example, drop in blood pressure, line separation, air in lines, decreased appetite, or infection) and offer immediate solutions (Table 80-2). Give the family the telephone number of the physician or nurse and the dialysis center.

2. Teach aseptic catheter care and dialysis protocol to the child and family and have them return the demonstration.

3. Reinforce principles of fluid and electrolyte balance. Show the child how to keep his or her own intake and output record. Reinforce correct behaviors, and provide instruction to modify incorrect behaviors.

4. Check menu planning and, with the dietitian, work to find new foods or new preparations of old ones that will give variety to a meal.

5. Assess self-medication schedule. Review medications, dose to be taken, and side effects. Show the child how to keep his or her own medication record.

6. Listen to the child's problems and feelings. Reassure the child and family that it is normal to feel discouraged, overwhelmed, and anxious. Help the family work out solutions to problems with the child. Explain that motivation is the single most important factor in a successful dialysis program.

7. Begin a training program when the decision is made to initiate CAPD or CCPD.

Table 80-2. Peritoneal Dialysis Complications

Complications	Indications	Considerations
1. Peritonitis	Fever, abdominal pain, abdominal cramping, cloudy drainage, swelling or drainage around the catheter, and slow dialysate drainage	Use scrupulous aseptic technique throughout entire procedure. Send culture of fluid to the lab.
2. Exit-site infection	Redness, swelling, drainage, rigidity, and tenderness around the catheter	Use aseptic technique throughout procedure. Obtain a culture of exit site drainage and send to the lab.
3. Perforation of bowel or bladder	Signs of peritonitis, bright yellow drainage, or feces in drainage	Have child empty bowel and bladder before catheter is inserted. Catheterization and enema may be necessary.
4. Bleeding through catheter	Minor trauma to abdomen or subcutaneous vessels versus perforation of major abdominal blood vessel	Bleeding usually stops, but if not, child may need to be transfused and taken to the operating room for exploration.
5. Leakage around catheter	Dressing wet after instillation of dialysate may be due to excessive instillation of fluid, incomplete healing around new catheter, catheter obstruction, or dislodged catheter	Instill less dialysate at exchanges. Drain the abdomen completely. Irrigate the catheter with normal saline. Physician replaces or revises the catheter.
6. Low back pain	Caused by the weight and pressure of the dialysate in the abdomen	Backrubs and frequent change of position may help. Also, exercises to strengthen muscles and improve posture may help.
7. Fluid overload	Increased weight, edema of eyelids, abdomen, and face; increased blood pressure (BP) and shortness of breath	Monitor the weight and BP. Decrease intake of sodium and oral fluid. Increase use of dialysate with 4.25% dextrose.
8. Excessive fluid loss	Decreased weight, signs and symptoms of dehydration, and decreased BP	Monitor the child's weight and BP. Increase intake of sodium and oral fluids. Decrease use of dialysate with 4.25% dextrose.
9. Cramping	Dialysate warmer or colder than 37°C (98.6°F); rapid infusion or drainage; chemical irritation, or air in the abdomen	Warm dialysate to 37°C (98.6°F) before infusion. Decrease infusion or drainage rate. Clamp tubing when bag empties, but before air fills the tubing. Use dialysate with less than 4.25% dextrose.

(Adapted from *Nursing photobook: Implementing urologic procedures.* (1981). Horsham, PA: Intermed Communications, Inc., 142–143.)

Teach one skill at a time and relate this new method to the old method and concepts. Proceed at a pace that is comfortable for the child and family.

References

Blatz, S., Paes, B., & Steele, B. (1990). Peritoneal dialysis in the neonate. *Neonatal Network, 8*(6), 41–44.

Fleming, L. (1984). Step-by-step guide to safe peritoneal dialysis. *RN, 47*(2), 44–47.

Lane, T. (1983). Standards of care for the CAPD patient. *Home Health Care Nurse, 4*(5), 34; 36; 41–45.

McFarland, K. (1988). Pediatric peritoneal dialysis. *Pediatric Nursing, 14*(5), 426.

Prowant, B.F., Schmidt, L. M., & Twardowski, Z. T. (1988). Peritoneal dialysis catheter exit site care. *American Nephrology Nurses Association, 15*(4), 219–222.

Sorrels, P. (1981). Peritoneal dialysis: A rediscovery. *Nursing Clinics of North America, 16*(3), 515–530.

Toper, M. (1981). Chronic renal disease in children. *Nursing Clinics of North America, 16*(3), 587–598.

Circumcision Care

81

Definition/Purpose

Circumcision is the removal of the foreskin. It may be performed at any age for disease, and it is a ritual requirement of Judaism and Islam, as well as many primitive tribes, and may be a sociocultural choice of many parents in the United States.

The medical indications for circumcision are phimosis, recurrent posthitis, and paraphimosis. *Phimosis* is excessive tightness of the foreskin preventing retraction behind the glans. It occurs in 1–2% of males. Because the foreskin normally cannot be retracted in infants, nonretractability of the foreskin is not pathologic until the age of 2 years. Forced retraction may cause phimosis by producing tears in the foreskin that heal with scarring and contraction. *Posthitis* is an inflammation of the foreskin caused by phimosis or poor hygiene. The foreskin is red and sore. *Paraphimosis* is used to describe the foreskin that is caught behind the glans. It results from phimosis or forcible retraction. The foreskin may be painful and swollen.

The 1971 edition of *Standards and Recommendations of Hospital Care of Newborn Infants* by the Committee on the Fetus and Newborn of the American Academy of Pediatrics stated that "there are no valid medical indications for routine circumcision in the neonatal period." In 1975 and 1983, an ad hoc task force reviewed this statement and concluded "that there is no absolute medical indication for routine circumcision of the newborn." However, recent large-scale studies have suggested possible medical benefits, including a decreased incidence of urinary tract infections in male infants, a decreased incidence of sexually transmitted diseases, and, in turn, a relationship between sexually transmitted diseases and cancers of the penis and cervix.

Newborn circumcision is a rapid and safe procedure when performed by an experienced operator. It is an elective procedure to be performed on stable healthy infants only, and is contraindicated in unstable sick infants or those with genital anomalies, including hypospadias, where the foreskin may later be needed for surgical correction of the anomalies.

Standard of Care

1. Obtain informed parental consent before the procedure.
2. Cleanse and reapply gauze with petroleum jelly to the tip of the penis with every diaper change.
3. Monitor for bleeding every 15–30 minutes for the first hour.
4. Monitor vital signs every 4 hours, with attention to an elevation in temperature.
5. Provide home instruction for proper care of the circumcised area to parent(s) before discharge.

Assessment

1. Assess maternal–infant history, with emphasis on bleeding disorders or congenital defects of the urinary tract.
2. Assess voiding immediately postoperatively and for the first 24 hours.

3. Assess for swelling or bleeding ever 2 hours for the first 12 hours after the procedure.

Nursing Diagnoses

The following is a list of possible diagnoses and could apply, depending on the child's age, clinical situation, and physical condition:

Pain

High risk for infection

High risk for injury

Impaired skin integrity

Planning

In planning to care for a child who has been circumcised, gather the following equipment:

Petrolatum gauze

1 disposable diaper

Basin with warm water

1 cloth diaper

Restraining board

Sterile scalpel, Gomco or Mogen clamp, or Plastibell

Interventions

PROCEDURE	**RATIONALE/EXPECTED OUTCOME (EO)**
1. Obtain informed consent.	Allows for the procedure to take place after all information on circumcision has been presented to the parents. *EO: The child's family will feel comfortable in their decision.*
2. Keep child NPO 2 hours prior to procedure (if done in a nursery) or 4 hours (if done in the operating room under anesthesia).	Keeping the stomach empty will decrease the risk of aspiration while supine. *EO: The child will not aspirate.*
3. Gather equipment.	
4. Prepare equipment.	
5. Administer sedative if ordered or hold child for local or caudal block.	The circumcision of infants has been used to study the physiologic response of newborns to pain. Adrenal cortical response, immediate postoperative behavior (for example, heart rate, respiratory rate, and PO$_2$ levels) and long-term behavior indicate that infants do feel pain and should be treated accordingly, with at least local anesthesia during circumcisions. *EO: The child will have relief of pain during the procedure.*
6. Take infant to his room.	
7. Restrain the child on a circumcision board, or assist the physician or anesthesiologist in positioning the child on the operating room table.	Prevents child from moving during the procedure, making it less possible for injury to occur. *EO: The child will not move during the procedure.*
8. Remove diaper.	
9. Assist physician during procedure which can be carried out in 1 of 3 ways:	

PROCEDURE   **RATIONALE/EXPECTED OUTCOME (EO)**

Gomco clamp. The rim of the prepuce is grasped
and a small round probe is used to separate the
adherent prepuce from the glans surface. A large
hemostat is used to crush the foreskin in the midline. After the foreskin is cut along the crush line, a
cone of adequate size is placed over the glans. The
top plate is bolted onto the baseplate. After 5 minutes, the redundant skin is cut away and the clamp
is removed (Fig. 81-1).

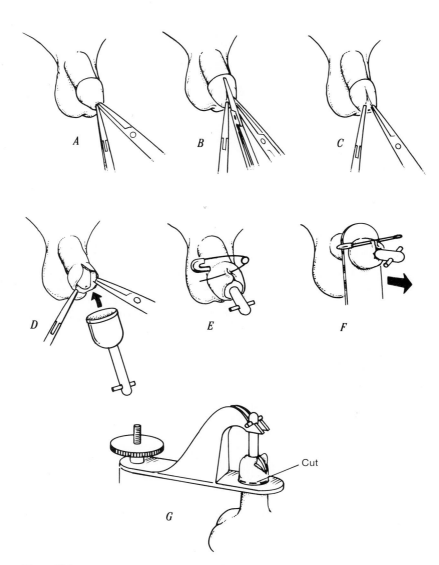

Figure 81-1.

Plastic cone. The adhesions are cleared, the prepuce is crushed, and the dorsal slit is cut as above.
The foreskin is then held open so that the cone can
be placed and a ligature tied tightly around the
cone, compressing the foreskin into the groove.
Break off the cone handle and discard. The tissue

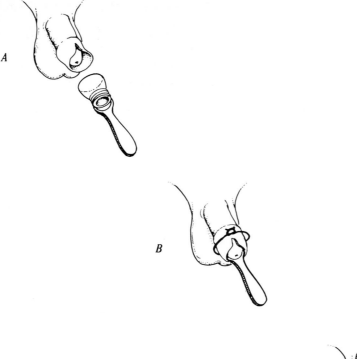

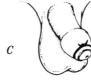

Figure 81-2.

PROCEDURE	**RATIONALE/EXPECTED OUTCOME (EO)**

under the ligature will atrophy and drop off with the cone in 5–8 days (Fig. 81-2).

Surgical excision. The adhesions are cleared, the prepuce is crushed, and a dorsal slit is cut. The foreskin is then cut, leaving 0.5 cm of skin at the sulcus. Each bleeding vessel is clamped and ligated.

10. Comfort the child, using a quiet voice, light touch, and a pacifier.

Provides the child with mechanisms to decrease painful stimuli by enhancing endorphin production.

EO: The child will have discomfort minimized.

11. Wrap the circumcised penis in lubricated gauze if the Gomco clamp or surgical excision method has been used.

Provides a waterproof barrier and lubrication to the surgical site.

EO: The child's penis will not become red and irritated or stick to the diaper.

12. Insert a cloth diaper inside disposable diaper and place on the infant.

Will apply steady pressure to the surgical site to prevent bleeding.

EO: The surgical site will have minimal or no bleeding.

13. Return the child to his mother and allow the infant to eat.

Provides reassurance for mother and infant. Allows for meeting infant's need to suck.

EO: The mother–child bond will be maintained. The child will be comforted.

PROCEDURE

RATIONALE/EXPECTED OUTCOME (EO)

14. With each diaper change:
    a. Assess voiding.

    Adequate voiding ensures patency of urinary tract during the initial period of swelling.

    EO: The child will maintain normal urine output.
    EO: The child will not have excessive blood loss.

    b. Assess for bleeding. If bleeding or swelling has increased, notify the physician immediately.
    c. Assess for infection at the suture line (for example, redness, drainage, excessive pain and swelling, or fever).

    EO: The child will not have an infected operative site.

    d. Place the child in a sitz bath for 10–15 minutes at least 3 times a day.

    Gentle cleansing of the area will prevent bacteria proliferation.

    EO: The child's surgical site will not become infected and will be cleansed in a nontraumatic manner (see Step 10 above).

    e. Reapply lubricated gauze and diaper if indicated.
15. Chart the procedure and the infant's tolerance of it. Describe the area after the procedure and with each diaper change.

    EO: The procedure will be documented in the medical record for future reference.

Patient/Family Education: Home Care Considerations

1. Instruct parents about home care of the circumcision:
   a. Remove soiled diaper every 4 hours (or as needed).
   b. Observe area for any swelling, bleeding, or discharge. Specify that a whitish–yellow discharge is normal up to 1 week after procedure, and that it is not to be rubbed off.
   c. Cleanse the area using a warm, wet soft cloth, making sure not to use diaper wipes, lotions, powders; or in a sitz bath as described above.
   d. Apply a small amount of petroleum jelly to the tip of the penis.
2. Inform the parents of ways to comfort the child:
   a. Positioning. Hold child close to the body, and place him side-lying or upright after feedings.
   b. Sucking. Use a pacifier or breast- or bottle-feed.
   c. Warmth. Wrap in a blanket.

References

Anderson, K.H. (1989). A method of analgesia for relief of circumcision pain. *Anesthesia, 44,* 118–120.

Bobak, I.M., Jensen, M.D. & Zolar, M.K. (1989). *Maternity and gynecologic care: The nurse and the family.* St. Louis: C.V. Mosby Co.

Leape, L. (1987). *Patient care in pediatric surgery.* Boston: Little, Brown & Company.

Lohr, J. (1989). The foreskin and UTIs. *The Journal of Pediatrics, 114*(3), 502–504.

Reeder, S.J., & Martin, L.L. (1990). *Maternity nursing: Family, newborn, and women's health care.* (17th ed.). Philadelphia: J.B. Lippincott Co.

Stange, H., Gunnar, M. R., Snellman, L., et al. (1988). Local anesthesia for neonatal circumcision. *Journal of the American Medical Association, 259*(10), 1507–1511.

Hemodialysis

82

Definition/Purpose

Hemodialysis is the most effective artificial method of removing toxic waste products and fluids from the systemic circulation and of restoring fluid, electrolyte, and acid–base balances when the kidneys are not functioning adequately.

The artificial kidney machine works on the principle of a semipermeable membrane separating the child's blood from the dialyzing fluid. Hemodialysis is based on three principles of fluid and particle movement: diffusion, osmosis, and ultrafiltration. Through diffusion and osmosis, the waste products pass from an area of low concentration (the child's blood) to an area of high concentration (the dialyzing fluid) until equilibrium is achieved. Molecules of the dialyzing fluid may also pass into the blood; thus the electrolyte content (glucose, sodium, calcium, and potassium) of the dialysate can be manipulated to meet the child's needs based on clinical and chemical determinations. Ultrafiltration involves the movement of fluid across a semipermeable membrane as a result of an artificially created pressure gradient.

The time involved for hemodialysis is 3 to 5 hours, depending on the condition of the child and the type of dialyzer used. It it usually performed 3 times a week at a dialysis center, or at home.

Hemodialysis requires removal of blood from the body through an artery and return of the blood and fluid through a vein. Types of access to the child's circulation include:

1. *External arteriovenous cannula.* A Silastic–Teflon cannula is surgically inserted and fixed in an artery, and another cannula is fixed in a nearby vein. Arterial blood is shunted through the artificial kidney and returned to the child through the venous cannula. After the dialysis cycle is completed, both cannulas are connected so that the flow of blood from the artery to the vein is continuous (Fig. 82-1).

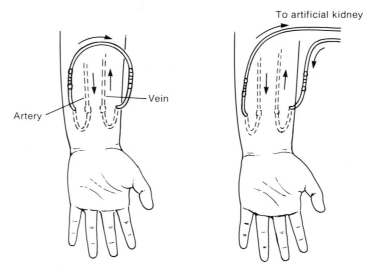

Figure 82-1.

2. *Internal arteriovenous graft.* A permanent dialysis access created by suturing an artificial device to the child's own vessels. At the time of dialysis, two needles are inserted: one to carry the blood to the dialysis machine, and one to return the blood to the child. The needles are removed and reinserted with each treatment. This is the most commonly used access for children because of the size of their blood vessels (Fig. 82-2).

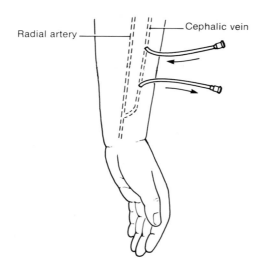

Radial artery ————— Cephalic vein

Figure 82-2.

3. *Subclavian vein catheterization.* A temporary access using a double-lumen catheter. This type of emergency catheter is being used in the pediatric population instead of the external arteriovenous cannula to preserve the peripheral vessels for long-term access.

Because the dialyzer must draw blood from the body and then return the blood, pumps are required. The dialyzer and tubing must be primed with fluid or blood and should not require a filling volume of more than 10% of the child's blood volume. As even the smallest dialyzer requires a priming volume of 60–75 mL, the smallest child suitable for hemodialysis is 8–10 kg. For smaller children, peritoneal dialysis is safe and effective.

Standard of Care

1. Hemodialysis should be performed only by trained professionals who are knowledgeable about the equipment, its use with children, and its potential complications. (These include trained parents and family).

Assessment

1. Assess the child's history and physical findings for lethargy, anorexia, confusion, restlessness, oliguria, anuria, edema, fluid and electrolyte disturbances, anemia, congestive heart failure, or drug toxicity.
2. Assess the psychosocial and developmental factors related to fear regarding the disease and treatment, body image, depression about long-term condition, and potential for death.
3. Assess the child and family's knowledge of the purpose and effects of the dialysis, the procedure for renal transplant, and community support resources for emotional and financial concerns.

Nursing Diagnoses

The following is a list of possible diagnoses and could apply, depending on the child's age, clinical situation, and physical condition:

Anxiety

Powerlessness

Body image disturbance

Altered growth and development

Pain

High risk for injury

High risk for infection

Fluid volume deficit

Decreased cardiac output

Impaired gas exchange

Planning

In planning the care of a child on hemodialysis, the following equipment must be assembled:

Thermometer

Sphygmomanometer

Monitor for cardiac rhythm

Stethoscope

Interventions

PROCEDURE	**RATIONALE/EXPECTED OUTCOME (EO)**
1. Explain in simple terms the reason for dialysis and the actual procedure. Encourage questions from the child and family.	The child and family will have anxiety related to limited understanding of the disease and its relationship to the need for dialysis and related therapy.
	EO: The child and family's behavior demonstrates decreased anxiety.
2. Review baseline vital signs, including weight, before initiating dialysis.	This will give a point of reference for comparison of pre- and post-dialysis values.
3. Review baseline laboratory values before initiation of dialysis.	This will give an indication of the effectiveness of the dialysis in eliminating metabolic waste products and toxic substances from the body.
	EO: The child's electrolytes and blood levels of metabolic waste products (BUN, uric acid, creatinine, and ammonia) are within normal limits.
4. Monitor pulse, respiration, and blood pressure every 15–30 minutes during and after dialysis.	Hypovolemia and hypotension may be related to kinked tubing, vessel spasm, blood leaks in the dialyzer, or volume depletion.
	EO: The child's vital signs are within normal limits.
5. Monitor the child for a fluid volume deficit: • Increased pulse • Decreased blood pressure • Vomiting • Dizziness.	With ultrafiltration, there is a risk of rapid volume depletion because too much fluid is removed too rapidly.
	EO: The child will remain hemodynamically stable.

PROCEDURE

6. Administer volume expanders or vasopressors as ordered. Report and record the effectiveness of the treatment. Watch for signs of fluid overload or hypertension (for example, headache, confusion, nausea, vomiting, convulsion, and disequilibrium syndrome).

7. If signs of shock are present (for example, decreased blood pressure, increased pulse, and poor peripheral perfusion), elevate the feet and give intravenous fluids as ordered.

8. If child is short of breath, elevate head 15–30° and administer oxygen.

9. Auscultate lungs every hour.

10. Assess for signs of decreased cardiac output hypoxia (for example, weak pulse, dizziness, and confusion).

11. Monitor blood gases; watch for decreased PO_2 and acidosis.

12. Monitor cardiac rhythm.

13. Inspect the access site every 15–30 minutes during dialysis for signs of bleeding.

14. Check the patency of the shunt or fistula every 4 hours:
    a. Observe blood flow through the shunt.
    b. Auscultate for bruit and palpate for thrill in internal fistula.

15. To prevent air from entering the system:
    a. Tape connections.
    b. Avoid infusing solutions in vented containers.
    c. Keep air detector on all tubing.
    d. Avoid kinks in tubing, because they can pull air into the system.

16. Ensure that no punctures are made in the external shunt. Do not draw blood or take blood pressure from the access extremity. Post a sign at the head of the bed to remind all staff of the proper precautions.

17. Monitor the child for signs of infection (increased temperature and respirations; decreased blood pressure; change in mental status; mottled skin color; swelling, redness, or warmth of the skin

RATIONALE/EXPECTED OUTCOME (EO)

Volume expanders (blood, blood products, and intravenous fluid) and vasopressor medication can reverse a hypovolemic hypotensive state.

EO: The child will have a disequilibrium syndrome recognized and treated.

Hypotension can be related to diversion of the child's blood into the dialysis machine.

EO: The child will have the signs of shock recognized and treated.

Congestion within the pulmonary circulation causes alterations in the ventilation/perfusion ratio, resulting in impaired gas exchange.

EO: The child will have the signs of respiratory distress recognized and treated.

The child will have normal respirations and breath sounds.

Congestive heart failure may be related to hypovolemia between dialysis treatments.

EO: The child will maintain cardiac output sufficient to promote normal gas exchange.

Anemia reduces the oxygen-carrying capacity of the blood, causing impaired gas exchange.

EO: The child's hemoglobin, hematocrit, and platelet levels are within normal levels.

Hyperkalemia causes changes in cardiac conduction, which may cause dysrhythmias.

EO: The child has an absence of arrhythmias and normal electrolyte levels.

EO: The child's shunt will remain in the site without dislodgment.

Bleeding may be caused by accidental dislodgement or rupture of a dialyzer disconnection of the shunt. Heparin, which is metabolized in 4 hours, also promotes bleeding.

EO: The child is free from injury.

An opening in the dialysis system can become a port of entry for air. A risk of air embolism develops when 3 mL of air enters the vascular system.

EO: The child's dialysis system will remain intact without air in the system.

Shunt or fistula closure related to clotting can be prevented by taking precautions as stated.

EO: The child's shunt or fistula will remain patent.

Local infection may lead to systemic infection, especially in children who have compromised immune systems.

EO: The child is free from infection.

PROCEDURE	RATIONALE/EXPECTED OUTCOME (EO)
around the shunt or fistula; drainage of exudate around insertion sites; and decreased circulation to the extremity).	
18. Administer antibiotics as prescribed.	Antibiotics are used to treat an infection.
	EO: The child will have a systemic infection treated.
19. Monitor liver function studies for elevations indicative of hepatitis. Assess for signs of hepatitis (for example, fatigue, fever, and jaundice). Institute isolation when indicated.	When frequent transfusions are required, the risk of hepatitis is increased. Hospital staff should exercise caution to protect themselves against blood-transmitted diseases.
	EO: The child will be free from injury from dialysis treatment.
20. Monitor hematology studies for indications of immunosuppression such as decreased as white blood cell count and lymphocytes. Initiate protective isolation as needed or ordered.	The risk of AIDS increases with frequent transfusions. Hospital staff should exercise caution to protect themselves.
21. Monitor for signs of increased intracranial pressure during and after dialysis (for example, nausea, vomiting, headache, restlessness, hypertension, bradycardia, and seizures).	A shift of fluid between blood and cells results in cerebral edema and possible seizures.
	EO: The child is free from seizure activity.
22. Assess the child for signs of discomfort and promote measures for relief of the pain.	
23. Assist the child in using distraction, imagery, and play to control pain.	
24. Apply heat and pressure to areas of discomfort. Explain to the child and family the reason for discomfort.	Fluid overload causing hypertension may lead to headache. Electrolyte imbalance may cause muscle cramps, nausea, vomiting, and abdominal pain.
	EO: The child is free from headache, cramping, and abdominal pain.
25. Assist in the evaluation of the child's degree of impairment in renal function which, together with age and activity, determines protein intake.	The child may be malnourished due to protein catabolism (negative nitrogen balance), loss of protein and fat stores, and the loss of body muscle mass and weight.
	EO: The child will have adequate nutrition to prevent protein catabolism, maintain and build body mass, preserve protein and fat stores with reasonable BUN and creatinine levels, and a reduction in uremic symptoms.
26. Assess the child's level of anxiety. Encourage the child to ask questions regarding the disease and treatment.	Lack of knowledge and fear of the unknown causes high anxiety and stress.
	EO: The child and parents will express a decreased level of anxiety. The child will express acceptance of the treatment.
27. Encourage independence in self-care activities. Allow the older child to participate in dialysis activities.	Changes in physical appearance and lifestyle may result in a lessened sense of self.
28. Allow the child and parents a degree of control over the planning and management of care (such as scheduling of meals and medications).	The child needs to feel a sense of control over some aspect of his or her life.
	EO: The child and parents will participate in decision making regarding the care plan.

Patient/Family Education: Home Care Considerations

1. Teach the child and family to check external shunt site for swelling, coolness, redness, or other discoloration of the skin.

2. Teach the child and family to check subclavian catheter dressing and the catheter itself for drainage or leakage.

3. Teach the child and family restrictions necessary for bathing and swimming when an external catheter is in place.

4. Teach the child and family what to do in case of an accidental separation of the cannulas. Be sure the child has two clamps present at all times.

5. Demonstrate to the child and family the skin cleansing technique at the shunt site, using aseptic technique and hospital procedure.

6. Instruct the child and family to check for patency by palpitating the thrill and listening for the bruit in the internal fistula. Teach the family to monitor the circulation in the shunt or fistula extremity.

7. Teach the child and family to protect the shunt by avoiding the following:
   a. Pressure on the arm (such as blood pressure cuff, tourniquet, or tight clothing)
   b. Using weights
   c. Sleeping on the arm
   d. Carrying a purse or packages in the affected arm
   e. Exposing the extremity to extremes of hot or cold.

8. Make a medication chart so that the child can learn names of medicines, dosages, times of administration, and reasons for the medications.

9. Ensure that the family has emergency phone numbers of the dialysis unit and the physician.

10. Encourage the family's participation in support groups through the local chapter of the Kidney Foundation.

References

David-Kasdon, J. (1984). Alterations in body image in the hemodialysis population. *Journal of Nephrology Nursing, 1,* 25–28.

Johanson, B.C., et al. (1981). *Standards for critical care.* St. Louis: C.V. Mosby Co.

Pitman, N. (1982). *Nephrology nursing standards of clinical practice.* American Association of Nephrology Nurses and Technicians.

Topor, M. (1981). Chronic renal disease in children. *Nursing Clinics of North America, 16*(3), 587–598.

Clean intermittent catheterization (CIC) is useful for children with various urologic or neurologic problems that result in inadequate bladder emptying (such as spinal cord injuries or meningiomylocele). CIC is helpful in controlling bedwetting and urinary tract infections. By emptying the bladder completely at regular intervals, the child should stay dry in between catheterizations and should have a decreased incidence of infections of the kidneys and bladder.

Children as young as 5 years of age are able to catheterize themselves. With the use of pictures, demonstrations, and return-demonstrations, the child can be successful and proud of this accomplishment. Children will start to learn this procedure by holding and opening the equipment and will gradually increase their degree of involvement until they can catheterize themselves.

Frequency of CIC

CIC is usually performed every 4 hours, beginning when your child wakes up and continuing every four hours until bedtime. Because of this schedule, CIC must be carried out during school hours. Your child's teacher and school nurse should be informed of your child's catheterization schedule.

Equipment Needed

Soft red rubber or plastic catheter (Size 8F [smallest]–16F [largest])

Water soluble lubricant

Mild soap and water

Cotton balls (6)

Collection jar

White vinegar

10-mL syringe

Plastic storage bag

Mirror

How to Catheterize a Boy

1. Wash hands with soap and water.
2. Wash the catheter with soap and water and rinse well with water.
3. Your child can either stand or sit.
4. Coat the catheter with water soluble lubricant.
5. While holding the penis upright so the urethra is straight, retract the foreskin (if the child is not circumcised) and wash the penis from the tip downward with soap and water and cotton balls. Use each cotton ball once only and discard. Do not wash back and forth over the opening.
6. Insert the catheter gently. You may feel some resistance when the catheter reaches the muscle just before the bladder. Use gentle but firm pressure on the catheter until the muscle relaxes. If the catheter cannot be inserted or causes pain, remove the catheter and try again (Fig. 1).

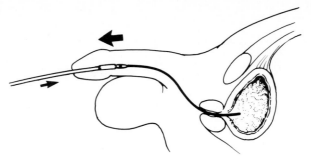

Figure 1.

7. Continue to insert the catheter until urine starts to flow.

8. Because of a lack of bladder tone, gently exert pressure with a hand over the bladder to ensure emptying of the bladder.

9. When the urine stops flowing, slowly remove the catheter.

10. Wash the catheter with soap and water. Use a syringe filled with white vinegar to clean and deodorize the inside of the catheter. Rinse well with water; dry and store in a plastic bag.

11. Note the amount, color, and odor of urine.

How to Catheterize a Girl

1. Wash hands with soap and water.

2. Wash the catheter with soap and water and rinse well.

3. Your child can either lie down, with knees bent in a frog-like position, or sit with legs spread apart. A mirror may be helpful to your child to visualize her anatomy.

4. Coat the catheter with water soluble lubricant.

5. Separate the labia with the thumb and forefinger and locate the opening above the vagina.

6. Wash the labia with soap and water and cotton balls from top to bottom. Use each cotton ball once only and discard.

7. Insert the catheter gently into the urethra until urine flows (Fig. 2).

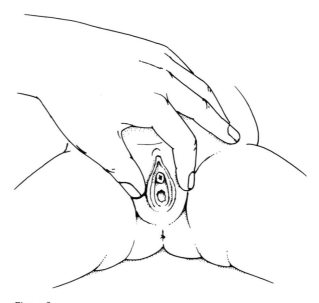

Figure 2.

8. Because of a lack of bladder tone, gently exert pressure with a hand over the bladder to ensure emptying of the bladder.

9. When the urine stops flowing, slowly remove the catheter.

10. Wash the catheter with soap and water. Use a syringe filled with white vinegar to clean and deodorize the inside of the catheter. Rinse well with water, dry and store in a plastic bag.

11. Note amount, color, and odor of urine.

Do not expect 100% success immediately. Be patient and supportive of your child. Consult your doctor or nurse if the following problems arise:

a. Catheter cannot be inserted

b. Pain with catheterization

c. Scant or no urine output

d. Foul-smelling urine

e. Bloody urine (red)

f. Brown urine

Important Telephone Numbers

Doctor's Name: _____

Telephone: _____

Nurse's Name: _____

Telephone: _____

References

Brown, J.P., & Reichenbach, M. B. (1989). Screening children with myelodysplasia for readiness to learn self-catheterization. *Rehabilitation Nursing, 11–12,* 334–337.

Dimmock, W. (1987). An approach to bladder and bowel management in children with spina bifida. *Urologic Nursing, 8*(1), 9–12.

Henderson, J.S. (1989). Intermittent clean self-catheterization in clients with neurogenic bladder resulting from multiple sclerosis. *Journal of Neurosurgical Nursing, 21*(3), 160–164.

Sugar, E. (1980). *Intermittent catheterization and your child.* Chicago: Children's Memorial Hospital.

PATIENT TEACHING CHECKLIST

All of the following skills must be learned before discharge. The nursing categories must be dated and signed by the nurse who has assumed responsibility for teaching. Parents are to sign and date each task as mastery is achieved. (See skills as outlined in "Clean Intermittent Catheterization ".)

Child and Parent Should Be Able to:	Nurse Demonstration (Initials & Date)	Parent Return-Demonstration (Initials & Date)
1. Verbalize the reason for CIC.		
2. Verbalize the frequency of catheterization.		
3. Assemble equipment needed.		
4. Catheterize the child, completely emptying the bladder.		
5. Clean used equipment and store for future use.		
6. Identify when to call the physician or nurse.		

Endocrine System Procedures

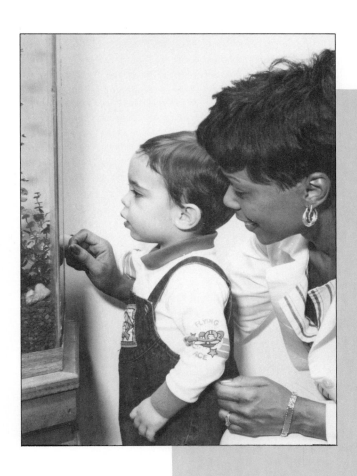

Unit XII

Blood Glucose Monitoring

83

Definition/Purpose

Hypoglycemia is defined as a serum glucose of less than 50–60 mg/100 mL, regardless of whether or not symptoms are present. A consistent supply of glucose is necessary to provide energy for cellular metabolism in most tissue; therefore, the maintenance of adequate blood sugar is critical for normal function. The serum glucose reflects a dynamic balance among glucose input from dietary sources, glycogenolysis and gluconeogenesis, and glucose utilization by muscle, heart, adipose tissue, brain, and blood elements. When there is adequate glucose intake, it is stored in the liver as glycogen. With fasting, this glycogen is degraded to glucose, which is released into the blood stream.

Insulin is the primary hormone that regulates the blood glucose level. It stimulates the uptake of glucose and amino acids into skeletal, cardiac, and adipose tissue, and promotes glycogen and protein synthesis.

Hypoglycemia is a common complication among high-risk infants, particularly among prematures, infants with intrauterine growth retardation, and infants born to mothers with poorly controlled diabetes. Most infants do not require complex evaluation unless the hypoglycemia persists for more than several days or an infusion of more than 10% glucose is needed for a period of days to correct the hypoglycemia.

The clinical manifestations of hypoglycemia are as follows:

1. Palpitations
2. Anxiety
3. Tremors
4. Hunger
5. Sweating
6. Irritability
7. Headache
8. Fatigue
9. Confusion
10. Seizures.

Hyperglycemia is a biochemical finding of elevated ketones in blood and urine and metabolic acidosis. Clinically, dehydration is always present and poses the most serious immediate risk to the child. Laboratory findings include a serum glucose that is greater than 200–250 mg/mL (usually 400–800 mg/mL), the presence of glucose and ketones in the urine, acidosis (pH < 7.3 and HCo_3 < 15 mEq/L), normal to high potassium, and an elevated BUN. Insulin deficiency is always accompanied by elevations of the counter-regulatory hormones, glucagon, catecholamines, corticosteroids, and growth hormone. These hormonal changes lead to hyperglycemia by reducing peripheral glucose utilization and increasing hepatic glyconeogenesis. Hyperglycemia promotes an osmotic diuresis that results in dehydration.

Hyperglycemia is not uncommon in low–birth-weight infants and is thought to result from insulin resistance and pancreatic beta cell immaturity. In these infants, hyperglycemia is exacerbated by asphyxia, intracranial hemorrhage, and infection. The onset is usually within the first few days of life and gradually returns to normal in 7 to 10 days. In most cases, insulin therapy is not needed; however, some infants with prolonged hypergly-cemia require insulin to correct weight loss and polyuria.

Clinical manifestations of hyperglycemia are as follows:

1. Polyuria
2. Polydipsia
3. Nausea and vomiting
4. Abdominal pain
5. Listlessness
6. Fatigue
7. Anorexia.

If hypoglycemia or hyperglycemia is suspected, blood should be obtained for a serum glucose determination. Rapid screening should be done with one of the glucose-specific, chemically coated plastic strips.

Standard of Care

1. Check the expiration date of the test strip vial label. Obtain new strips if the date has passed.
2. When using the Accu-Check II Blood Glucose Monitor, be sure the instrument has been programmed with the correct programming strip.
3. Keep the test strips in their original capped vial, which contains a drying agent. Store at room temperature—below 30°C (86°F)—and away from excess humidity or freezing temperatures.

Assessment

1. Assess the history and physical findings for the child's age, behavior, unusual di-etary pattern or inactivity level, medications ingested, vital signs, current weight and recent weight loss, abdominal pain, blurred vision, excessive thirst, or hunger, changes in amount or pattern of urination, or enuresis in a previously toilet-trained child.
2. Assess the child's developmental level, interests, hobbies, usual coping mecha-nisms, and supportive family and friends.
3. Assess the family's knowledge of the reason for glucose monitoring, recognition and management of hypo- or hyperglycemia, the long-term nature of the disease, if applicable, and their readiness and willingness to learn.

Nursing Diagnoses

The following is a list of possible diagnoses and could apply, depending on the child's age, clinical situation, and physical condition:

High risk for injury

Impaired skin integrity

High risk for infection

Fluid volume deficit

Pain

Planning

When planning to test the blood glucose of a child, the following equipment should be gathered:

Non-sterile gloves

Alcohol swab
Watch or timer
Lancet or autolet
Dextrostix
2 × 2 gauge
Adhesive bandage

Interventions

| **PROCEDURE** | **RATIONALE/EXPECTED OUTCOME (EO)** |

Testing with Chemstrips

1. Prepare the child in a developmentally appropriate manner.

The child and family will tend to cooperate with the procedure if they understand what to expect.

EO: The child and family will describe the blood glucose test correctly.

EO: The child will cooperate with the procedure as developmentally able.

2. Gather necessary equipment.
3. Wash hands.
4. Remove one strip from the vial, replacing the cap immediately.

Protect the remaining strips from light and moisture, which would affect the readings. Do not cut or alter the strips in any way.

5. Put on gloves.
6. Cleanse the child's finger and heel with the alcohol swab and allow to dry completely. If child is old enough, allow child to choose the site.

Alcohol will change the test result, as will water.

Give the child some sense of control.

7. Prick the side of the child's finger or heel with a lancet or autolet (Fig. 83-1).

The sides of fingers and heels are more vascular and have fewer nerve endings than the bottoms.

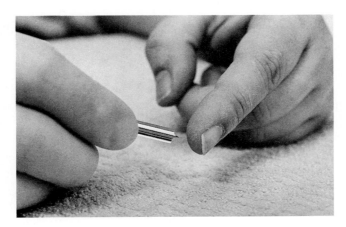

Figure 83-1.

8. Squeeze the finger or heel proximal to the site. Place a large droplet of blood on both reagent pads. Do not smear. Note the time (Figs. 83-2 and 83-3).

Smearing or adding additional blood after initial contact will alter the results.

EO: The child will have the glucose test performed accurately.

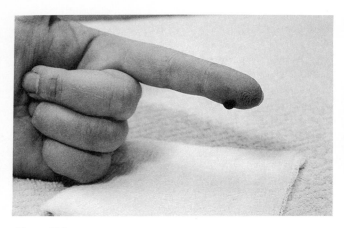

Figure 83-2.

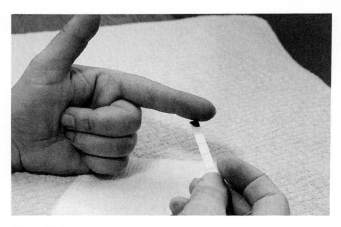

Figure 83-3.

PROCEDURE

9. After exactly 60 seconds, wipe the blood from the test pad with a gauze. Do not stop timing (Fig. 83-4).

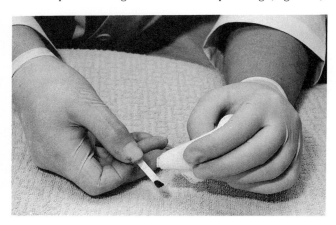

Figure 83-4.

10. After another 60 seconds (for a total of 2 minutes), match the colors on the test strip to the color scale on the vial:
    a. Find the closest match to the lower pad (for example, 80 mg/dL).
    b. Find the closest match to the upper pad (for example, 120 mg/dL).
    c. Add the two numbers together (example: 120 + 80 = 200 mg/dL).
    d. Divide by 2 to obtain the glucose level (for example, 200 ÷ 2 = 100 mg/dL).

11. While timing the chemstrip, place pressure on the puncture site to stop bleeding.

12. Record blood glucose level and notify the physician.

Testing with a Glucometer

13. Follow steps 1–6 above.

14. Turn meter on by pushing on/off button.

RATIONALE/EXPECTED OUTCOME (EO)

If the color on the strip is darker than those for 240 mg/dL, wait another 60 seconds and then compare final colors to the scale.

EO: The child's skin at the puncture site will stop bleeding and will remain infection-free.

The number 888 will appear on the display followed by three more numbers. The numbers should match the

PROCEDURE	**RATIONALE/EXPECTED OUTCOME (EO)**
	code on the vial. If not, reprogram the meter, using the operator's manual.
15. Select a test strip and prick the finger or heel with a lancet as before.	
16. Apply the drop of blood to the test strip, completely covering the two test pads. Immediately press the timer button.	The meter will begin counting and will beep at 57, 58, 59 and 60 seconds.
17. At the 60-second mark, wipe blood from the test pad.	
18. Before the timer reaches 120 seconds, put the test strip into the slot with pads facing toward the on/off button.	Inserting the strip incorrectly will create false readings.
19. After 120 seconds, the blood glucose reading will appear on the display window.	Check the strip visually after getting the meter reading. *EO: The child will have his or her glucose measured accurately by use of the glucometer.*
20. Turn meter off. Record results and notify physician.	

Patient/Family Education: Home Care Considerations

1. Instruct the child and family how to do a blood glucose test and how to determine the results.
2. Review the signs and symptoms of hypo- or hyperglycemia with the child and family.
3. Instruct the family to call a physician to report symptoms described earlier in this chapter or a glucose test result of <40 or >240 mg/dL.
4. Instruct the family on comfort measures:
   a. Reassure the child that he or she has not been "bad" and is not being punished by the lancet sticks.
   b. Allow the child to perform as much of the procedure as possible to develop a sense of control.
5. Instruct the child and family on how frequently and when during the day the glucose testing should be done. To maintain strict control, test glucose levels 4 times a day—before meals, at bedtime, and any time a hypo- or hyperglycemic episode is suspected. Record results on the flow chart.

References

American Diabetes Association. (1989–1990). Clinical practice recommendations: Self-monitoring of blood glucose. *Diabetes Care*, (January Suppl.) *1*, 41–46.

Daniels, D.R. (1988). A guide to pediatric diabetes for the home health nurse. *Home Healthcare Nurse*, 6(5), 22–26.

Fleischer, G., & Ludwig, S. (1988). *Textbook of pediatric emergency medicine.* Baltimore: Williams & Wilkins.

Fow, S. (1983). Home blood glucose monitoring in children with insulin-dependent diabetes mellitus. *Pediatric Nursing, 9*(6), 368–373.

Heenan, A. (1990). Blood glucose measurement. *Nursing Times, 1*, 24–30; 65–68.

Jenkins, C.A., Powers, M. A., & Molitch, M. E. (1988). Comparison of ease of learning of four glucose meters. *Diabetes Educator, 14*(4), 313–315.

Montana, J.A. (1989). Glucose meters. *Journal of Pediatric Nursing, 4*(2), 132–136.

Continuous Insulin Infusion

84

Definition/Purpose

Continuous insulin infusion is used in the treatment of moderate-to-severe diabetic ketoacidosis, which is a state of hyperglycemia hypertonic dehydration and ketotic acidemia. Diabetic ketoacidosis exists when:

1. The glucose is > 300 mg/dL.
2. Ketonemia is present, and ketones are strongly positive at > 1 : 2 dilution of serum.
3. The patient is acidotic (pH < 7.30 and bicarbonate < 15 mEq/L).
4. Glucosuria and ketonuria are present.

   Rapid initial evaluation is needed to confirm the diagnosis and assess the extent of metabolic abnormality. This should be followed by starting the initial phase of treatment—continuous insulin infusion. Treatment is vigorous initially, to halt and begin to reverse the metabolic disturbances, but once the situation is more controlled, over-vigorous medication can produce too rapid changes in glucose, osmolarity, and pH, and can possibly contribute to development of cerebral edema.

Standard of Care

1. Only registered nurses may draw up and mix the insulin infusion. Most institutions require that the dose be checked by 2 RNs.
2. An insulin syringe must be used to measure the insulin dose.
3. The physician must write the order for the insulin dose and infusion rate. All changes must be in writing; accept no verbal orders.
4. An infusion pump is necessary to maintain the accuracy of the infusion.
5. A fresh insulin infusion should be mixed every 24 hours.
6. Continuous insulin infusion:
   Regular insulin 0.2 U/kg/hr made up of 100 U regular insulin in 100 mL of normal saline to yield a solution containing 1 U of insulin/1 mL of fluid.

Assessment

1. Assess pertinent history and physical findings for age, behavior, medications (including type of insulin, dosage, and time), glucose monitoring techniques used, vital signs, height, weight (current and previous), serum glucose levels, polydipsia, polyuria, polyphagia, abdominal pain, or blurred vision.
2. Assess psychosocial and developmental concerns regarding school history, interests, hobbies, usual coping mechanisms, and supportive friends and family members.
3. Assess the child and family's knowledge in relation to the reason for hospitalization, dietary planning, insulin administration, recognition and management of hypo- or hyperglycemia, long-term complications, glucose monitoring, follow-up care needed, and use of community resources.

Nursing Diagnoses

The following is a list of possible diagnoses and could apply, depending on the child's age, clinical situation, and physical condition:

Anxiety

Fear

High risk for injury

Impaired adjustment

Ineffective, compromised family coping

Planning

When planning to initiate a continuous insulin infusion, the following equipment must be gathered:

Infusion pump

Appropriate IV fluid, as ordered

U100 Insulin syringe

U100 Regular insulin

IV tubing

Interventions

PROCEDURE	**RATIONALE/EXPECTED OUTCOME (EO)**
1. Explain to the child and family the goals of the current therapy. Provide opportunities for family members to discuss their concerns.	When confronted with a chronic disease, the child and family may be overwhelmed and feel unable to control their situation. *EO: The child and family will have an opportunity to verbalize fears and anxieties about a change in previous abilities.*
2. Document baseline vital signs, blood glucose, and admission assessment of level of consciousness, dietary history, etc.	To properly integrate the data, an up-to-the-minute flow sheet must be maintained. *EO: The child's ongoing clinical course will be documented in the medical record.*
3. Assemble equipment.	
4. Check IV site for patency.	
5. Check the physician's order. It should include: a. Type of insulin b. Amount of insulin c. Type and amount of IV solution d. Rate of infusion in mL/hr.	*EO: The child will have an insulin infusion mixed and infused according to the physician's order.*
6. Using the insulin syringe, draw up the ordered dose. Have another nurse check the dose.	
7. Inject insulin into the appropriate IV fluid.	
8. Allow 50 mL to run through the IV tubing to saturate the insulin binding sites before starting the infusion.	Insulin will bind to the plastic IV tubing, so flush tubing with 50 mL to stabilize the insulin in the solution.
9. Attach mixture to primary IV line and begin infusion on a pump.	

PROCEDURE	**RATIONALE/EXPECTED OUTCOME (EO)**

10. Monitor the child as follows:
  a. Blood sugar every 1–2 hours
  b. Electrolytes every 1–2 hours initially
  c. BUN, creatinine, calcium, and phosphate every 4 hours
  d. Venous pH every 1–2 hours until stable (> 7.30)
  e. Urine and serum ketone dilutions every 2–4 hours until negative at $1:2$.
	EO: The child's response to the insulin infusion will be monitored.

Patient/Family Education: Home Care Considerations

1. Assist the family with efforts toward planning for adaptation required by the child's changing health status.

2. Reinforce family teaching specific to a child with diabetes.

3. Provide information on resources available regarding respite care, summer camp, and other facilities to provide short-term care if a crisis arises.

4. Provide contact resources for an advocacy group so the family can explore ongoing support with individuals who share the same health problems.

References

_____ (1989). *Guidelines for management of pediatric patients with diabetic ketoacidosis.* Chicago: Michael Reese Hospital and Medical Center—Pediatric Intensive Care.

Balik, B., Haig, B., & Monjihan, P. (1986). Diabetes and the school-age child. *American Journal of Maternal Child Nursing, 11*(5), 324–330.

Turco, S.J. (1985). Absorption of insulin to infusion bottles and tubing. *Canadian Intravenous Nurses' Association Journal,* Fall, 6.

Musculoskeletal and Integumentary System Procedures

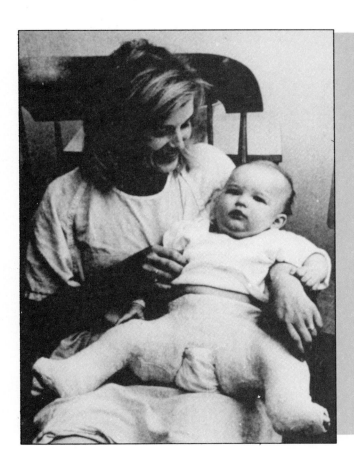

Unit XIII

Cast Care

85

Definition/Purpose

A cast is applied to immobilize and support a body part in a specific position to provide healing of a fracture or to prevent a deformity. Casts are also used to permit earlier weight bearing on an extremity after an injury.

Standard of Care

1. Circulation and nerve function will be observed and recorded every 30 minutes for the first 4 to 8 hours after cast application; then every two hours for the next 24 hours; and every 4 to 8 hours thereafter.
2. Inspect and record the skin condition around the cast edges every 8 hours.
3. Turn the child every 2 hours.
4. Auscultate breath sounds every 4 hours, with attention to respiratory rate, pattern, skin color, mental status, and abdominal girth.

Assessment

1. Assess the medical history of the child, with emphasis on neuromuscular, musculoskeletal, respiratory, renal, or elimination problems. Also assess the child for congenital defects or impairment of circulation.
2. Assess physical findings such as the type of cast, its fit on the affected body part, signs of drainage, sensation, motion, temperature, color, pain sensation, capillary refill, pulse, and edema.
3. Assess the child's developmental level, coping mechanisms, adjustment to loss of body functioning, and previous experience in a hospital environment and with a cast (such as crutch walking and cast care).

Nursing Diagnoses

The following is a list of possible diagnoses and could apply, depending on the child's age, clinical situation, and physical condition:

Altered tissue perfusion

High risk for injury

Pain

Impaired skin integrity

Ineffective breathing pattern

Self-care deficit

Impaired physical mobility

Diversional activity deficit

Body image disturbance

Planning

When planning to care for a child with a cast, the following equipment is needed:

Alcohol

1-inch adhesive tape

Pillows

Scissors

Cast cutter (available on unit)

Interventions

PROCEDURE	**RATIONALE/EXPECTED OUTCOME (EO)**
1. Assess and document the neurovascular status of the extremity (color, capillary refilling, pulses above and below the injury, temperature, sensation, and motion).	Disruption of tissues and blood vessels caused by trauma or surgery results in bleeding and release of plasma. Swelling may occur, compressing the blood vessels and interrupting circulation to the surrounding area and the distal extremity (compartment syndrome). *EO: The child will maintain adequate peripheral tissue perfusion.* *EO: The skin will be intact and warm to touch, with good perfusion and pink color.*
2. Note and record the amount of edema.	
3. Observe and record complaints of burning, twitching, tingling, or facial expression denoting discomfort.	
4. Note the amount of bleeding on cast; circle and time the area.	A child may lose a considerable amount of blood under the cast before it is visible through the cast material. *EO: The child will remain hemodynamically stable.*
5. Monitor vital signs for signs of excessive bleeding (such as rapid pulse and low blood pressure).	
6. Monitor hemoglobin and hematocrit results.	
7. Apply icepacks beside the casted area.	
8. Position the child using proper alignment to minimize pressure on dependent areas. Have child use trapeze for self-positioning.	
9. Elevate the involved extremity (elevate leg on a pillow without rubber or plastic) or suspend an arm in a stockinette from an IV pole. Support the child with pillows to prevent excessive weight on a damp cast (Figs. 85-1 and 85-2).	Plastic or rubber inhibits cast drying and cooling.
10. Be aware that the drying time varies with size and type of cast. (Plaster of Paris takes 10–72 hours and synthetic plaster takes 8–10 hours.) Handle the wet cast with the palms of the hands, not with the fingers.	This will prevent indentations in the cast which may compress underlying tissues. *EO: The cast will be free from indentations.*
11. Promote drying by leaving the cast uncovered and turning the child.	Turning allows all sides of the cast to dry.

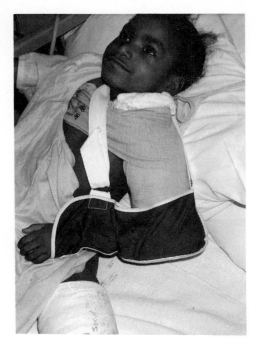

Figure 85-1.

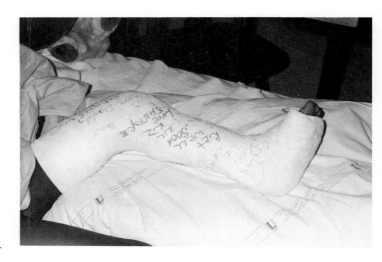

Figure 85-2.

PROCEDURE

12. Monitor and record the child's complaints of pain. Notify physician if pain is unrelieved by analgesics.

13. Report any abdominal discomfort resulting in nausea or vomiting.

14. Keep skin dry and clean. Cleanse excess plaster from skin, and dry well.

15. Inspect skin around cast edges for signs of irritation.

16. Peel rough edges of the cast. Pull the stockinette lining taut over the edge of the cast and petal the cast edge with tape (Fig. 85-3).
    a. Take 1-inch adhesive tape and cut it into 1½- to 2-inch strips.

RATIONALE/EXPECTED OUTCOME (EO)

Excessive pain may indicate the start of compartment syndrome, necessitating the removal or splitting of the cast.

EO: The child will maintain adequate comfort.

These are symptoms of cast syndrome or superior mesenteric artery syndrome caused by a body cast pressing on the mesenteric artery and causing a decreased blood supply to the bowel.

EO: The child has no occurrence of cast syndrome.

EO: The child maintains skin integrity.

Immobility places skin over bony prominences at risk for local irritation, due to pressure of the cast.

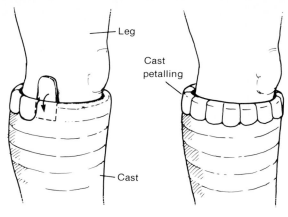

Leg

Cast petalling

Cast

Figure 85-3.

PROCEDURE	**RATIONALE/EXPECTED OUTCOME (EO)**

PROCEDURE

    b. Place one end of a strip of tape on the inside of the cast, sticky side against the cast.

    c. Bring other end up over the cast edge and tape down on the outside of the cast.

    d. Tape ends should overlap each other slightly.

17. Change moist linen as needed; keep bed free of wrinkles.

18. Reposition child every 2 hours during the day and every 4 hours at night. Support major joints while turning. Do not use abductor bar (if present on cast) to turn the child. The child can be positioned on his or her back, stomach, or on either side if in a body cast. Those sitting should push up or shift their position frequently. In a nonwalking leg cast, the cast may be placed on a pillow on the floor or on a chair in front of the child. For the child who cannot walk, use a stroller, wagon, or scooter board as means of transportation.

19. To protect the cast from body excrement, tuck waterproof material around the perineal edge (for example, plastic wrap, disposable diaper, or sanitary napkin.)

20. Clean and dry the child's skin after each diaper change or use of the bedpan or urinal.

21. Remove stains from the outer cast with a damp cloth.

22. Inspect the cast for cracks, softening, or excessive flaking.

23. Avoid covering cast with varnish.

24. Monitor complaints of pain. Palpate cast over painful area, inspect for drainage, and smell cast edges to detect foul odor.

RATIONALE/EXPECTED OUTCOME (EO)

Avoid long periods of sitting or lying in one position, which causes unnatural pressure over body areas.

EO: The child is mobile within the limitations set by the cast and the orthopedic problem.

EO: The cast will be clean and intact.

Varnish inhibits evaporation of body moisture.

Foul odor may indicate infection or necrosis. The warm dark environment under the cast is a good medium for bacteria.

EO: The child is free of wound infection and purulent drainage on cast.

PROCEDURE	**RATIONALE/EXPECTED OUTCOME (EO)**
25. Place call bell and frequently used items within reach.	Immobilization of a body part will interfere with performing functions independently. *EO: The child will perform activities of daily living (ADL) when able.*
26. Observe which activities the child is able to perform, and reinforce those behaviors.	
27. Medicate for pain before potentially painful ROM exercises.	
28. Teach the older child to perform ROM on all unaffected joints.	Disuse of unaffected muscles and joints will result in atrophy, stiffness, and loss of function. *EO: The child exhibits full ROM of unaffected joints.*
29. Provide for safe ambulation as soon as possible.	*EO: The child will ambulate safely.*
30. Auscultate breath sounds when vital signs are taken.	Immobility results in the pooling of secretions. Hip spica body casts limit abdominal movement and chest excursion. *EO: The child maintains an effective breathing pattern free of pulmonary congestion.*
31. Instruct child to take deep breaths. Observe child's ability to fully expand lungs and inform the physician of any problem related to a restricted cast.	
32. Give small frequent feedings to prevent abdominal distention.	
33. Monitor elimination pattern.	Immobility may cause constipation. *EO: Child will maintain a normal elimination pattern.*

Patient/Family Education: Home Care Considerations

Instruct the family about the following aspects of caring for a child in a cast.

Skin Care

1. Give child a daily sponge bath, washing only the areas not under the cast. Do not get the cast wet.
2. Clean toes, fingers, and the skin around the edges of the cast with rubbing alcohol 2–3 times a day to toughen the skin and prevent skin breakdown. Lotion may be used if the alcohol is cracking the skin. Do not use oils or powders under or around the edges of the cast, because powders "cake" and oils soften the skin, making it easier for the skin to break down.
3. If the child spends a great deal of time in a chair or in bed, rub the elbows, knees, heels, ankles, or base of the spine (if exposed) with alcohol to toughen the skin at those locations.
4. Make sure the child does not pull small objects (such as food, toys, buttons, pins, coins, or bottle caps) down into the cast. Do not place any item down into the cast (such as sticks, coat hangers, or rulers) in an attempt to retrieve anything that has fallen into the cast, or to relieve itching. You may reach inside the cast with fingertips only.
5. If there is a problem with the cast, do not remove the child's cast at home. Call the physician and he or she will advise the family on what to do.

Daily Observations

1. Using a flashlight, look inside the cast as far as possible. If you see any reddened areas that you can reach, rub the skin with alcohol. If you find skin breakdown or sores, notify the physician.
2. Check the cast for rough edges where the petals might have become loosened. Re-petal the cast if necessary.
3. Ask the child to move fingers or toes if they are in a leg or arm cast. If they could move them before and cannot now, notify the physician.
4. If the child complains of numbness or tingling, notify the physician.
5. Check the color and warmth of the extremity in the cast. If the color is blue, pale, or reddened, or if it feels unusually warm or cold, notify the physician.
6. If fingers or toes on the extremity swell, elevate them on a pillow. Notify the physician if the swelling persists.
7. If the child is unusually irritable or complains of persistent pain in an area, or if the child has a fever, there may be an infected area under the cast that needs the physician's attention.
8. If there is a foul odor or foul-smelling drainage on the cast, it could mean an open sore or infection that needs the physician's attention.
9. Also notify the physician if:
   a. A cast is soft, cracks, or breaks.
   b. A cast is loose and slips up and down easily.

Activity

1. Small children should be held as often as possible, regardless of the fact that they are in a cast (Fig. 85-4).

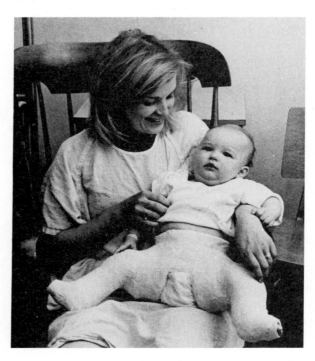

Figure 85-4. Reprinted from Pillitteri, A. (1987). Child health nursing, ed 3. Boston: Little, Brown and Company, p. 1195.

2. For the child who cannot walk, use a stroller or wagon to take him or her outside.

3. Place a rug or blanket on the floor so the child can get out of bed and be allowed to play.

4. Never leave an immobile child home alone.

Cast Removal

1. Support the joints immediately after the cast is removed to prevent pain and discomfort.

2. The skin under the cast will be caked with a yellow material that is dead skin and oil. This material should be soaked off in a tub of warm water. It may take several days for the material to soak off—*Do not scrub it off.*

3. Lotion or oil may be applied to the skin to prevent itching.

References

Cuddy, C.M. (1986). Caring for a child in a spica cast: A parent's perspective. *Orthopedic Nursing, 5*(3), 17–21.

Dunn, B. (1977). Cast care. *Pediatric Nursing (4)*, 41–42.

Feller, N.G., Stroup, K., & Christian, L. (1989). Helping staff nurses become mini-specialists. . . cast care. *American Journal of Nursing, 89*(7), 991–992.

Mather, M.L.S. (1987). The secret to life in a spica. *American Journal of Nursing, 87*(1), 56–58.

Pellino, T.A., Mooney, N.E., & Safmond, S.W. (1986). *Care Curriculum for Orthopedic Nursing.* Pitman, N.J.: Anthony Jannetti, Inc.

Shesser, L.K., & Kling, F.T., Jr.. (1986). Practical consideration in caring for a child in a hip spica cast: An evaluation using parental input. *Orthopedic Nursing, 5*(3), 11–15.

Wise, L. (1986). A comparison of orthopedic casts: Breaking the mold. *MCN: American Journal of Maternal Child Nursing, 11*(3), 174–176.

Traction

86

Definition/Purpose

Traction is the application of a pulling force to an injured or diseased part of the body or to an extremity while a countertraction pulls in the opposite direction. The purpose of the traction is to:

1. Reduce fractures or dislocations and maintain alignment.
2. Decrease muscle spasms and relieve pain.
3. Correct, lessen, or prevent deformities.
4. Promote rest of a diseased or injured part.

The classifications of traction are discussed below.

Skin Traction

Technique

The various forms of skin traction use the following techniques:

1. Attaches to the skin and soft tissue, providing a light pull
2. May be removed and reapplied intermittently
3. Usually uses 5–8 pounds of weight applied with skin adherents or elastic bandages.

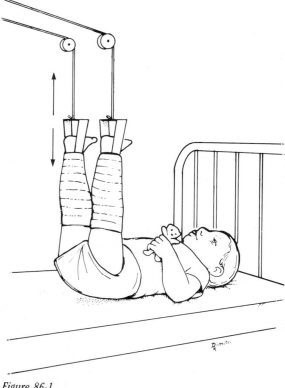
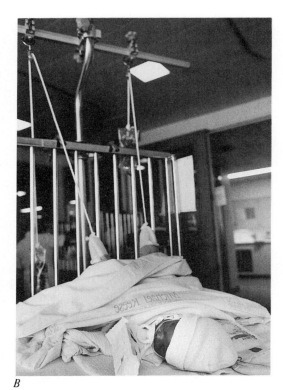

A

B

Figure 86-1.

Types

There are five types of skin traction:

1. Bryant traction is used for treating fractures of the femur in children under 2 years old, and in congenital hip dislocations in children less than 3 years old and less than 30 pounds. It is always applied bilaterally and distributes the same amount of traction to both legs. The traction is applied to the legs by elastic bandages over the adhesive traction strips, which are wrapped from the foot to the thigh or the groin. The hips are flexed at a 90° angle and the legs are extended by ropes through pulleys that are attached to the bed frame. Weights hold the legs in position and the weight of the child provides countertraction. The buttocks should clear the bed slightly, while the shoulders and upper back rest on the bed (Fig. 86-1).

2. Buck extension traction is used to reduce fractures of the hip or pelvis or to immobilize knee and hip contractures. The lower leg is pulled directly away from the body by weights that hang at the foot of the bed. Countertraction is achieved by the weight of the child (Fig. 86-2).

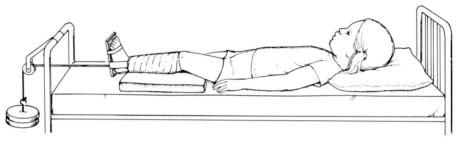

Figure 86-2.

3. Russell traction is used to treat knee injuries and fractures of the femur and hip. It is similar to Buck extension applied to the lower leg, except that a padded sling is held under the knee by means of a pulley attached to the bed frame (Fig. 86-3).

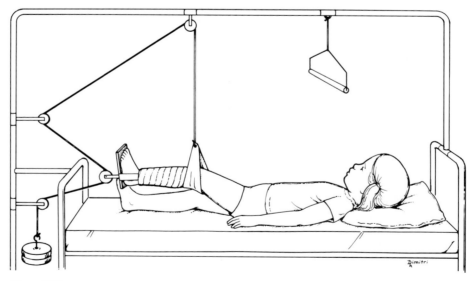

Figure 86-3.

4. The cervical head halter is used for children with spinal fractures, muscle spasms, or spinal injuries to provide immobilization in a neutral position, which causes the least pressure on the spinal cord (Fig. 86-4).

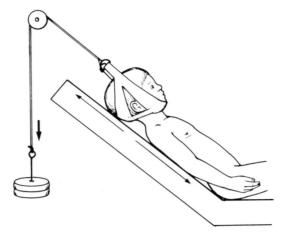

Figure 86-4.

5. Dunlop traction is used for fractures of the humerus. The arm is suspended horizontally with the elbow flexed, using skin or skeletal traction. Adhesive straps are placed on the upper and lower arms so that pull can be exerted in two directions (Fig. 86-5).

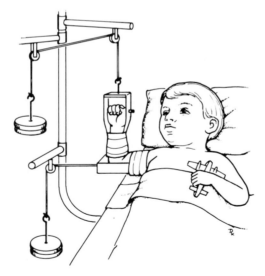

Figure 86-5.

Skeletal Traction

Technique

Skeletal traction employs the following techniques:

1. Attaches directly to the bone, providing a strong, steady continuous pull.
2. Weight is applied to the extremities with Steinmann pins or Kirschner wires.
3. A range of 15–40 pounds of weight is used, depending on:
   a. Injury
   b. Body size
   c. Muscle spasm.

4. Should not be removed without a physician's order.

5. Skeletal traction is frequently used in conjunction with balanced suspension.

Types

1. Ninety–ninety skeletal traction, with a boot cast on the lower leg and a Steinmann pin through the distal femur, is used for children over 2 years old for treatment of fractures of the femoral shaft. It maintains 90° flexion of both the knee and the hip. As with Bryant traction, the pelvis is lifted from the bed (Fig. 86-6).

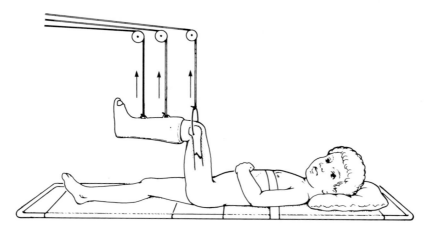

Figure 86-6.

2. Balanced suspension traction with Thomas leg splint and Pearson attachment is used to suspend the leg in a flexed position to relax the hip and hamstring muscles. A Thomas splint is a ridged frame that fits around the leg and has a ring that encircles the groin. The splint extends to midair above the bed. Countertraction is provided by the friction of the thigh against the splint and the pressure of the groin ring. Weights pull the leg toward the foot of the bed. A Pearson attachment is used to lift the Thomas splint by means of ropes and pulleys attached to the overbed frame to flex the knees and balance the lower leg (Fig. 86-7).

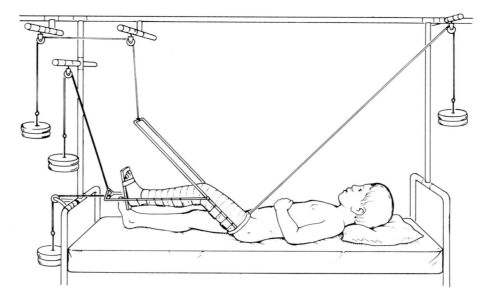

Figure 86-7.

3. Halo traction with Crutchfield tongs is used to immobilize the child with a spinal fracture or to place traction and countertraction on a severe curvature of the spine (scoliosis). Traction may be accomplished by making small burr holes in the skull into the outer layers of the parietal bones on each side and inserting tongs that then are connected with a pulley and weights (Fig. 86-8).

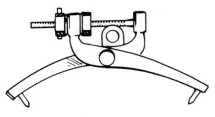

Figure 86-8.

4. A halo device with body cast or vest is used to immobilize the child with cervical injuries. An adjustable steel hoop is placed around the child's head and secured to the skull with two occipital and two temporal screws. Steel bars anchor the device to the child's body cast or vest. This halo device allows the child greater mobility, with minimal risk of disturbing the spinal alignment (Fig. 86-9).

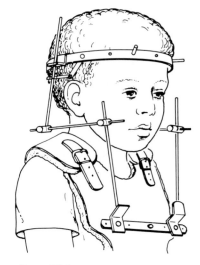

Figure 86-9.

Manual Traction

Technique

The following techniques are used in manual traction:

1. Applied with hands
2. Steady pull is maintained
3. Used during casting, fracture reduction, and halo application.

Standard of Care

1. Verify desired position of the ropes, pulleys, supports, and amount of weight to be used.
2. Verify activities and amount of movement permitted.

3. Maintain proper alignment. Place child on a firm mattress with a bedboard, footboard, and overhead trapeze if necessary.

4. Ensure that ropes and pulleys are in straight lines, at correct angles, and unobstructed (for example, not resting on the bed, on the floor, or on any other objects that prevent the weights from hanging freely).

5. Ensure that ropes are well-knotted and not frayed.

6. Keep slings clean, dry, and secure.

7. Place toys, call light, phone, bedside table, and other necessary items within reach of the child.

Assessment

1. Assess onset of symptoms, type of injury, musculoskeletal history, allergies, and medication history.

2. Assess physical findings such as muscle spasms, level of pain, range of motion, and skin condition.

3. Assess the child's developmental level, living situation, and usual coping mechanisms, as well as the child's and family's understanding of the purpose of traction, its potential complications, and their willingness to learn.

Nursing Diagnoses

The following is a list of possible diagnoses and could apply, depending on the child's age, clinical situation, and physical condition:

Fear

Anxiety

High risk for injury

High risk for infection

Altered tissue perfusion

Impaired skin integrity

Diversional activity deficit

Body image disturbance

Altered constipation urinary elimination

Pain

Planning

The following equipment must be gathered to care for a child in traction:

Egg crate mattress or sheepskin

Povidone-iodine solution or hydrogen peroxide

Sterile gloves

Diversional activities (such as toys, TV, or music)

Interventions

PROCEDURE	**RATIONALE/EXPECTED OUTCOME (EO)**
1. Orient the child and parents to the environment. Explain the traction setup, the equipment to be	Children placed in traction experience fear and anxiety about the equipment used and how successful the trac-

PROCEDURE

used, and the purpose of traction. If possible, introduce the child to another child in similar traction.

2. Explain which activities are permitted while in traction:
   a. Suspension traction—The child may sit, turn slightly, and move head as desired.
   b. Running traction—The head of the bed may be elevated to the point of countertraction.

3. Discuss with the child and parents how they can help with care (bathing, turning, etc.)

4. Teach child how to call for assistance and ensure that calls are answered promptly.

5. Assess bony prominences, especially the heels and elbows, every 2 hours for signs of impaired circulation (such as reddened areas or broken skin). Massage bony prominences with lotion.

6. Use an eggcrate mattress or sheepskin to protect bony areas.

7. Avoid pillows or pads under the knees or calves. Monitor for signs of thromboembolus (pain in chest or leg, tenderness in calf, shortness of breath, coughing up blood).

8. For skeletal traction:
   a. Clean pin sites every 8 hours with povidone-iodine solution or hydrogen peroxide. After thoroughly cleaning around each pin, apply pov-

RATIONALE/EXPECTED OUTCOME (EO)

tion will be. Demonstrations and explanations will help alleviate some of these feelings.

EO: The child and parents will verbalize their feelings and will be able to cope with the traction. The child and parents will verbalize an understanding of the type of traction used and the activities it permits.

Due to immobilization of the child by traction, the pressure exerted on blood vessels compromises circulation to an area and causes decreased perfusion to the tissues. The tissues are destroyed when the blood supply falls below what is required for survival. Also, clots form in vessels that have decreased blood flow.

EO: The child is free from signs or symptoms of pressure sores.

EO: The child is free from signs or symptoms of thromboembolus.

Pins, wires, and tongs are surgically placed on skeletal structures. There is a risk of introducing pathogens through the sites, and thus potential for a local infection.

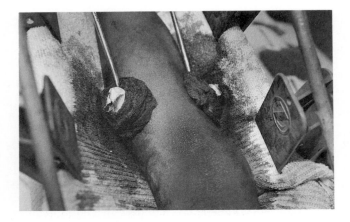

Figure 86-10.

PROCEDURE

      idone-iodine ointment at the site and wrap the site with gauze. (Wear sterile gloves for this procedure.) (Fig. 86-10)

    b. Observe pin site for redness, edema, or discharge. Notify the physician if any of these occur.

    c. If a pin becomes detached from the tongs or halo, stabilize the child's head with pillows or sandbags and call the physician.

9. For skin traction:

    a. Take the child out of traction for 10–20 minutes every 8 hours, or twice a day for fractures. Two people are needed to unwrap and rewrap to exert manual traction.

    b. Check skin for redness. If redness lasts longer than 20 minutes, rewrap more loosely.

    c. Clean skin with soap and dry thoroughly. Do not apply oil or creams to soften skin.

10. Check splints and wraps for tightness and bunching. Remove and replace wraps as ordered.

11. Check the skin and affected extremity for temperature, color, sensation, capillary refill, and movement every hour. Monitor for signs of Volkmann's syndrome, which is characterized by severe pain, absent pulse, pallor, cyanosis, paralysis, and paresthesia.

12. Note amount of edema in the affected extremity.

13. Note amount of bleeding from injured area. Monitor hemoglobin and hematocrit.

14. Observe for neurologic impairment specific to the location of the traction. Observe eye movements, pupillary changes, blurred vision, difficulty swallowing, speech, and tongue control.

15. Ask verbal child to describe level of discomfort using a 0–10 scale or a picture scale. Assess preverbal child by a change in behavior, decreased appetite, irritability, or inability to sleep.

16. Medicate child for pain, using the ordered medication and route. Determine the medication's effectiveness after 30 minutes.

17. Reposition the patient or adjust the traction to decrease pain. Never turn or lift the child by grabbing the halo. Avoid letting anything hit the halo or tongs.

18. Instruct older child in relaxation techniques, such as deep breathing.

19. Provide diversional activities that the child can do in bed. Place the child in a multibed room. Move child out of room, in bed (when possible) for a change of environment. Encourage family and friends to visit.

RATIONALE/EXPECTED OUTCOME (EO)

EO: The child has no drainage or odor from pin sites, and maintains a temperature within normal limits.

Oils will allow the traction to slip off easily and increase the risk of skin breakdown.

This is an ischemic process that progresses from arterial occlusion to muscle anoxia and vasospasm, resulting in contractures, muscle necrosis, and paralysis.

EO: The child had normal neurovascular checks.

Incorporate signs and symptoms of cranial nerve impairment with vascular checks for patients in halo or cervical tong traction. An abnormal neurologic exam with a patient in halo traction may indicate increased intracranial pressure or compression of nerves.

Children in traction are frequently in acute pain from an injury or the traction itself.

EO: The child will maintain an adequate level of comfort. The traction will maintain alignment and decrease long-term pain.

Children with tongs or halo are sensitive to any noise made by striking the metal because it is an excellent sound detector.

The immobile child requires activities that provide diversion so the necessary traction can be maintained. Allow for flexibility in visiting hours to maintain family contact.

EO: The child participates in unit activities and care.

PROCEDURE	**RATIONALE/EXPECTED OUTCOME (EO)**

20. Provide age-appropriate activities:
    a. All ages—Decorate room with colorful posters and cards; push child and bed into the playroom or hall to prevent isolation, and arrange for child to eat meals with family or other children.
    b. School-age—Provide books and puzzles; encourage calls or visits from classmates; hang a punching bag or bell overhead, and arrange for continuation of school activities by contacting the child's teacher.
    c. Preschool—Provide video programs, coloring books, modelling clay, puppets, storytelling, and music.
    d. Infant to toddler—Provide a mobile, music, stuffed animals, rattles, or a "busy box."

21. Record intake and output during each shift. Note urinary frequency, distention, and complaints of burning. Encourage fluids. Promote roughage, and bulk in the diet. Maintain a steady diet. Use a fracture urinal and bedpan, providing privacy while the child is on the bedpan.

Decreased physical activity and less than adequate dietary intakes and bulk can lead to constipation and urinary tract infections. Also, lack of privacy will make it more difficult for the child to use a bedpan or urinal.

EO: The child maintains a normal bowel and urinary elimination pattern.

Patient/Family Education: Home Care Considerations

1. Explain to the parents and the child the use of the traction, its purpose and application, as well as the care of the child in traction, and what will happen when the traction is removed (casting, bracing, etc).

2. The nurse should determine with the family members which aspects of care can be given to the parents, the child, and the nurse. Some degree of self-care by the child will increase the child's sense of responsibility and enhance his or her self-esteem.

3. Assess the need for referral to a home health agency for continued physical therapy and to assess the home for needed equipment, such as a special bed.

4. Instruct the child and parents about the use of pain medications, their side effects, and possible alternatives for pain control, such as relaxation exercises.

5. Instruct the child and parents in care of incisions until they are completely healed.

6. Inform the child and parents about the signs and symptoms of infection and the appropriate persons to notify if they appear:
    a. Odor from pin or incision site
    b. Pain, swelling, or drainage at a pin or incision site
    c. Elevated temperature.

7. Review activity limitations and suggest diversional activities.

References

Cohen, S. (1979). Nursing care of the patient in traction. *American Journal of Nursing, 79*(10), 1771–1778.

Evans, M.J. (1989). *Neurologic–neurosurgical nursing.* Springhouse, PA: Springhouse Corporation.

Hansen B., & Evans, M. (1981). Preparing a child for a procedure. *American Journal of Maternal Child Nursing, 6*(6), 194–199.

Shriners' Hospital for Crippled Children—St. Louis Unit. (1984). *Standards for nursing care.* St. Louis: Shriners' Hospital for Crippled Children.

Continuous Passive Motion Device

87

Definition/Purpose

A continuous passive motion device (CPM) is a machine that passively moves a child's joints or extremities through a predetermined range of motion. It is constructed in two parts: an orthosis that supports the anatomy surrounding the joint to be mobilized, and a controller. The controller can be programmed for speed, a pause, the length of treatment, and ranges of motion for flexion and extension. The device can be used on the hand, wrist, elbow, shoulder, hip, knee, and ankle. (Devices for the toe and jaw will soon be available.)

CPM is passive, not active. It is not an exercycle, nor is it intended for muscle strengthening. CPM is not meant to replace active exercise. CPM has been shown to stimulate healing of articular cartilage and to reduce the development of adhesions during healing. Clinical benefits include preservation of range of motion, reduction in pain and edema, and facilitation of total end-range time (TERT)—the total amount of time the joint spends at or near the end of its available range.

Standard of Care

1. CPM devices are categorized as durable medical equipment and require a prescription for use in the hospital or at home.

Assessment

1. Assess the pertinent history, with emphasis on the description of an acute injury, or chronic, developmental, or congenital conditions requiring treatment with CPM.
2. Assess for a previous history of treatment with CPM.
3. Assess hand dominance if the upper extremity is involved.
4. Assess developmental factors such as age, habits, living situations, and usual coping mechanisms.
5. Assess the child's and family's understanding of the purpose of CPM, how it works, its potential complications, and its benefits.

Nursing Diagnoses

The following is a list of possible diagnoses and could apply, depending on the child's age, clinical situation, and physical condition:

Anxiety

Fear

Pain

High risk for injury

Impaired physical mobility

Self-care deficit; feeding, bathing, pressing, toileting

Impaired skin integrity

Planning

When planning to set up a CPM, the following equipment is needed:

CPM device for the appropriate joint (Fig. 87-1)

Padding for pressure points.

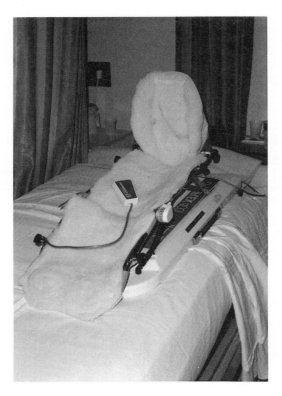

Figure 87-1.

Interventions

PROCEDURE	**RATIONALE/EXPECTED OUTCOME (EO)**
1. Explain to the child and family the purpose and expected duration of treatment with CPM.	The child and family will need instruction about activity restrictions, mobility, safety, pain management, and further rehabilitation that may be necessary. *EO: The child and family verbalize the purpose and correct use of the CPM machine.*
2. Assist the child into the CPM machine.	
3. Set the speed, degree of ranges of motion, time of pause, and length of treatment as ordered by the physician.	
4. Check the neurovascular status of the involved extremity every 2–4 hours (feeling, pulses, color, and sensation).	Impaired blood circulation and edema lead to interrupted vasomotor pathways, which affect oxygenation and nutritional support to the tissues. *EO: The child's neurovascular status remains stable.*
5. Maintain correct alignment in CPM machine. a. Assess the involved extremity for signs of skin breakdown (redness, edema, blisters, and abrasions). Pay special attention to areas coming in contact with the machine.	*EO: The child will maintain correct alignment of the extremity and will be free from injury.* Immobility fosters muscle disuse and decreased circulation to soft tissues. Prolonged pressure on a body area leads to disrupted nerve impulses and decreased circulation.

PROCEDURE	**RATIONALE/EXPECTED OUTCOME (EO)**
b. Pad any areas that rest against parts of the machine.	Friction produces blisters. This will decrease friction between the skin and the machine.
	EO: The child's skin integrity will be maintained.
c. Assess the incision for signs of infection (redness, tenderness, swelling, and drainage).	*EO: The child will not exhibit signs of infection.*
6. Assess the affected joint for increased swelling, redness, tenderness, or unusual pain:	
a. Provide comfort measures.	
b. Position the child as comfortably as possible.	
c. Use the time that the child is out of the machine for rest and comfort measures, such as repositioning or massaging bony prominences.	*EO: The child's comfort is maintained.*
7. Organize the child's environment to facilitate independence while in the CPM machine. Allow the child to structure the time spent out of the machine.	*EO: The child participates in self-care.*
8. Provide age-appropriate toys from the child's own environment.	*EO: The child will participate in age-appropriate activities to decrease fear and anxiety.*

Patient/Family Education: Home Care Considerations

1. Assess the need for referral to a home care agency for a progressive ambulation program and continuation of the CPM program.
2. Instruct the child and parents in the care of incisions.
3. Teach signs and symptoms of infection or skin breakdown.
4. Review activity restrictions and suggest diversional activity that is age-appropriate.

References

Diehn, S.L. (1989). The Powers of CPM: Healing through motion. *Continuing Care, 11*, 28–36.

Pellino, T.A., Mooney, N.E., & Safmond, S.W., et al. (1986). *Core curriculum for orthopaedic nursing*. Pitman, NJ: Anthony J. Jannette, Inc.

Wound Care

88

Definition/Purpose

Understanding the pathophysiology of wound healing and the factors that influence wound healing provides the basis for nursing care, particularly wound care. When cells are injured, tissue repair may result either in regeneration of the tissue with little evidence that injury occurred, or in scar formation. The type of cells that constitute the tissue determines the end result.

There are three types of cells: labile cells, stable cells, and permanent cells. Labile cells multiply and constantly replace similar cells that are destroyed. Examples of these cells are those of the skin and mucous membranes and blood cells. Stable cells do not normally multiply vigorously, but will do so if injured. Examples of these cells are those of the bone and glandular organs. Both labile and stable cells require an underlying structure; they will not grow across an empty space. Because of this, if there is an underlying structure there will be regeneration of normal structure. If there is no underlying structure, scarring will occur. Permanent cells constitute muscle and nerve tissue. Because they are unable to regenerate, destruction of permanent cells results in scarring. A surgical incision cuts into muscle tissue and destroys permanent cells, so although the epithelial cells regenerate over the scar tissue, the epithelial layer is thin and scar tissue will remain visible underneath.

Tissues heal in one of three ways: primary, secondary, or tertiary intention. Wounds that are created surgically, with a minimum of tissue destruction or reaction, heal through primary intention. Healing by primary intention takes place under the following conditions (Fig. 88-1):

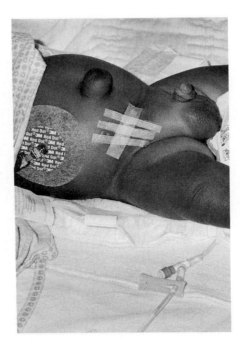

Figure 88-1.

1. Minimal drainage from the wound
2. Minimal trauma to the wound
3. Minimal contamination of the wound
4. Prompt and accurate approximation of edges of the wound
5. No dead space left to become a site of infection after suturing

Wounds that are characterized by tissue loss with the inability to approximate wound edges heal by secondary intention (granulation tissue). This type of wound is left open and allowed to heal from the inside toward the outer surface. The area of tissue loss will fill with granulation tissue (fibroblasts and capillaries).

Healing by third intention takes place when approximation of wound edges is delayed by 3 to 5 days or more. Conditions requiring delayed closure include a heavily contaminated wound or the removal of an inflamed organ.

Some factors that affect a child's response to surgery are directly related to wound healing. Wounds in children heal more rapidly than those in adults because of increased metabolism and good circulation. Adequate circulation to injured tissue is important to provide the white blood cells, fibroblasts, and nutrients needed for healing and to remove the debris after phagocytosis. Nutrients are also important for wound healing. Vitamin C is necessary to form collagen and to maintain the integrity of the capillary walls. Vitamin A is important for epithelial growth. Protein insufficiency will also delay wound healing, because collagen is a protein. All of these nutrients, and others as well, become depleted in the surgical child because of inadequate dietary intake and stress. Other factors that delay healing of a wound include infection, foreign bodies in the wound, radiation of areas near the wound, and the administration of corticosteroids.

The Centers for Disease Control (CDC) has established four surgical wound classifications: clean wounds, clean contaminated wounds, contaminated wounds, and infected wounds. Clean wounds are primarily closed and can be drained with a closed drainage system. They show no signs of infection. The respiratory, alimentary, and genitourinary tracts were not entered. Clean contaminated wounds are those in which the respiratory, alimentary, or genitourinary tract is entered under controlled conditions. There is no sign of infection or break in surgical technique. Contaminated wounds, however, are open, fresh, accidental wounds with signs of infection or where spillage of gastrointestinal contents has occurred. Infected wounds include traumatic wounds with retained devitalized tissue and wounds that involve an existing infection or perforated viscera.

For psychologic reasons and to prevent trauma, a wound is usually covered with a dressing (Fig. 88-2). A dressing serves the following purposes:

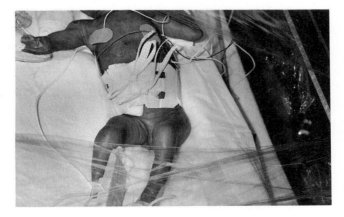

Figure 88-2.

1. To apply medications
2. To cushion and protect the wound from trauma and contamination
3. To absorb drainage

4. To support, splint, or immobilize the body part and incisional area

5. To aid in hemostasis and minimize edema

6. To maintain a moist environment and prevent cell dehydration.

Dressings are grouped into two categories: primary and secondary. Primary dressings are placed directly over the wound and function to absorb drainage and allow it to wick away from the wound. Secondary dressings are placed over the primary dressing and function to absorb excessive drainage, provide hemostasis by compression, and protect the wound from trauma.

Standard of Care

1. Always wash hands before and after wound care.

2. Use aseptic technique to change the dressings.

3. Take a culture of any suspected wound drainage.

Assessment

1. Assess the pertinent history and physical findings for fever, pain, anorexia, dehydration, changes in vital signs, elevated white blood cell count, and type of trauma to the tissue.

2. Assess the psychosocial and developmental factors for age, the meaning of hospitalization to the child and the family, and previous hospital experiences and habits.

3. Assess the child's and family's knowledge of the disease and the need for immediate attention, past experience with family members who have had wounds or required wound care, and their willingness to learn.

Nursing Diagnoses

The following is a list of possible diagnoses and could apply, depending on the child's age, clinical situation, and physical condition:

Altered skin integrity

Pain

Anxiety

Fear

Body image disturbance

High risk for infection

Planning

When planning to care for a child with a wound,
the following equipment must be gathered (Fig. 88-3):

Sterile gloves

Disposable, clean gloves

Sterile dressings

Tape

Betadine

70% alcohol

3% hydrogen peroxide

Sterile normal saline

Plastic bag for soiled dressings

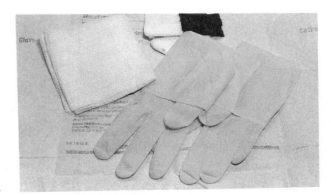

Figure 88-3.

Interventions

PROCEDURE	**RATIONALE/EXPECTED OUTCOME (EO)**

General Assessment

1. Assess the appearance of the wound:
   a. Approximation of wound edges

   b. Color of the wound and surrounding tissue

   c. Presence of drains and tubes.

The wound edges should be clean and well-approximated with a crust along the wound edges.
Initially the wound edges will be red and slightly swollen and will return to normal in a week.
Drains and tubes are inserted near a wound when fluid is anticipated to collect in the wound and delay healing.
EO: The child will demonstrate progressive healing of the wound.

2. Assess for signs of dehiscence or evisceration:
   Dehiscence—Partial or total disruption of wound layers
   Evisceration—Protrusion of viscera through the incisional area
   If either occurs, cover the wound with sterile gauze soaked with saline and notify the physician.

3. Assess the wound for drainage:
   a. Amount
   b. Color
   c. Odor
   d. Consistency.
   Assess the drainage on dressings, and in bottles or reservoirs.

Drainage described as:
a. Serous—Clear and watery; consists of the serous portion of the blood
b. Sanguineous—Looks like blood; consists of a large amount of blood cells
c. Purulent—Thick with a musty foul odor; consists of WBCs, liquified dead tissue debris, and bacteria.
EO: The child will remain free of infection with normal WBC, temperature, and absence of purulent drainage.

4. Assess the wound for pain.

Pain with palpation and an increase in incisional drainage signal delayed healing or infection. Incision pain is most severe in the first 1 to 2 days, and then becomes milder.
EO: The child will have decreased wound pain.

5. Assess the child's nutritional status (see Nutritional Assessment).

Inadequate nutrition delays healing and increases the risk of infection.

6. Assess the child for other factors that will affect healing:
   a. Obesity

   b. Poor circulation
   c. Anemia
   d. Emotional stress
   e. Postoperative radiation

Large amounts of subcutaneous and tissue fat take longer to heal, are difficult to suture, and are more prone to infection because of decreased blood vessels.

Oxygenation is decreased in children with anemia.

7. Monitor the child's vital signs (temperature, pulse, respiration, and blood pressure) at least every 4 hours, or more often if condition warrants.

Elevated pulse rate and temperature may indicate a wound infection. Hemorrhage may be indicated by a drop in blood pressure and an increase in pulse and respiratory rate.
EO: The child will maintain normal vital signs for age.

PROCEDURE	**RATIONALE/EXPECTED OUTCOME (EO)**
8. Monitor the child's intake and output every 8 hours, or more often if condition warrants.	Decreased urinary output may indicate hemorrhage or fluid depletion due to drainage from the wound. *EO: The child will maintain adequate urinary output (0.5–1.0 mL/kg/hr).*
9. Monitor the child's hemoglobin, hematocrit, and white blood cell count.	Decreased hemoglobin and hematocrit may indicate hemorrhage. An elevated white blood cell count may indicate an infection.

Cleaning Wound and Applying Dressing

PROCEDURE	**RATIONALE/EXPECTED OUTCOME (EO)**
10. Explain the dressing change procedure to the child and family.	An explanation reduces anxiety and encourages cooperation.
11. Gather equipment. Wash hands.	
12. Position the child in a comfortable position, keeping him or her warm with a blanket.	Provide privacy and warmth for the child.
13. Open a plastic bag near the work area.	Soiled dressings will be placed in the bag to prevent contamination of other surfaces.
14. Loosen tape on the dressing.	
15. Put on clean disposable gloves and remove soiled dressings, being careful not to dislodge drains or tubes.	The gloves protect the nurse from touching contaminated dressings.
16. Assess amount, type, and odor of drainage.	
17. Discard old dressings in the plastic bag. Remove gloves.	*EO: The child's soiled dressing is removed and discarded in a way that prevents the spread of microorganisms.*
18. Open sterile dressings and supplies.	
19. Open sterile cleaning solution and pour over gauze sponges, being careful not to touch the dressings with the solution bottle.	
20. Put on sterile gloves.	Maintain asepsis throughout dressing change.

21. Clean the wound:
  a. Clean from the center outward or from top to bottom.
  b. Use one gauze for each wipe, discarding the wipe in the plastic bag.
  c. Clean around drains from drain site outward in a circular motion.
  d. Dry wound with a gauze sponge with same motion as above.
	Move from the least contaminated area to the most contaminated.
	
	EO: The child shows normal wound healing.

22. Apply a layer of dry, sterile dressings over the wound.	Primary dressing serves as a wick for drainage to be pulled away from the wound.
23. Apply a second layer of sterile gauze to wound.	
24. Remove gloves and apply tape or ties to secure dressings.	*EO: The child will have a sterile dressing applied to the wound.*
25. Wash hands.	
26. Document the dressing change in the medical record.	This provides accurate documentation of the procedure in the record.
27. Check dressing every 8 hours, or more often as the condition warrants.	

Patient/Family Education: Home Care Considerations

1. Teach the child and family home care of the incision.
2. Provide the family with sources for supplies.
3. Teach handwashing and the correct disposal of contaminated dressings.
4. Reinforce the need for a high protein and vitamin C diet if not contraindicated.
5. Instruct the family in the administration of medications.
6. Teach the family the signs of infection (for example, fever, redness, pain or warmth at the incision site, and change in behavior).
7. Reinforce the need to keep follow-up appointments.

References

American Association of Operating Room Nurses. (1990). *AORN standards and recommended practices for perioperative nursing.* Denver, CO: Author

Brunner S., & Suddarth, D.S. (1988). *Textbook of medical–surgical nursing.* Philadelphia: J.B. Lippincott Company.

Meeker, M., & Rothrock, J. (1991). *Alexander's care of the patient in surgery.* St. Louis: Mosby Yearbook.

Neuberger, G.B., & Richling, J.B. (1985). A new look at wound care. *Nursing '85, 15*(2), 34–41.

Taylor, C., Lillis, C., & LeMone, P. (1989). *Fundamentals of nursing—The art and science of nursing.* Philadelphia: J.B. Lippincott Company.

Wysochi, A. (1989). Surgical wound healing: A review for perioperative nurses. *Journal of the American Association of Operating Room Nurses, 49*(2), 502–518.

Burn Care

89

Definition/Purpose

Burn wounds are a common cause of injury, disability, and disfigurement in childhood. Burns are second only to automobile accidents as a cause of death during childhood. An estimated 1500 to 2500 children die from thermal injury in the United States each year.

The majority of thermal injuries in childhood result from an accident in the home. Toddlers, for example, tend to be burned when they pull over a container of hot liquid on themselves (Fig. 89-1). The resultant scald affects the head, face, shoulders, and arms.

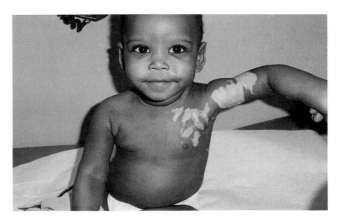

Figure 89-1.

These burns are usually partial thickness in depth. Young children also suffer from immersion in hot water. Older children are fascinated by matches and may set flammable liquids on fire. These wounds are usually full thickness in depth, involving much of the body surface area. The majority of fatal burns come from this group.

Although thermal burns may result from a variety of causes, including scald, flame, contact, electrical, radiation, or chemical, all injuries involve denaturation of cellular protein, either as a result of increased temperature or as a result of oxidation reactions with the cutaneous protoplasm. The pathophysiologic alterations seen in the following thermal injuries include:

1. Rapid development of increased capillary permeability resulting in loss of intravascular fluid and the development of hypovolemia. The degree of hypovolemia is proportional to the size and magnitude of the burn injury.

2. Gradual development of hypermetabolism, resulting in increased energy expenditure. In the most severely burned individual, the basal metabolic rate may increase 100%.

3. Development of pulmonary dysfunction induced by the inhalation of smoke.

The severity of the burn wound is determined by its length, width, and depth. First degree burns (partial thickness) are defined as injuries of the epidermis and most frequently are the result of excessive exposure to ultraviolet radiation from the sun (sunburn). These burns require little medical attention and heal rapidly. The epithelium is replaced in 3–5 days.

A second degree burn (partial thickness) involves destruction of the epidermis and dermis. These injuries do not extend through the dermis. Re-epithelialization of the wound may take place spontaneously if infection is prevented. If infection is present, a second degree wound may result in further tissue destruction and conversion of a partial thickness injury into a full thickness injury. Superficial partial thickness burns heal in less than 3 weeks, whereas deep injuries heal in 4 to 5 weeks.

Third degree or full thickness burns result from destruction of all of the epidermal and dermal layers of the skin (Fig. 89-2). Spontaneous re-epithelialization is impossible. These wounds close with the development of scar tissue. Such wounds exhibit contraction and functional disability; therefore, these wounds are covered by skin grafts to achieve wound closure.

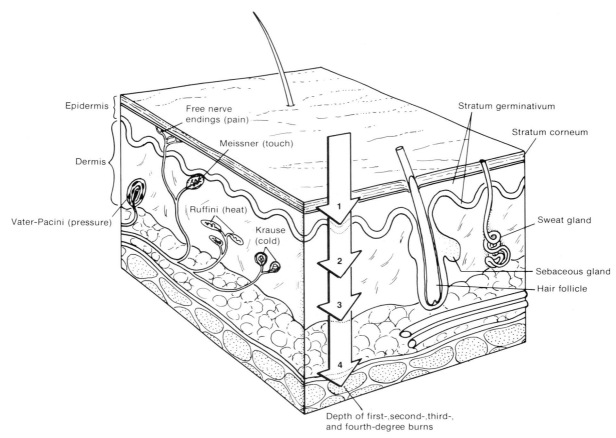

Figure 89-2.

Burns are also classified according to the extent of the burn on the body. A minor burn involves less than 10% of the body surface, is partial thickness, and does not involve the face, hands, perineum, or feet. Also excluded from this category are electrical or inhalation injuries. A 10%–20% burn is considered moderate if less than 10% of the burn area is full thickness. Any burn of 20% thickness or more in children is severe. Likewise, any burn in a child under 2 years old is more serious because of the fragile skin and the difficulties in preventing infection.

Burns involving less than 10% of the total body surface in children over 1 year old usually can be managed on an outpatient basis. Exceptions are made for burns involving the hands, feet, face, and perineum. If there is any question of child abuse or the family's ability to follow instructions, the child should be admitted and the family response evaluated.

Standard of Care

1. The child will be maintained in a sterile environment using sterile supplies and equipment.
2. Dressing changes will be carried out using sterile technique.

Assessment

1. Assess the pertinent history and physical findings for the mechanism of the injury, loss of function of the body parts, past medical history, vital signs, depth and extent of the burn, fluid status, level of pain, serum electrolytes, and bowel sounds.
2. Assess the psychosocial and developmental factors such as age, ethnic background, usual coping mechanisms, child and family interaction, acceptance of altered body image, compliance with treatments, and family and peer support.
3. Assess the child's and family's knowledge of the disease condition, perception of the health status, and their willingness to learn.

Nursing Diagnoses

The following is a list of possible diagnoses and could apply, depending on the child's age, clinical situation, and physical condition:

High risk for infection

Anxiety

Fear

Hypothermia

Impaired skin integrity

Impaired gas exchange

Fluid volume deficit

Altered nutrition: less than body requirements

Pain

Ineffective family and individual coping

Impaired physical mobility

Self-esteem disturbance

Planning

In planning to care for a child who is burned, the following equipment must be gathered:

Intake/Output sheet

Nasogastric tube of appropriate size

Urinary catheter of appropriate size

Oxygen equipment and source

Splints

Masks

Sterile gloves

Sterile gowns

Sterile sheets

Emergency tray (intubation equipment)

Stethoscope

Thermometer

Supplies for intravenous access
Appropriate medications (pain relief, antibiotics)
Isolation cart

Interventions

| PROCEDURE | RATIONALE/EXPECTED OUTCOME (EO) |

Initial Management

1. Maintain patent airway with high flow of oxygen and humidity and intubation if necessary.

Humidity and supplemental oxygen are provided to any child suspected of having an inhalation injury.

EO: The child will maintain a patent airway and adequate oxygenation.

2. Auscultate breath sounds every hour or more often to detect decreased aeration.

3. Monitor arterial blood gases for acid–base abnormalities.

EO: The child's ABGs are within normal limits.

4. Monitor respiratory rate and depth every hour or more often as condition warrants.

The first stage of inhalation injury is acute pulmonary insufficiency, the second is pulmonary edema, and the last is bronchopneumonia.

5. Monitor for stridor, hoarseness, dyspnea, or wheezing.

Most children with inhalation injuries do not wheeze or produce carbonaceous sputum for 24–48 hours after the injury.

EO: The child is free from stridor, hoarseness, or wheezing.

6. Monitor level of consciousness every hour or more often to determine cerebral oxygenation.

EO: The child exhibits lucid level of consciousness.

7. Provide chest physical therapy.

8. Turn, cough, and deep breathe every 1–2 hours to mobilize secretions.

Inability to expectorate secretions as a result of a decreased cough reflex may lead to an altered respiratory status.

9. Monitor carboxyhemoglobin level for possible carbon monoxide poisoning. Symptoms include:
   a. Headache
   b. Fatigue
   c. Weakness
   d. Nausea or vomiting
   e. Impaired judgment
   f. Tachycardia
   g. Hyperventilation
   h. Seizures
   i. Coma.

Symptoms rarely develop until the carboxyhemoglobin is greater than 10%. Levels greater than 10% usually are fatal.

Fluid Resuscitation

10. Weigh child on admission and daily in same clothes and on the same scale at the same time every day.

EO: The child's weight changes less than .25–1 kg in 24 hours.

11. Monitor vital signs hourly or more often as condition warrants.

12. Start intravenous fluid through a large-bore needle.

13. Titrate fluid replacement based on urine output, central venous pressure, LOC, etc., as ordered by physician.

Adequate replacement of intravascular volume is indicated by return of a normal blood pressure, pulse rate, and cardiac output.

PROCEDURE	**RATIONALE/EXPECTED OUTCOME (EO)**

14. Administer crystalloid or colloid fluid as ordered by physician.

15. Insert Foley catheter if greater than 20% of the child's total body surface is burned or if genital burns are present.

16. Insert nasogastric tube for major burn.

> This can be used to remove gastric contents and prevent vomiting and pulmonary aspiration.

17. Record accurate fluid intake (oral, IV) and output (nasogastric drainage, urine) every hour.

> The best monitor of fluid resuscitation is the measurement of hourly urine output.
>
> *EO: The child excretes at least .5–2.0 mL/kg/hour of urine.*

18. Observe urine for hematuria or a red–brown color.

> This is indicative of intravascular hemolysis related to thrombosis or hemomyoglobinuria.

19. Assess for signs and symptoms of inadequate fluid replacement or shock.
    Symptoms include:
    a. Increased pulse
    b. Disorientation
    c. Decreased blood pressure
    d. Decreased urine output
    e. CVP less than 5 mL water.

> Capillary destruction initiates a shift from plasma to interstitial fluid, causing hypovolemia.

20. Assess for signs and symptoms of excessive fluid replacement or pulmonary congestion.
    Symptoms include:
    a. Increased blood pressure
    b. Venous engorgement
    c. Dyspnea
    d. Moist rales
    e. CVP greater than 15 mL water.

> *EO: The child maintains a CVP between 5 and 15 mL water.*

21. Assess ECG.

22. Monitor laboratory results (for example, hemoglobin, hematocrit, glucose, protein, potassium, sodium, BUN, creatinine, and urinalysis).

> *EO: The child maintains electrolytes within normal levels.*

23. Monitor distal peripheral pulses. Notify physician if pulses are unobtainable.

> Circumferential burns of an extremity or thorax cause the burn eschar to compromise circulation by becoming unyielding to movement and blood flow.
>
> *EO: The child will maintain optimum peripheral circulation.*

24. Elevate burned areas to allow for venous return.

Pain Control

25. Assess the child's level of pain using a rating scale (see Appendix 5).

> Pain receptors left intact will respond to pressure and edema resulting in pain.

26. Record the amount, time, and type of medication administered.

> Intravenous morphine (0.1 mg–0.2 mg/kg) given slowly, or (0.02 mg–0.03 mg/kg) given every 10–15 minutes, can be titrated to achieve analgesia. Ketamine produces analgesia and preserves airway reflexes.

27. Administer sedation or pain medication 30–60 minutes before a treatment, debridement, or application of topical agents.

28. Record the effectiveness of the medication.

> *EO: The child verbalizes decreased pain.*

29. Provide diversional activity to distract the child from the pain experience.

PROCEDURE

30. Maintain the environmental temperature of 24.4–28.8°C (76°–84°F).

Infection

31. Monitor temperature hourly or more often as condition warrants.

32. Administer tetanus immunization.

33. Determine the type of isolation to be used.

34. Observe for signs and symptoms of infection or sepsis.
    Symptoms include:
    a. Fever
    b. Foul-smelling wound
    c. Increased WBCs
    d. Disorientation
    e. Intolerance to feedings.

35. Administer antibiotics and record response.

36. Apply antimicrobials and bacteriostatic agents (Table 89-1).

RATIONALE/EXPECTED OUTCOME (EO)

This will ensure warmth and comfort of the child who is without the protective layer of skin that maintains body heat.

The child's body temperature may be elevated if infection is present or decreased because of the loss of skin integrity.

EO: The child maintains a temperature within normal limits.

During the first few days after a burn, the likely source of contaminating bacteria is the child. Previously it was thought that the major source of contamination was the eschar. Both sources do contribute to the problem, so children with greater than 40% total body surface area (TBSA) burned are placed in reverse isolation until wound closure has occurred.

If burn wound sepsis is suspected, three steps are taken:
a. Change the topical agent being used
b. Begin systemic antibiotics. They are not effective in

Table 89-1. Topical Agents

Drug	Preparation; Wound Care	Pain Caused by Drug	Side Effects
Silver sulfadiazine (Silvadene)	Cream; Apply 2×/day with a light layer of dressing.	None	Fungal overgrowth frequent; absorbed into fetal circulation
Mafenide (Sulfamylon)	Cream; Apply 2×/day with one light layer of dressing.	Severe	Fungal overgrowth frequent; may develop rash; carbonic anhydrase inhibition leading to acidosis
Silver nitrate solution	Aqueous solution; Apply 2×/day with a light layer of gauze.	None	Significant loss of Na and K into wet dressings; stains tissues
Iodophors (Efodine)	Foam; Apply 2×/day with a light layer of gauze dressing.	Moderate	Fungal overgrowth frequent; iodine absorption; tissue staining
Bacitracin	Cream; Apply to small areas of cosmetic importance 2×/day and leave open.	None	Rapid development of resistance; conjunctivitis

PROCEDURE	**RATIONALE/EXPECTED OUTCOME (EO)**

<table>
<tr><td></td><td>treating a wound infection since there is little blood supply to the eschar but transient sepsis can be controlled.
c. Excise the wound.</td></tr>
<tr><td>37. Obtain cultures from wounds.</td><td></td></tr>
<tr><td>38. Shave or clip body hair that may harbor bacteria.</td><td>This will prevent autocontamination.</td></tr>
<tr><td>39. Prevent skin surfaces from touching.</td><td>*EO: The child will be free from wound infection.*</td></tr>
</table>

Nutrition

<table>
<tr><td>40. Auscultate bowel sounds every 4 hours.</td><td>The child may initially have a paralytic ileus.</td></tr>
<tr><td>41. Monitor bowel movements for diarrhea or constipation.</td><td></td></tr>
<tr><td>42. Insert a soft Silastic catheter via the nose into the stomach.</td><td>For burns of 15% TBSA or greater, a feeding tube is passed.</td></tr>
<tr><td>43. Administer tube feedings as ordered when bowel sounds return.</td><td>Enteral feedings are usually begun within 48 hours of the burn.</td></tr>
<tr><td>44. Keep an accurate daily caloric count with a determination of protein intake.</td><td>Formula for required calories:
calories per day = (25 × kg or body weight)
+ (40 × % BSA burned).</td></tr>
<tr><td>45. Monitor serum proteins, transferrin, retinol-binding protein, and prealbumin.</td><td>Concentrations of serum proteins can be used as indicators of visceral protein status. Visceral proteins are necessary for wound healing, oncotic pressure, and host-defense mechanisms.</td></tr>
<tr><td>46. Monitor child for gastrointestinal bleeding.</td><td>Stress ulceration (Curling's ulcer) of the stomach or duodenum is found in 90% of burned children.</td></tr>
<tr><td>47. Administer antacids as ordered.</td><td>*EO: The child will maintain adequate nutrition.*</td></tr>
<tr><td>48. Do not schedule painful procedures prior to meals.</td><td></td></tr>
<tr><td>49. Provide an environment conducive to eating (for example, have the family eat with the child or bring the child's favorite foods from home).</td><td></td></tr>
</table>

Burn Wound Scars

<table>
<tr><td>50. Have the child evaluated by occupational and physical therapists.</td><td>Joint contractures can be minimized with early splinting.</td></tr>
<tr><td>51. Provide proper positioning and immobilization of the burn wound and graft site.</td><td></td></tr>
<tr><td>52. Provide active and passive range of motion (ROM) every 4 hours.</td><td>ROM is taught to the child, parents, and caregivers and monitored daily by the therapist.</td></tr>
<tr><td>53. Turn the child every 2 hours to prevent pressure areas.</td><td></td></tr>
<tr><td>54. Make the therapy enjoyable for the child (for example, let the child play with toys in the bath).</td><td></td></tr>
<tr><td>55. Keep the healed burns moisturized with a cream such as cocoa butter.</td><td>During the healing phase, the child may complain of itching. Scratching results in loss of epithelium and scar formation.
EO: The child will be free from complications associated with immobility.</td></tr>
</table>

PROCEDURE	**RATIONALE/EXPECTED OUTCOME (EO)**

Psychosocial/Coping

56. Arrange for continued schooling.

57. Encourage participation and cooperation in care. (Give the child acceptable ways to vent his or her feelings).

58. Allow the child to control appropriate care (such as the time of dressing changes).

59. Provide explanations of all procedures.

60. Convey a positive attitude about the child; reinforce positive aspects about the child's appearance.

Children will demonstrate fear, anxiety, regression, and concerns regarding painful procedures and abandonment. They are also concerned with disfigurement.

EO: The child and family will cope effectively.

EO: The child will achieve a degree of control over the care needed.

Patient/Family Education: Home Care Considerations

1. Inform the child and family of all indications of continued progress.
2. Provide for financial counseling as needed or requested.
3. Provide for spiritual counseling as needed or requested.
4. Discuss the impact of returning to home or school: Peer reaction, physical change, and emotional change.
5. Instruct the family about medications and treatments that need to be continued after discharge.
6. Assist the family in making follow-up appointments. Stress the need for adherence to medical treatment.

References

Carvaijal, H.F., & Parks, D.H. (1988). *Burns in children: Pediatric burn management.* Chicago: Yearbook Medical Publishers.

Greenberg, C.S. (1988). *Nursing care planning guides for children.* Baltimore: Williams & Wilkens.

Hurt, R. (1985). More than skin deep: Guidelines for caring for the burn patient. *Nursing '85, 15*(6), 52–57.

Lushbough, M. (1981). Critical care of the child with burns. *Nursing clinics of North America, 16*(4), 435–436.

Polk, H.C., Stone, H.H., & Gardner, B. (1987). *Basic surgery.* Norwalk, CT: Appleton-Century-Crofts.

Raffensperger, J.G. (1990). *Swenson's pediatric surgery.* Norwalk, CT: Appleton & Lange.

Robertson, K.E., Cross, P.J., & Terry J.C. (1985). CE burn care: The crucial first days. *American Journal of Nursing, 85*(1), 29–45.

Rogers, M. (1989). *Handbook of pediatric intensive care.* Baltimore: Williams & Wilkins.

Rosequest, C., & Shepp, P. (1985). CE burn care: The nutritional factor. *American Journal of Nursing, 85*(1), 45–47.

PARENT TEACHING GUIDE
Cast Care

The nursing staff would like you to feel comfortable in caring for your child while it is necessary for him or her to be in a cast. We would like you to read this pamphlet, which discusses all aspects of cast care, so you can help make the cast effective and comfortable for your child.

What Is the Purpose of the Cast?

A plaster or fiberglass cast is applied to immobilize and support a body part in a specific position, to provide healing of a fracture, or to prevent a deformity. A cast is also used to permit early weightbearing on an extremity after an injury or surgery.

How Should You Handle a Wet Cast?

It will take 28 to 48 hours, depending on the type of material used, after the cast is applied for it to dry. Because circulating air is the best method of drying, the cast should be kept uncovered. A fan can be placed in the room to facilitate air movement. When touching a wet cast, use only the palms of your hands. Fingertips will cause dents in the cast, which may cause pressure areas on the skin. When moving your child, support the joints, because these are points of stress and a wet cast may crack at these areas.

Does Your Child Need to Be Turned?

Your child will need to be turned frequently to avoid any pressure areas. This can be done every 4 hours at night and every 2 hours during the day. Also, turn your child whenever he or she complains of discomfort, or whenever you notice any reddened areas. Use pillows to position your child's cast and to provide good body alignment.

What Type of Skin Care Is Necessary?

Give your child a daily sponge bath, washing only the areas not under the cast. Do not wet the cast. Clean the skin around the edges of the cast with rubbing alcohol 2 to 3 times a day to toughen the skin and prevent skin breakdown. If a reddened area around the edges of the cast is noted, the frequency of skin care should be increased to every 1 to 2 hours until the reddened area disappears. Do not use oils or powders under or around the edges of the cast, because powders cake and oils soften the skin, making it easier for skin to break down.

If your child spends a great deal of time in a chair or in bed, rub his or her elbows, knees, heels, ankles, and the base of the spine with alcohol to toughen the skin.

Make sure your child does not put small objects (for example, food, toys, buttons, coins, pins, or bottle caps) into the cast. Do not place any item (such as a stick, ruler, or coat hanger) down into the cast in an attempt to remove anything or to scratch (Fig. 1). You may reach inside the cast with fingertips only.

What Types of Daily Observations Need to Be Made to Ensure Your Child's Comfort and Safety?

Look inside the cast as far as you can see using a flashlight. If you see any reddened or sore areas, call your doctor.

Check the cast for rough edges where the petals might have become loosened. Re-petal the cast with white tape and moleskin if necessary to prevent skin breakdown and increase the cast life (Fig. 2).

To re-petal the cast, peel rough edges of the cast. Pull the stockinette lining taut over the edge of the cast and petal the cast edge with tape:

1. Take 1-inch adhesive tape and cut it into $1\frac{1}{2}$- to 2-inch strips.

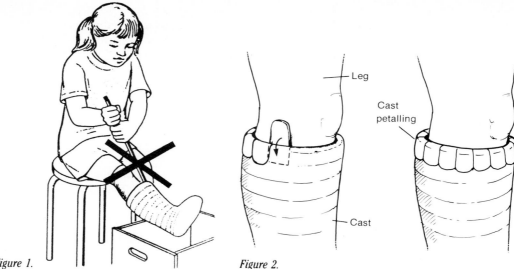

Figure 1.

Figure 2.

2. Place one end of a strip of tape on the inside of the cast, sticky side against the cast.

3. Bring the other end up over the cast edge and tape down on the outside of the cast.

4. Tape ends should overlap each other slightly.

Ask your child to move his or her fingers and toes if they are inside the arm or leg cast. If they could move them before and cannot now, call your doctor.

Check the color and warmth of the extremity in the cast. If the color is blue, pale, reddened, or feels unusually warm or cold, or if the child complains of numbness or tingling, call your doctor.

If fingers or toes swell, elevate the extremity on a pillow. Call the doctor if the swelling persists.

If your child is unusually irritable or complains of persistent pain in an area, or if there is a foul odor or foul-smelling drainage on the cast, there may be an infected area under the cast that needs a doctor's attention.

Also notify your doctor if:

- The cast is soft, breaks, or cracks.
- The cast is loose and slips up and down easily.
- Your child has a fever.

How Do You Care for the Cast?

The cast should be kept clean and dry. If the cast becomes wet, it may soften and crack. If the cast becomes soiled, use a damp cloth to clean the area, allowing it to air-dry afterwards.

If your child wears diapers, they need to be changed as soon as they become wet. Plastic wrap may be put around the edges of the cast to protect it from urine and stool. Sanitary napkins may be placed inside the diaper for extra nighttime protection.

If your child can use a bedpan, first place plastic wrap around the edges of the cast; then have the child turn to the unaffected side, slipping the bedpan under them while they turn back to a lying position. Elevate your child's head so the urine will flow into the pan and not inside the cast.

What Kind of Activity Can Your Child Participate In?

Small children can be held as often as they would be held if they did not have a cast in place. For children who cannot walk, use a stroller or wagon with safety ties to take the child outside, or place a rug, towel, or blanket on the floor so he or she can get out of bed and be allowed to play.

What Should You Anticipate When the Cast is Removed?

The skin under the cast will be caked with a yellow material that is dead skin and oil. This material should be soaked off in a tub of warm water. It may take several days for the material to soak off—*do not scrub it off.* Lotion or oil may be applied to the skin to prevent itching.

Special Considerations for the Care of the Child in a Spica Cast

All of the previously discussed care principles apply to the care of a child in a hip spica cast. There are additional considerations directed toward mobilizing your child and keeping the cast dry that need to be addressed.

What Is the Purpose of the Bradford Frame?

A split Bradford frame is used for any child in a hip spica cast who is not toilet trained (Fig. 3). When properly positioned, your child can urinate and defecate through the split and maintain a dry cast.

Front view   Back view

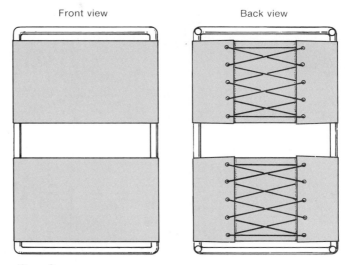

Figure 3.

Setting Up the Frame

1. Place a piece of plywood over the mattress.
2. Set the frame on the plywood.
3. Elevate the head of the frame as ordered by the physician. You may use books or magazines to raise the frame.
4. Strap the frame to the bed.
5. Cover the canvas with pillowcases.

Daily Care of the Frame

1. Check the canvas daily to make sure it is tight. Tighten the ropes as necessary.
2. Change the pillowcases as needed to prevent odor from soiled linen.
3. Check the straps for wear and replace them as needed.

Putting Your Child on the Frame

1. Position your child on the frame so that the top of the perianal cutout of the cast is just below the bottom edge of the canvas on the top frame.
2. Strap your child in place as demonstrated.

Care of the Cast

1. Keep the cast clean and dry. If anything accidentally wets the cast, keep the area uncovered until it is dry. Cover the cast with a towel when your child eats or drinks.
2. Use plastic petals around the perianal cutout. Funnel the plastic into a bedpan below. Replace the plastic petals when soiled.
3. If a bar is placed between the legs of the cast, it is there to stabilize the legs. Do not use this bar to turn your child, because it can break.

Mobilization of Your Child

- The entire Bradford frame can be positioned on a child's play wagon when the principles of maintaining a dry cast can be accomplished (Fig. 4).

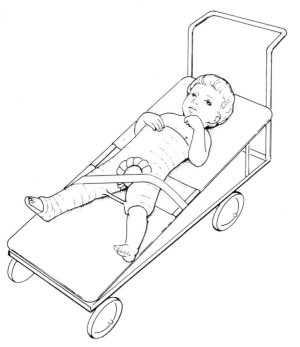

Figure 4.

- A Spica skateboard (a padded platform larger than the child) sits on casters several inches off the floor (Fig. 5). If your child is placed on the skateboard on his or her stomach, they may push themselves by means of hands and arms.

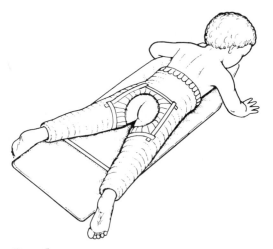

Figure 5.

PATIENT TEACHING CHECKLIST

All of the following skills must be learned before discharge. The nursing categories must be dated and signed by the nurse who has assumed responsibility for teaching. Parents are to sign and date each task as mastery is achieved.

(See skills as outlined in "Cast Care Teaching Guide".)

Parent Should Be Able to:	Nurse Demonstration (Initials and Date)	Parent-Return Demonstration (Initials and Date)
1. Verbalize an understanding of the purpose of the cast		
2. Verbalize how to handle a wet cast		
3. Verbalize how to reposition the child		
4. Perform basic skin care and daily observations		
5. Demonstrate how to care for the cast		
6. Know reasonable activities for the child		
7. Demonstrate safety precautions to be taken		
8. Verbalize what signs and symptoms to report immediately to the physician		
9. Anticipate the care needed after the cast is removed		
10. Verbalize when to return for the next visit		

References

Benz, J. (1986). The adolescent in a spica cast. *Orthopedic Nursing, 5*(3), 22–23.

Dunn, B. (1977). Cast care. *Pediatric Nursing,* (4), 1977.

Feller, N.G., Stroup, K., & Christian, L. (1989). Helping staff nurses become mini-specialists . . . cast care. *American Journal of Nursing, 87*(7), 991–992.

Mather, M.L.S. (1987). The secret to life in a spica. *American Journal of Nursing, 87*(1), 56–58.

Pellino, T.A., Mooney, N.E., Safmond, S.W., et al. (1986). *Care curriculum for orthopedic nursing.* Pitman, NJ: Anthony Jennetti, Inc.

Shesser, L.K., Kling, F.T., Jr., et al. (1986). Practical considerations in caring for a child in a hip spica cast. *Orthopedic Nursing, 5*(3), 11–15.

Shriners' Hospitals for Crippled Children. *Cast Care.* Chicago: Shriners' Hospitals for Crippled Children—Chicago Unit.

Approved Nursing Diagnostic Categories

This list represents the NANDA approved nursing diagnostic categories for clinical use and testing.

Pattern 1: Exchanging

Altered Nutrition: More than body requirements
Altered Nutrition: Less than body requirements
Altered Nutrition: Potential for more than body requirements
High Risk for Infection
High Risk for Altered Body Temperature
Hypothermia
Hyperthermia
Ineffective Thermoregulation
Dysreflexia
Constipation
Perceived Constipation
Colonic Constipation
Diarrhea
Bowel Incontinence
Altered Urinary Elimination
Stress Incontinence
Reflex Incontinence
Urge Incontinence
Functional Incontinence
Total Incontinence
Urinary Retention
Altered (Specify Type) Tissue Perfusion (Renal, cerebral, cardiopulmonary, gastrointestinal, peripheral)
Fluid Volume Excess
Fluid Volume Deficit
High Risk for Fluid Volume Deficit
Decreased Cardiac Output
Impaired Gas Exchange
Ineffective Airway Clearance
Ineffective Breathing Pattern
High Risk for Injury
High Risk for Suffocation
High Risk for Poisoning
High Risk for Trauma
High Risk for Aspiration
High Risk for Disuse Syndrome
Altered Protection
Impaired Tissue Integrity
Altered Oral Mucous Membrane
Impaired Skin Integrity
High Risk for Impaired Skin Integrity

Pattern 2: Communicating

Impaired Verbal Communication

Pattern 3: Relating

Impaired Social Interaction
Social Isolation
Altered Role Performance
Altered Parenting
High Risk for Altered Parenting
Sexual Dysfunction
Altered Family Processes
Parental Role Conflict
Altered Sexuality Patterns

Pattern 4: Valuing

Spiritual Distress (distress of the human spirit)

Pattern 5: Choosing

Ineffective Individual Coping
Impaired Adjustment
Defensive Coping
Ineffective Denial
Ineffective Family Coping: Disabling
Ineffective Family Coping: Compromised
Family Coping: Potential for Growth
Noncompliance (Specify)
Decisional Conflict (Specify)
Health Seeking Behaviors (Specify)

Pattern 6: Moving

Impaired Physical Mobility
Activity Intolerance
Fatigue
High Risk for Activity Intolerance
Sleep Pattern Disturbance
Diversional Activity Deficit
Impaired Home Maintenance Management

Altered Health Maintenance
Feeding Self-Care Deficit
Impaired Swallowing
Ineffective Breastfeeding
Effective Breastfeeding
Bathing/Hygiene Self-Care Deficit
Dressing/Grooming Self-Care Deficit
Toileting Self-Care Deficit
Altered Growth and Development

Pattern 7: Perceiving

Body Image Disturbance
Self-Esteem Disturbance
Chronic Low Self-Esteem
Situational Low Self-Esteem
Personal Identity Disturbance
Sensory/Perceptual Alterations (Specify) (Visual, auditory, kinesthetic, gustatory, tactile, olfactory)
Unilateral Neglect
Hopelessness
Powerlessness

Pattern 8: Knowing

Knowledge Deficit (Specify)
Altered Thought Processes

Pattern 9: Feeling

Pain
Chronic Pain
Dysfunctional Grieving
Anticipatory Grieving
High Risk for Violence: Self-directed or directed at others
Post-Trauma Response
Rape-Trauma Syndrome
Rape-Trauma Syndrome: Compound Reaction
Rape-Trauma Syndrome: Silent Reaction
Anxiety
Fear

Normal Laboratory Values

Blood

Acetone
  1–6 mg/100 mL

Acid–Base Measurements

	Neonate	Child
pH	7.32–7.42	7.35–7.45
pCO_2	30–40 mm Hg	35–45 mm Hg
pO_2	60–80 mm Hg	80–100 mm Hg
HCO_3	20–26 mEq/L	22–28 mEq/L

Alkaline Phosphatase
  30–205 IU/L

Ammonia

Premature	100–200 μg/100 mL
Newborn	90–150 μg/100 mL
Child	45–80 μg/100 mL

Amylase
  28–108 IU/L at 37°C (98.6°F)

Bilirubin

Total	Less than 1.5 mg/dL
Direct	0.2–0.4 mg/dL
Indirect	0.4–0.8 mg/dL

Bleeding Time
  1–3 minutes

BUN
  4–8 mg/100 mL

Calcium
  9–11 mg/100 mL

Chloride
  97–104 mEq/L

Cholesterol

Full-term newborn	45–167 mg/100 mL
Infant	70–190 mg/100 mL
Child	135–175 mg/100 mL
Adolescent	120–210 mg/100 mL

Complete Blood Count (CBC)

	Hb (gm/dL)	Hct (%)	WBC (per UL)	RBC (millions/μL)	Retic (%)	Plat (μL)
Newborn	14–24	54 + 10	8–38,000	4.1–7.5	2–8	350,000
1 month	11–17	35–50	5–1,500	4.2–5.2	0–0.5	300,000
1 year	11–15	36	1–15,000	4.1–5.1	0.4–1.8	260,000
8–12 years	13–15.5	40	5–12,000	4.5–5.4	0.4–1.8	260,000

	Lymphocytes (%)	Eosinophils (μL)	Monocytes (%)
Newborn	20	20–1000	10
1 month	56	150–1150	7
1 year	53	70–550	6
8–12 years	31	100–400	7

MCV (mean corpuscular volume) (cu)

Newborn	85–125
1 month	90
1 year	78
8–12 years	82

MCHC (mean corpuscular hemoglobin concentration) (%)

Newborn	36
1 month	34
1 year	33
8–12 years	34

MCHgb (mean corpuscular hemoglobin)

Newborn	35–40
1 month	30
1 year	25
8–12 years	28

Copper

0–6 months	<70 µg/100 mL
6 months–5 years	27–153 µg/100 mL
5–17 years	94–234 µg/100 mL

CPK

0–70 IU/L

Creatinine (mg/dL)

Age	Female	Male
Newborn	0.2–1.0	0.2–1.0
1 year	0.2–0.5	0.2–0.6
2–3 years	0.3–0.6	0.2–0.7
4–7 years	0.2–0.7	0.2–0.8
8–10 years	0.3–0.8	0.3–0.9
11–12 years	0.3–0.9	0.3–1.0
13–17 years	0.3–1.1	0.3–1.2

Fibrinogen

200–400 mg/dL

Glucose

Newborn	20–80 mg/dL
Child	60–110 mg/dL

Immunoglobulin Levels

	IgG (mg/dL)	IgM (mg/dL)	IgA (mg/dL)
Newborn	831–1231	6–16	0–5
1–3 months	310–549	20–40	8–34
4–6 months	240–613	26–60	10–46
7–12 months	442–880	31–77	19–55
13–25 months	553–970	27–73	26–74
26–36 months	710–1075	40–80	35–108
3–5 years	700–1257	38–74	66–120
6–8 years	667–1180	40–90	80–170
9–11 years	890–1359	45–112	70–190
12–16 years	822–1563	70–126	85–210

Iron- total (µg/dL)

Newborn	20–157
6 weeks–3 years	20–115
3–9 years	20–141
9–14 years	21–151
14–16 years	20–181

Iron binding capacity (μg/dL)
Newborn	59–175
Children/Adolescents	250–400

Lead
<30 μg/dL whole blood

LDH
Birth	290–501 IU/L
1 day	185–404 IU/L
1 month–2 years	110–244 IU/L
3–17 years	80–165 IU/L

Magnesium
1.2–1.8 mEq/L

Osmolality
275–295 mOsm/L

Phenylalanine (mg/100 mL)
Premature —	0–5 days	1–6
	5–21 days	3–27
	>21 days	2–7
Newborn —	0–1 day	<6
	2–10 days	1–7
Children		0.7–3.5
Adolescent		<4

Phosphorus
Premature —	Birth	5.6–8.0 mg/dL
	6–10 days	6.1–11.7 mg/dL
	20–25 days	6.6–9.4 mg/dL
Full term —	Birth	5–7.8 mg/dL
	3 days	5.8–9.0 mg/dL
	6–12 days	4.9–8.9 mg/dL
Children —	1 year	3.8–6.2 mg/dL
	10 years	3.6–5.6 mg/dL

Potassium (mEq/L)
Premature	4.5–7.2
Full term	3.7–5.2
Child	3.5–5.8
Adolescent	3.5–5.8

Proteins
Premature —	Total	4.3–7.6 g/100 mL
	Albumin	2.8–3.9 g/100 mL
Full term —	Total	4.6–7.4
	Albumin	2.3–5.1
Infant —	Total	4.8–7.7
	Albumin	—
Child —	Total	6.0–8.0
	Albumin	3.2–5.5

PT
13 + 2 seconds

PTT
Premature	<120 seconds
Newborn	<90 seconds
Thereafter	24–40 seconds

SGOT (Alt) (IU/L)
1–5 days	5–120
Infant	8–40
Preschool–Adolescent	8–40

SGPT (AST) (IU/L)

1–5 days	5–90
Infant	5–35
Preschool–Adolescent	5–35

Sodium

135–144 m Eq/L

Triglycerides (mg/dL)—(blood collected after 12–16 hour fast, except cord blood)

Cord	14–61
Children	10–175
Adolescent	30–135

Uric Acid

2.6 mg/dL

Zinc

Newborn	25% adult value
1 year	50% adult value
Adult	80–165 ug/100 mL

Urine

Urinalysis

pH	Newborn	5.0–7.0
	Thereafter	4.8–7.8
SG	Newborn	1.001–1.020
	Thereafter	1.001–1.030
Sugar	Negative	
Protein	Newborn	240 mg/day
(Quantitative)	Child	30–50 mg/day
	Adolescent	25–70 mg/day
(Qualitative)	Negative	
Leukocytes	0.4	
Casts	rare	
Erythrocytes	rare	

Addis Count (12-hour specimen)

Red cells	<1 million
White cells	<2 million
Casts	<10,000
Protein	<55 mg

Catecholamines

0.4–2.0 μg/kg/day

Chloride

170–254 mEq/day

Creatinine

Newborn	7–10 mg/kg/day
Child	20–30 mg/kg/day

Lead

<400 ug/day

Osmolality

Infant	50–600 mOsm/L
Child	50–1400 mOsm/L

Potassium

25–123 mEq/day

Sodium

Infant	0.3–3.5 mEq/day
Child	5.6–17 mEq/day

Urobilinogen

<3 mg/day

VMA (vanillymandelic acid)

1st day	Full term	606 + 429 μg/day
	Premature	187 + 111 μg/day
15th day	Full term	471 + 196 μg/day
	Premature	2506 + 1319 μg/day
<2 years	0.1–8.6 mg/L	
2–14 years	0–10.2 mg/L	

Sweat

Sodium

5 weeks–11 months	5–24 mEq/L
1–9 years	3–36 mEq/L
10–16 years	6–52 mEq/L

Chloride

<45 mEq/L

Fibrocystic disease > 50 mEq/L

Cerebrospinal Fluid

Pressure	40–200 mm H_2O
Appearance	Clear
WBC	Neonates—8–9; >6 months–0
Glucose	Neonates—50–52; >6 months–>40 (40–60% of blood glucose level)
Protein	Neonates—90–115; >6 months–<40
Chloride	110–128 mEq/L
Sodium	138–150 mmol/L
SG	1.007–1009

Bone Marrow

Myeloblasts	0–4%
Promyelocytes	0–6%
Myelocytes	7–25%
Metamyelocytes	7–30%
Polymorphonuclear neutrophils	5–30%
Eosinophils	1–10%
Lymphocytes	5–45%
Monocytes	0–7%
Pronormoblasts	0–8%
Normoblasts	4–35%

Stool

Fecal fat	0–6 years	<2 g/day
	Thereafter	2–6 g/day
Fecal urobilinogen	2–12 months	0.03–14 mg
	5–10 years	2.7–39 mg
	10–14 years	7.3–99 mg

(Normal values may differ, depending on the laboratory method used in processing the specimen.)

Normal Growth and Development

Age 1–6 Months

General Considerations

Weight: Gains 5–8 oz/week
    Doubles birth weight by $4\frac{2}{3}$ months
Height: Grows 1 in/month
Posterior fontanelle: Closes by 2 months
Skin: Diaper rash common
    Infantile acne on face common at 4–5 weeks
      (lasts 4–6 weeks).
    Associated with disappearance of mother's hor-
      mones and activation of oil and sweat glands.
Teething: Begins at 5–6 months.
    Salivation increases at 3 months when salivary
      glands mature.
Reflexes: Palmar grasp–reaches to mouth
    Mouths fist at 2 months
    Chews at 4–6 months.
    Moro–startle reflex present from 0–4 months
    Tonic neck–preference for one side of head
      reaches peak at approximately 3 months, then
      gradually disappears.

Play	Cry/Socialization	Movement	Vision	Feeding/Sleep
2 Months				
Likes brightly colored, large toys of varied shapes and textures.	Opens eyes, alert smile. Responds to others' smiles. Cry differentiates cause (such as pain or cold).	Moves in crib; holds head erect in mid-position, still wobbly.	Can follow bright moving objects. Prefers people to objects. Stares at surroundings	18–20 hours a day of sleep. 115 cal/kg/day. Eats every 4 hours (breast-feeders more frequently).
3 Months				
	Cries less. More spontaneous smile. Babbles coos. Locates sounds.	Moves arms and legs. Raises head and chest. Reaches for objects. Puts hands and objects in mouth.		Needs 16–20 hours of sleep per day.

(continued)

Play	Cry/Socialization	Movement	Vision	Feeding/Sleep
4 Months				
Likes brightly colored rings, spoons, keys, or noisemakers.	Likes attention; becomes fussy or demanding if ignored. Enjoys sitting up. Recognizes voices. Attentive to music. Makes sounds, laughs, gurgles, shrieks.	Hold head steady. Supports body with hands. Rolls from back to abdomen.	Eyes focus at different lengths. Discriminates familiar and strange faces.	10–11 hours of sleep per day. 110 cal/kg/day. Learning to eat from a spoon.
5–6 Months				
Enjoys unrestricted movement; likes to look at self in mirror; enjoys bath and water toys; likes large soft balls; can roll and play; has longer attention span; shows interest in books, paper, and pictures.	Distressed around strangers; utters syllables; grunts, squeals, babbles, purrs.	Sits momentarily without support in forward leaning position; begins creeping; touches knees; brings feet to mouth; tonic neck reflex disappears; likes to sit in a high chair and watch surroundings; rolls from stomach to back to stomach. No head lag when pulled to a sitting position. Bears some weight on lower extremities.	20–24 oz formula/day. Begins finger foods; and holds bottle and spoon.	

Age: 7–12 Months

General Considerations

Weight: Gains 4–5 oz/week
Height: Grows $\frac{1}{2}$ inch/month
     Approximately 26–28 inches
Teething: Teeth begin to erupt at 6 months
     (two central lower incisors first, followed by the
       two central upper incisors, then upper and
       lower laterals.)

Play	Cry/Socialization	Movement	Vision	Feeding/Sleep
7–9 Months				
Likes large blocks, rings, water toys, bowls, cups, and paper to crumple. Enjoys peak-a-boo and pat-a-cake.	Giggles in anticipation of play; performs for audience; fear of strangers reaches peak; learns the meaning of "no"; shows affection for family; understands disappearance concept; imitates adult movements. Responds to own name.	Toe sucking common; sits alone; raises self to sitting position; may pull to standing position; bears weight in standing position.		14–16 hrs of sleep per day, with 1 or 2 naps. Eats three meals a day; drinks from a cup; holds spoon; retains strong sucking need—may show readiness to wean from bottle.

(continued)

Play	Cry/Socialization	Movement	Vision	Feeding/Sleep
10–12 Months				
Likes riding toys; likes to rock and sway to music; likes to push, rather than pull, toys, bangs blocks together.	Begin temper tantrums; not always cooperative; shows moods. Responds to name; may say two or three words.	Crawls and creeps well; climbs on furniture; climbs up stairs; pulls self to feet; begins to help dress self; can bend to pick up objects. Manipulates all objects.		11–12 hrs of sleep per day, with 1 nap. Will eat solid food if formula is reduced; gains less weight as activity increases.

Age: 12–18 Months

General Considerations

Weight: Gaining 2–6 pounds in next six months
    Average 20–24 pounds
    Triples birth weight by 12 months
Height: Growth to 33 inches by 18 months
Head/chest circumference: Are equal at 12 months
Reflexes: Babinski reflex disappears
Anterior fontanelle: closes by 10–24 months
Body proportions: abdomen protrudes
Teething: 10–14 primary teeth by 18 months; good
    chewing, sucking, and swallowing

Play	Cry/Socialization	Movement	Vision/Elimination	Feeding/Sleep
12–18 Months				
Likes large cars and trucks, dolls, stuffed animals; Likes to throw and retrieve objects, and push and pull toys. Likes picture books. Scribbles spontaneously.	Explores everything; curious; enjoys new skills; shows pride in achievements; mimics household chores; displays rapid attention shifts. Has 3–6 word vocabulary. Uses gestures.	Able to walk alone; climbs up stairs one step at a time; turns pages of book; builds tower of 3 objects.	May be able to control bowels or void at will on a potty chair (although usually not interested).	Needs 100 cal/kg/day. Feeds self with spoon; appetite decreases with decreasing growth rate. Drinks well from a cup.

18 Months–3 Years

General Considerations

Weight: Average weight 28–30 pounds
    Quadruples birth weight by 2½ years
Height: Growth to 33–37 inches
    Approximately 50% of eventual adult height by 2
      years
Teething: 16 teeth by 2 years
    20 primary teeth by 3 years

Body proportions: abdomen protrudes,
    arms and legs lengthen rapidly,
    trunk and head growing slowly
Vision: acuity 20/70 in 2-year-old.
    Poor depth perception
    Good ability to assess size and location of ob-
      jects by age of 3 years

Play	Cry/Socialization	Movement	Vision/Elimination	Feeding/Sleep
2 Years				
Has short attention span; needs motor activities and quiet play; enjoys TV, music, clay, finger painting; likes cars, trucks, and wagons; enjoys playground equipment; and likes musical instruments.	Is egocentric; treats other children as objects; may bite in anger; sucks thumb; engages in ritualism.	Gait is steady; walks, runs, jumps; can open doors; turns knobs; can kick a ball; can throw objects; begins to use scissors; can scribble; washes and dries hands; uses toothbrush.	May become toilet trained at least during day.	10–14 hrs of sleep a day. Prolongs process of going to bed. Drinks and feeds self without spilling. Plays with food. 2–3 glasses of milk a day. Foods from 4 basic food groups.
3 Years				
Uses blackboard and chalk; likes wind-up musical toys, tape player; likes a variety of books and puzzles.	Tolerates short periods of separation. Speech intelligible.	Goes to bathroom with minimal help.	Feeds self.	

Age: 3–6 Years

General Considerations

Weight: Average 44 pounds
    4–6 year olds require 36–41 cal/lb (80–90 cal/kg)
Height: Growth to 44 inches
    Double birth length by 4 years
    Height and weight are even at 5 years
Teething: Begins losing primary teeth at 5–7 years
Body proportion: Loses baby fat and protruding abdomen
    Legs continue to grow rapidly, equaling 44% of
      total length
Vision: Acuity 20/40 in 3-year-old.
    Acuity 20/30 in 4-year-old
    Acuity 20/20 by age 6
    Developing depth perception
    Color vision established

Play	Cry/Socialization	Movement	Feeding/Sleep
4 Years			
May have imaginary companion; likes jump ropes; likes boxes to climb around in;	Brags; shows off; looks for praise; tattles; common age for nightmares; fears	Adult stride; walks backwards; runs well; hops; can draw a picture of a	11–12 hours of sleep a day, napping only when tired or ill. Rarely needs assistance

Play	Cry/Socialization	Movement	Feeding/Sleep
enjoys swimming and group exercises, likes to cut and paste.	scary objects and animals. Has a vocabulary of 1500 words expanding 600 words/year. Talks and questions constantly; knows phone number; knows primary colors, numbers, and letters.	person with head, eyes, and two other parts. Climbs a ladder. Walks on tiptoes.	to eat. Pours from a pitcher.
5 Years			
Can use roller skates; ice skates; skateboards; likes building sets; likes doll houses, plastic people, and toy soldiers. Can identify coins. Plays cooperatively.	Takes some responsibility for actions; increased respect for the truth; wish for privacy; interested in family relationships. Has a vocabulary of 2000+ words. Can give explanations.	Can run and play games. May ride 2-wheel bike. May print first name. Draws person with body and 4 other parts. Counts to 20.	Uses fork and knife.
6 Years			
Plays well alone; likes simple games with basic rules; likes to make things; high energy level; active, can draw a flower and house, can paint, paste and cut. Likes tag games; plays house. Skates, bounces a ball 4–6 times.	Boisterous; bossy; assertive; outgoing; sometimes whiny; moods and feelings expressed in extremes. Can use telephone. Aware of teacher's attitude. Begins reading; learns coinage, days of the week, months of the year. Knows right from left.	Large muscle ability exceeds fine motor coordination. Girls ahead of boys in fine motor skills. Dresses self with no help; can master shoelaces. Draws a person with six body parts.	Needs 2000 calories/day. Eats 3 meals and several snacks.

Age: 7–11 Years

General Considerations

Weight: Gains 5–7 pounds/year
   45 pounds at 6 years
   62 pounds at 7–10 years
   7–10 year olds require 32–36 cal/lb (70–80 cal/kg)
Height: Growth appears in spurts
   Increases 3 inches per year to 52 inches at 7–10 years
Teething: First permanent molars at 6–7 years
   Has 10–11 permanent teeth by 10–11 years
Body proportions: Early sexual development begins in girls as early as 8 years and in boys by 10 years.

Play	Cry/Socialization	Movement	Feeding/Sleep
7 Years			
Begins to prefer to play with own sex. Peer group important. Collects things. Likes table and card games. Enjoys magic tricks; likes books, records, TV. Girls ready for lessons in piano, dance.	Less impulsive and boisterous. Can count by 2s, 5s and 10s. Can add and subtract. Can tell time, days, months, and seasons. Thinks before acting; thought is more flexible. Wants to be friends. Likes school.	Motor control improved. Has fine motor hand control.	

Play	Cry/Socialization	Movement	Feeding/Sleep
8 Years			
Makes detailed drawings; reads comic books; likes board games, craft kits, and sports of all types. Can tell time.	Gregarious; self-assured; eager to absorb the world; curious; selective in choice of companion; likes group projects; has a sense of humor. Is concerned with fair vs. unfair. Can take responsibility for home chores.	Movements are graceful. Active, vigorous.	Needs 2100 calories a day.
9 Years			
Peer activities dominate. Both sexes like sports. Girls like crafts, boys like war games, tag, and fort building. Time spent watching TV increases to 20 hours per week.	Rules are a guiding force in all aspects of life. Concerned with peer-imposed rules. Interested in family life. Rivalry between siblings. Interest in how things are made.	Constantly on the go; plays and works hard, often to fatigue. Uses both hands independently.	
10 Years			
Likes gangs and secret codes, rules and rituals. Enjoys crafts. Parental involvement to encourage participation of child in groups.	Happy, cooperative, relaxed, casual, well-mannered. Capacity for thought and conceptual organization. Discusses problems. Companionship is the most important.	Good coordination. Boys surpass girls in strength. Girls exceed boys in flexibility and graceful movement.	
11 Years			
Enjoys working with hands. Likes to run errands that will earn money. Involved in sports, dancing, and talking on the telephone.	Rebels at routines, doing homework or chores. Mood swings—may cry or lose temper. Peers are significant. Wants unreasonable amounts of freedom. Wants to be given responsibility. Boys begin to tease girls. Hero worship prevalent.	Differences between sexes more noticeable.	Needs 8–10 hrs of sleep a day. Boys need 2500 cal per day; girls need 2250 cal per day.

Age: 12–19 Years

General Considerations

Weight: (girls) 11–14 years—101 pounds
              15–19 years—120 pounds
     (boys) 11–14 years—99 pounds
              15–19 years—145–147 pounds
Height: (girls) 11–14 years—62 inches
              15–19 years—64 inches
     (boys) 11–14 years—62 inches
              15–19 years—69–70 inches
Teething: Wisdom teeth come in at 18–20 years.
Body proportions: Primary and secondary sex characteristics develop (increase in size of genitalia, change in body hair distribution)

Play/Leisure	Cry/Socialization	Movement	Feeding/Sleep
12–15 Years			
Peer group activities important. Enjoys school-related activities. Likes shopping and talking on the telephone. Wants unsupervised free time. Shows interest in part-time jobs.	Interest in the opposite sex. Dating begins. Peer pressure to conform. Strong bonds formed with 1–2 close friends. Increasing hostility against parents. Concerned with morality, ethics, and religion. Reasoning is mature. Daydreaming is common.	Awkward and uncoordinated. May demonstrate poor posture. Physically active but tires easily.	Needs 7–9 hrs. of sleep a day. Prefers "junk" foods. Girls need 1500–3000 cal per day. Boys need 2000–3700 cal per day.
16–19 Years			
Works for altruistic causes. Likes beach activities. May explore volunteer work, summer jobs.	Refines language, reasoning and thinking skills. Parental advice and support is sought. Dates in pairs and groups. Effort to be self-supportive. Plans for career. Balances responsibility and pleasure.	Increased energy as growth spurts taper. Coordination increases.	Needs 6–8 hrs of sleep a day. Girls need 1200–3000 cal per day. Boys need 2100–3900 cal per day.

References

Committee on Psychosocial Aspects of Child and Family Health. (1988). *Guidelines for Health Supervision, vol. II*. Elk Grove Village, IL: American Academy of Pediatrics.

Haynes, U. (1967). *A Developmental Approach to Casefinding*. U.S. Department of Health, Education, and Welfare; Social and Rehabilitation Service, Children's Bureau.

Yoos, L. (1981). A developmental approach to physical assessment. *American Journal of Maternal Child Nursing*, June, 168–170.

Dilution Chart for Reconstitution of Infant Formula (20, 22, and 24 calories/fluid ounce)

Calories	Concentrated Liquid (oz)	Plus Water (oz) Equals	Ounces of Feedings
From Concentrated Liquid			
20 cal/fl oz	1	1	2
22 cal/fl oz	5.5	4.5	10
24 cal/fl oz	3	2	5

Calories	Scoop	Plus Water (oz) Equals	Ounces of Feedings
From Powder			
20 cal/fl oz	1	2	2.2
22 cal/fl oz	3	5.5	6.2
24 cal/fl oz	3	5	5.7

Use the scoop in the can of powder.

Young, T.E., & Mangum, O.B. (1990). A manual of drugs used in neonatal care. Columbus, OH: Ross Laboratories, pp. 9-20.

Pain Rating Scales

The ability to assess pain and provide comfort is an important skill for nurses. Pain measurement is based on three components: behavioral responses, physiologic changes, and the child's report of pain. For a complete picture of the child's pain, all three need to be assessed. Children are, however, at a disadvantage because their vocabulary does not permit them to describe a painful experience. By using pain assessment scales that do not rely on verbal descriptions of pain, nurses can more readily assess the intensity of a child's pain and treat accordingly.

The following is a description of five tools used to assess a child's pain:

1. *Chips scale.* This scale uses five plastic chips to describe the intensity of pain. Zero chips represents no pain. One chip represents a little hurt. Children select the number of chips needed to describe their pain (Hester, 1979). This is appropriate for ages 3 years to adolescence.

2. *Descriptive scale.* This scale uses words to denote intensities of pain. The child points to the word that most describes the amount of pain felt (Fig. 1). This is appropriate for ages 7 years to adolescence.

3. *Numeric scale* (visual analogue scale). This scale uses a straight line with marks indicating no pain to the worst pain. The child chooses the number that describes the pain (Fig. 2). This is appropriate for ages 7 to adolescence.

4. *Faces scale.* This scale consists of six faces. The first picture is of a smiling face and the last is of a frowning tearful face. The child chooses the face that most describes the pain he or she is feeling. (Beyer, 1984; Fig. 3). This is appropriate for ages 7 years to adolescence.

5. *Color scale.* This scale requires the child to arrange a number of different crayons in order to represent intensities of pain. The child then chooses the color that most closely matches the pain felt (Eland, 1977). This is appropriate for ages 4–10 years.

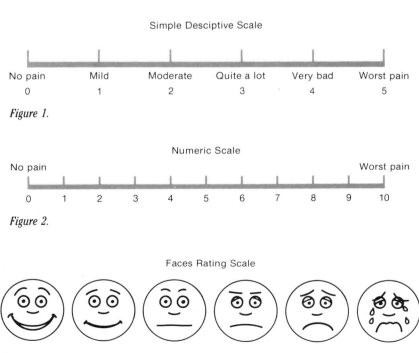

Simple Desciptive Scale

| No pain | Mild | Moderate | Quite a lot | Very bad | Worst pain |
| 0 | 1 | 2 | 3 | 4 | 5 |

Figure 1.

Numeric Scale

No pain   Worst pain

0   1   2   3   4   5   6   7   8   9   10

Figure 2.

Faces Rating Scale

Figure 3.

Newborn Pain Assessment Flow Sheet

(Check observed responses)	Date/Time		Date/Time		Date/Time		Date/Time	
Physiologic Response ↑ heart rate								
↑ respirations								
↑ blood pressure								
Attention/Anxiety Sleeplessness								
Restlessness								
Fussiness								
Facial Grimacing								
Wrinkling of forehead								
Vocal Crying								
Whimpering								
Groaning								
Movement Kicking								
Rigidity								
Wiggling								
Twisting								
Clenching of fist								
Medication Record type, dose/route								
Response to medication								

Figure 4.

Pain Scale 0–3
0—No pain
1—Slight pain
2—Moderate pain
3—Severe pain

Color Scale
—yellow
—blue
—orange
—red

Mood: Socializing
Quiet
Crying
Whining
Asleep
Anxious

Character: The pain is
Dull
Tingling
Sharp
Pressure
Nagging

Activity:
In bed—IB
In chair—IC
Out of room—OOR
In bathroom—IBR
On telephone—OT
Watching TV—WTV

Date/Time	Vital Signs				Medication	Pain Rating	Nurse			Child			Comments
	T	P	R	BP			Mood	Character	Activity	Mood	Character	Location	

Figure 5. Pain assessment flow sheet.

The nurse needs to choose the tool according to the child's age and developmental level, and consistently use it throughout hospitalization.

References

Ellis, J. (1988). Using pain scales to prevent under-medication. *Maternal/Child Nursing, 13*(3), 180–186.

Jones, M.A. (1989). Identifying signs that nurses interpret as indicating pain in newborns. *Pediatric Nursing, 15*(1), 76–79.

McGuire, L., Dizard, S., & Panayotoff, K. (1982). Managing pain in the young patient. *Nursing '82, 12*(8), 52–56.

Page, G.G., & Halvorson, M. (1991). Pediatric nurses: The assessment and control of pain in preverbal infants. *Journal of Pediatric Nursing, 6*(2), 99–106.

Wong, D., & Baker, C.M. (1988). Pain in children: Comparison of assessment scales. *Pediatric Nursing, 14*(1), 9–17.

Appendix 6

Basic Reflex Patterns

Rooting/Sucking

A hungry infant will turn the head to the right or left when the cheek is brushed by the hand. When the child is being fed, if the nipple is touched to the face, the lip and tongue tend to follow in that direction.

Moro

Sometimes called the startle reflex, the Moro reflex is a series of movements that begins with extension and abduction of the upper extremities and extension of the spine and retraction of the head. The forearms are supinated and the digits tend to extend and fan out. There may be slight tremor or rhythmic shaking of the limbs. The movement of the lower extremities is less pronounced.

Asymmetrical Tonic Neck

This reflex appears when the infant, lying on the back, turns his or head to one side with increased tone in the extensors of the chin extremities and with a decreased tone in the occiput extremities. The infant assumes a fencer position with the face turned toward the extended arm. The lower limbs respond in a similar manner.

Neck-Righting

Passive or active rotation of the infant's head to one side is followed by rotation of the shoulders, trunk, and pelvis in the same direction. There should be a momentary delay between the head rotation and the following of the shoulders.

Ventral Suspension and Landau Reflex

As a newborn infant is turned to prone, with trunk and abdomen supported, the legs should be flexed. The head may sag below the horizontal and the spine may be convex, but the infant should not become completely limp and collapse into an inverted U. As the infant becomes older, the head and spine are maintained in a more horizontal plane.

Parachute

This response consists of extending the arms over the head and out—as if to break a fall—when the infant is suspended and then plunged downward toward a flat surface.

Palmar and Plantar Grasp

These are both automatic reflexes of full-term newborns and are elicited by placing the observer's finger firmly in the palm or in back of the child's toes. The responses are strong and symmetrical.

Table 1. Normal Milestones of Development

Reflex	Months										
	1	2	3	4	6	9	12	15	18	24	36
Palmar grasp	+	+	±	±	0*	0	0	0	0	0	0
Tonic neck	+	+	±	±	0	0	0	0	0	0	0
Moro	+	+	±	±	0	0	0	0	0	0	0
Rooting/sucking	+	+	+	+	+	±	0**	0	0	0	0
Neck righting	0	0	0	±	±	+	+	+	+	+	+
Parachute	0	0	0	0	±	+	+	+	+	+	+
Landau	0	0	0	0	0	0	+	+	±	+	0

* May be present at sleep
** May be present when hungry or asleep
+, reflex present; 0, reflex absent; ± reflex evolving or diminishing.

Index

Page numbers followed by *f* indicate figures; those followed by *t* indicate tabular material.

A

abdomen, protrusion of
  at three to six years, 558
  at twelve to eighteen months, 557
abuse. *See* child abuse
acetaminophen, in pain, 66
acetone, serum, normal laboratory
      values for, 550
acid-base measurements, serum, nor-
      mal laboratory values for,
      550
acidemia, ketotic, hyperglycemia hyper-
      tonic dehydration and, 504
acidosis, metabolic, postoperative, 61
acne, infantile, 555
activity, cast care and, 514f, 514–515,
      544
addis count, urine, normal laboratory
      values for, 553
administration procedures, 1–21. *See
      also* names of specific pro-
      cedures
admission, procedures for, 3–11
  allergies and, 3f
  assessment in, 7–8
  communicable diseases and, 4f, 7
  definition of, 3
  development history and, 5f, 8
  discharge plans and, 5f–6f
  family education and, 11
  family history and, 4f, 7, 8
  form for, 3f–6f
    current problem and, 4f
    diet and, 4f
    elimination and, 4f
    medications and, 4f
    physical impairment and, 4f
    previous admission and, 4f
  health history and, 4f, 7
  immunization and, 5f, 7
  informed consent and, 19
  interventions in, 9f, 9–10
    for adolescent, 10
    for infant, 9, 9f
    for preschooler, 10
    for school-age child, 10
    for toddler, 10
  nursing diagnoses in, 8
  planning in, 8
  purpose of, 3
  review of system and, 8
  social history and, 7

standard of care in, 7
temperature measurement and, 98
adolescent
  admission procedures for, 10. *See
      also* admission
  blood pressure measurement for. *See
      also* blood pressure
    cuff size in, 42
    normal range in, 46t
  intravenous therapy for, 336. *See also*
      intravenous therapy
  medication administration for,
      119t–120t. *See also* medica-
      tion, administration of
Aerochamber, parent teaching guide
      for, 166f, 166–167
aerosol drug, holding chambers for,
      parent teaching guide for,
      165f, 165–167, 166f
air embolism, as transfusion reaction,
      275t
albumin
  serum, 438, 440
  in transfusion therapy, 273t. *See also*
      transfusion therapy
alkaline phosphatase, serum, normal
      laboratory values for, 550
allergy
  in admission form, 3f
  immunization and, 157
  as transfusion reaction, 275t
American Cancer Society, 150
ammonia, serum, normal laboratory
      values for, 550
amylase, serum, normal laboratory
      values for, 550
analgesia, patient-controlled, 151–154,
      152f, 153f
  assessment in, 151–152
  contraindications to, 151
  definition of, 151
  family education in, 153
  home care considerations in, 153
  interventions in, 152f, 152–153, 153f
  limitations in, 151
  nursing diagnoses in, 152
  patient education in, 153
  planning in, 152
  purpose of, 151
  standard of care in, 151
  supplemental techniques and, 153
anemia, sickle cell, 74

ankle, veins of, venoclysis and, 334,
      334f
antigen testing, specimen collection in,
      respiratory syncytial virus
      and, 143
antineoplastic drug therapy. *See* chemo-
      therapy
antipyretic
  family education in, 33
  immunization and, 159
anxiety, preoperative, interventions in,
      56f, 56–58, 57f
Apgar score, 25–27, 26t
  in asphyxia, 25
  assessment in, 25
  definition of, 25
  family education in, 27
  home care considerations in, 27
  implication of, 26, 26t
  interventions in, 26t, 26–27
  nursing diagnoses in, 25
  planning in, 26
  purpose of, 25
  standard of care in, 25
apnea
  definition of, 39t, 227
  end-tidal carbon dioxide in, 218,
      218f
  etiology of, 39t
  parent teaching guide for, 227–230,
      229f
artery
  blood, collection of in. *See also*
      blood, collection of
  blood collection in, 286, 290f,
      290–291
  popliteal, in blood pressure mea-
      surement, 44, 44f
asphyxia, description and etiology of,
      39t
asplenia, immunization and, 157
Assess peak flow meter, 239f
asthma
  end-tidal carbon dioxide in, 219,
      219f
  peak flow meter in, parent teaching
      guide for, 239f, 239–240
auscultation measurement, of blood
      pressure, 42, 43f, 43–44
Ayala's index, in lumbar puncture, 302